COVID-19 and Perinatology

Daniele De Luca • Alexandra Benachi
Editors

COVID-19 and Perinatology

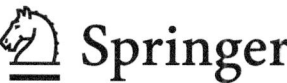

Editors
Daniele De Luca
Neonatology Department
APHP-University of Paris-Saclay
Le Kremlin-Bicêtre, France

Alexandra Benachi
Obstetrics and Gynecology Department
APHP-University of Paris-Saclay
Le Kremlin-Bicêtre, France

ISBN 978-3-031-29135-7   ISBN 978-3-031-29136-4 (eBook)
https://doi.org/10.1007/978-3-031-29136-4

© The Editor(s) (if applicable) and The Author(s), under exclusive license to Springer Nature Switzerland AG 2023

This work is subject to copyright. All rights are solely and exclusively licensed by the Publisher, whether the whole or part of the material is concerned, specifically the rights of translation, reprinting, reuse of illustrations, recitation, broadcasting, reproduction on microfilms or in any other physical way, and transmission or information storage and retrieval, electronic adaptation, computer software, or by similar or dissimilar methodology now known or hereafter developed.

The use of general descriptive names, registered names, trademarks, service marks, etc. in this publication does not imply, even in the absence of a specific statement, that such names are exempt from the relevant protective laws and regulations and therefore free for general use.

The publisher, the authors, and the editors are safe to assume that the advice and information in this book are believed to be true and accurate at the date of publication. Neither the publisher nor the authors or the editors give a warranty, expressed or implied, with respect to the material contained herein or for any errors or omissions that may have been made. The publisher remains neutral with regard to jurisdictional claims in published maps and institutional affiliations.

This Springer imprint is published by the registered company Springer Nature Switzerland AG
The registered company address is: Gewerbestrasse 11, 6330 Cham, Switzerland

Preface

The COVID-19 pandemic changed our lives in many ways. Initially we thought that this would not have touched pregnancy, delivery, and the early life.

We were wrong.

We soon realized how disruption of routine healthcare was affecting hospital organization and, unavoidably, perinatal care. Then, in a rush where new discoveries were coming up every day, we learnt a lot about SARS-CoV-2 in a short time and we demonstrated its perinatal transmission, whose first case had been observed by our group in Paris. We knew that this was a turning point: if the virus could pass the placenta the possible consequences on maternal and neonatal healthcare would have been many.

In fact, over the months we have studied and increased our knowledge about these consequences both from a pathophysiological or biological perspective and from the healthcare organization point of view. This was not all, since the mental consequences of SARS-CoV-2 in the perinatal period also became evident.

Overall, COVID-19 has been clinically more dangerous for the elderly than for young women and neonates; however its consequences are very important from the pathophysiology point of view and have ethical consequences since, although rarely, severe and life-threatening cases can occur in women and neonates. We could not remain blinded to these issues that are so relevant although relatively uncommon. This pushed us to increase our knowledge investing in research on perinatal COVID-19 and eventually to edit this book.

We felt the need for a place where to present the knowledge about the crossroad between COVID-19 and perinatology. This book, written thanks to many esteemed colleagues who shared the same need, would like to represent that place. We can only thank all the colleagues who contributed to this endeavor.

We hope this can be useful to summarize everything that is known from the perspective of different specialists. We hope this can push us to advance even more for maternal and neonatal well-being.

Le Kremlin-Bicêtre, France Daniele De Luca
Le Kremlin-Bicêtre, France Alexandra Benachi

Introduction: The Importance of European Perinatology During COVID-19 Pandemics

Hon. Mrs. Stella Kyriakides
EU Commissioner for Health and Food Safety

The COVID-19 pandemic has had far-reaching consequences for our health, our lives, and our communities. This is especially true for the most vulnerable among us.

So I am delighted to introduce this unique book, which focuses on some of the most important and fragile moments in life—pregnancy and early childhood.

And I want to thank Prof. De Luca for the invitation and the European Society for Paediatric and Neonatal Intensive Care (ESPNIC), the Union of European Neonatal and Perinatal Societies (UENPS), and the European Association of Perinatal Medicine (EAPM) for shining a light on this vital topic.

We know that pregnant women that have been infected with SARS-CoV-2 and show symptoms are at higher risk of hospitalization and death, compared to non-pregnant women and to pregnant women without COVID-19.

Thankfully, for small children, such severe outcomes are rare. However, there are newborns experiencing severe respiratory disease or even severe consequences due to COVID-19.

The bottom line is simple—we are still learning about this virus and its long-term consequences.

We need to develop our understanding of these issues, and to raise awareness in the European Union among health professionals and beyond. This book aims to do exactly that.

First, it focuses on how COVID-19 can impact women and children, including trans-placental transmission, increased severity in pregnant women, the risk of miscarriage and prematurity, psychological consequences, and rare but severe pediatric cases.

And let me say that I am delighted to also see a focus on women's psychological well-being and mental health.

Second, this book brings together world-renowned experts in these fields, as well as health professionals and scientists who are helping to manage the pandemic across the EU.

This is exactly the type of collaboration we need to address this pandemic.

The availability of COVID-19 medicines and vaccines that are safe and effective for pregnant women and children is particularly important.

The European Commission, together with the European Medicines Agency and Member States, has taken a proactive approach in this respect.

I know that there is a varied approach to vaccination of pregnant women across Europe. However, we should remember that the WHO currently recommends vaccination in pregnant women only when the benefit of vaccination outweighs the potential risk.

Our EU agencies, the European Medicines Agency and the European Centre for Disease Prevention and Control, are jointly coordinating observational studies to monitor the safety and effectiveness of COVID-19 vaccines, including in pregnant women.

In parallel, we are supporting efforts to get pediatric indications for COVID-19 medicines.

Before you delve into the wealth of information presented in this book, let me finish by assuring you that the European Commission is working in all fronts to tackle the pandemic.

The insight, expertise, and experience of the authors are essential to this effort. So I thank them all for their commitment.

I urge you to speak up, speak loudly, and speak often, and I look forward to overcoming this pandemic together.

Contents

Part I Obstetrics

1. **Clinical Management of COVID-19 During Pregnancy** 3
   Alexandre J. Vivanti and Alexandra Benachi

2. **Complications of COVID-19 in Pregnant Women** 13
   Charles Egloff and Olivier Picone

3. **Peculiarities of ARDS Induced by COVID-19
   in Pregnant Patients** 19
   Matteo Di Nardo, Francesco Alessandri, Maximilian Fischer,
   Maria Grazia Frigo, Fabrizia Calabrese, and V. Marco Ranieri

4. **Miscarriage and Fetal Death** 33
   Baptiste Tarasi and David Baud

5. **COVID-19 in Perinatology: Obstetrical Counseling
   to Pregnant Women During Pandemics** 39
   Inês Martins and Diogo Ayres-de-Campos

Part II Perinatal Medicine

6. **Biological Mechanisms of Transplacental SARS-COV-2
   Transmission** 49
   Serena Pirola and Luisa Patanè

7. **Placental Pathology During COVID-19** 63
   David A. Schwartz

8. **Perinatal Diagnostic of SARS-CoV-2 Infection** 77
   Christelle Vauloup-Fellous

9. **Vertical SARS-CoV-2 Transmission** 91
   Daniele De Luca and Maurizio Sanguinetti

10 Transplacental Transfer of SARS-COV-2 Antibodies 105
    Dominique A. Badr and Jacques C. Jani

Part III Neonatology

11 COVID-19 in Neonates: Mechanisms, Clinical Features,
    and Treatments 131
    Lucilla Pezza, Shivani Shankar-Aguilera, and Daniele De Luca

12 Impact of COVID on Prematurity............................... 155
    Helena Blakeway and Asma Khalil

13 Management of Neonatal Care During COVID19 Pandemics 173
    Manuel Sánchez Luna and Belén Fernández Colomer

Part IV Public Health

14 Research Networks and Accelerated Research Pathways
    for Perinatal Health 187
    Mark A. Turner

15 Impact of COVID-19 Lockdowns on Maternal
    and Perinatal Health... 207
    Jasper V. Been, Marijn J. Vermeulen, and Brenda M. Kazemier

16 Prevention of Future Pandemics and Impact
    on Perinatology 229
    Fidelia Cascini, Alberto Lontano, Giovanna Failla, Valeria Puleo,
    and Walter Ricciardi

Part V Psychology and Ethics

17 Perinatal Psychological and Psychiatric Impact of the
    SARS-CoV-2 Pandemic Health Crisis........................... 247
    Alexandra Doncarli, Catherine Crenn-Hebert, Sarah Tebeka,
    and Nolwenn Regnault

18 Collateral Damage of the COVID-19 Pandemic for the
    Next Generation: A Call to Action............................ 257
    Sam Schoenmakers, Roseriet Beijers, and E. J. (Joanne) Verweij

19 Management of Mental Health in Pregnant Women
    During COVID-19.. 269
    Sara Molgora and Monica Accordini

20 Ethical Issues of COVID-19 During Pregnancy and Childhood 281
    Daniele De Luca, Alexandra Benachi, and Renzo Pegoraro

Contributors

Monica Accordini Università Cattolica del Sacro Cuore di Milano, Milan, Italy

Francesco Alessandri Department of Emergency Medicine, Critical Care Medicine and Trauma, Sapienza Università di Roma, Policlinico Umberto I, Rome, Italy

Diogo Ayres-de-Campos Department of Obstetrics and Gynecology, Santa Maria University Hospital, Lisbon, Portugal

Department of Obstetrics and Gynecology, Medical School, University of Lisbon, Lisbon, Portugal

Dominique A. Badr Department of Obstetrics and Gynecology, University Hospital Brugmann, Université Libre de Bruxelles, Brussels, Belgium

David Baud Materno-Fetal and Obstetric Research Unit, Obstetric service, Woman-Mother-Child Department University Hospital of Lausanne, Lausanne, Switzerland

Jasper V. Been Division of Neonatology, Department of Paediatrics and Department of Obstetrics and Gynaecology, Erasmus MC Sophia Children's Hospital, University Medical Centre Rotterdam, Rotterdam, The Netherlands

Roseriet Beijers Social Development, Behavioural Science Institute, Radboud University, Nijmegen, The Netherlands

Cognitive Neuroscience, Donders Institute, Radboud University Medical Center, Nijmegen, The Netherlands

Alexandra Benachi Obstetrics and Gynecology Department, APHP-University of Paris-Saclay, Le Kremlin-Bicêtre, France

Helena Blakeway Fetal Medicine Unit, Department of Obstetrics and Gynaecology, St. George's Hospitals NHS Foundation Trust, London, UK

Fabrizia Calabrese Anaesthesia and Intensive Care Unit, Department of Medicine, Padua University Hospital, Padua, Italy

Fidelia Cascini Section of Hygiene and Public Health, Department of Life Sciences and Public Health, Università Cattolica del Sacro Cuore, Rome, Italy

Belén Fernández Colomer Pediatrics, Oviedo University, Oviedo, Spain

Neonatology Unit, HUCA, Oviedo, Spain

Infection Workgroup of the Spanish National Society of Neonatology (SENEO), Barcelona, Spain

Catherine Crenn-Hebert Department of Gynecology and Obstetrics, Louis Mourier University Hospital, AP-HP, Colombes, France

Alexandra Doncarli Direction of Non-Communicable Diseases and Trauma, Santé Publique France, Saint-Maurice, France

Charles Egloff Department of Gynecology and Obstetrics, Hôpital Louis Mourier, AP-HP, Colombes, France

Giovanna Failla Section of Hygiene and Public Health, Department of Life Sciences and Public Health, Università Cattolica del Sacro Cuore, Rome, Italy

Maximilian Fischer Department of Anesthesiology and Critical Care, Azienda Ospedaliero-Universitaria Careggi, Florence, Italy

Department of Health Sciences, Section of Anaesthesiology, Intensive Care and Pain Medicine, University of Florence, Florence, Italy

Maria Grazia Frigo Obstetric Anesthesia and Intensive Care Unit, Fatebenefratelli Hospital, Rome, Italy

Jacques C. Jani Department of Obstetrics and Gynecology, University Hospital Brugmann, Université Libre de Bruxelles, Brussels, Belgium

Brenda M. Kazemier Department of Obstetrics, Amsterdam Reproduction and Development Research Institute, Amsterdam UMC, Amsterdam, The Netherlands

Asma Khalil Fetal Medicine Unit, Department of Obstetrics and Gynaecology, St. George's Hospitals NHS Foundation Trust, London, UK

Vascular Biology Research Centre, Molecular and Clinical Sciences Research Institute, St George's University of London, London, UK

Fetal Medicine Unit, Liverpool Women's Hospital, University of Liverpool, Liverpool, UK

Alberto Lontano Section of Hygiene and Public Health, Department of Life Sciences and Public Health, Università Cattolica del Sacro Cuore, Rome, Italy

Daniele De Luca Neonatology Department, APHP-University of Paris-Saclay, Le Kremlin-Bicêtre, France

Manuel Sánchez Luna Pediatrics, Complutense University of Madrid, Madrid, Spain

Research Institute Gregorio Marañón, Madrid, Spain

Spanish National Society of Neonatology (SENEO), Barcelona, Spain

Neonatology Division and NICU, Hospital General Universitario "Gregorio Marañón", Madrid, Spain

Inês Martins Department of Obstetrics and Gynecology, Santa Maria University Hospital, Lisbon, Portugal

Sara Molgora Università Cattolica del Sacro Cuore di Milano, Milan, Italy

Matteo Di Nardo Pediatric Intensive Care Unit, Ospedale Pediatrico Bambino Gesù, IRCCS, Rome, Italy

Luisa Patanè Department of Gynecology and Obstetrics, ASST Papa Giovanni XXIII, Bergamo, Italy

Renzo Pegoraro Pontifical Academy for Life, Vatican State, Rome, Italy

Lucilla Pezza Paediatric Intensive Care Unit, Department of Anaesthesiology and Critical Care, University Hospital "A. Gemelli" - IRCCS, Rome, Italy

Olivier Picone Department of Gynecology and Obstetrics, Hôpital Louis Mourier, AP-HP, Colombes, France

IAME, INSERM, Université Paris Cité, Paris, France

Groupe de Recherche sur les Infections pendant la Grossesse, Paris, France

Serena Pirola Department of Gynecology and Obstetrics, ASST Papa Giovanni XXIII, Bergamo, Italy

Valeria Puleo Section of Hygiene and Public Health, Department of Life Sciences and Public Health, Università Cattolica del Sacro Cuore, Rome, Italy

V. Marco Ranieri Alma Mater Studiorum University of Bologna, Dipartimento di Scienze Mediche e Chirurgiche (DIMEC), Anesthesia and Intensive Care Medicine, Policlinico di Sant'Orsola, IRCCS, Bologna, Italy

Nolwenn Regnault Direction of Non-Communicable Diseases and Trauma, Santé Publique France, Saint-Maurice, France

Walter Ricciardi Section of Hygiene and Public Health, Department of Life Sciences and Public Health, Università Cattolica del Sacro Cuore, Rome, Italy

Maurizio Sanguinetti Catholic University of the Sacred Heart, Rome, Italy

Department of Laboratory Medicine, "A. Gemelli" University Hospital, Rome, Italy

European Society for Clinical Microbiology and Infectious Diseases (ESCMID), Basel, Switzerland

Sam Schoenmakers Division of Obstetrics and Fetal Medicine, Department of Obstetrics and Gynaecology, Erasmus MC, University Medical Center Rotterdam, Rotterdam, The Netherlands

David A. Schwartz, MD, MS Hyg, FCAP Perinatal Pathology Consulting, Atlanta, GA, USA

Shivani Shankar-Aguilera Division of Pediatrics and Neonatal Critical Care, Paris Saclay University Hospitals, Paris Saclay University, Paris, France

Baptiste Tarasi Materno-Fetal and Obstetric Research Unit, Obstetric service, Woman-Mother-Child Department, University Hospital of Lausanne, Lausanne, Switzerland

Sarah Tebeka Direction of Non-Communicable Diseases and Trauma, Santé Publique France, Saint-Maurice, France

Université Paris Cité, INSERM U1266, Paris, France

Department of Psychiatry, AP-HP, Louis Mourier Hospital, Colombes, France

Mark A. Turner Department of Women's and Children's Health, University of Liverpool, Liverpool, UK

Liverpool Neonatal Partnership, Liverpool, UK

Liverpool Women's NHS Foundation Trust, Liverpool, UK

Christelle Vauloup-Fellous Division of Virology, Department of Biology Genetics and PUI, APHP-Paris Saclay University, Villejuif, France

INSERM U1193, Université Paris Saclay, Villejuif, France

Marijn J. Vermeulen Division of Neonatology, Department of Paediatrics and Department of Obstetrics and Gynaecology, Erasmus MC Sophia Children's Hospital, University Medical Centre Rotterdam, Rotterdam, The Netherlands

Care4Neo, Dutch Neonatal Patient and Parent Organisation, Rotterdam, The Netherlands

E. J. (Joanne) Verweij Department of Obstetrics, Leiden University Medical Center, Leiden, The Netherlands

Alexandre J. Vivanti Division of Obstetrics and Gynecology, Paris Saclay University Hospitals, APHP- Paris Saclay University, Clamart, France

Part I
Obstetrics

Chapter 1
Clinical Management of COVID-19 During Pregnancy

Alexandre J. Vivanti and Alexandra Benachi

1.1 Introduction

On 31 December 2019, the Chinese health authorities informed the WHO (World Health Organization) of the appearance of a new coronavirus in Wuhan province. Initially named 2019-nCoV, then SARS-CoV-2, it is responsible for COVID-19. This virus spread rapidly around the world, and the first Italian and then French clusters were reported in February 2020. The speed of viral spread mandated the establishment of successive lockdowns in all affected countries. At the end of the first wave, the seroprevalence of SARS-CoV-2 in patients who gave birth during the pandemic was estimated at between 4% and 8% in France [1, 2]. Health-care providers from all disciplines were faced with a major difficulty in managing their patients, linked to lack of knowledge of the pathophysiology of SARS-CoV-2 infections. These difficulties did not spare obstetricians worldwide. Many questions remained when the pandemic hit the European continent. A major issue was the potential impact of SARS-CoV-2 infection on pregnancy and maternal health. Many teams had to manage their patients step-by-step due to lack of information. The little data of interest available at the time was from Wuhan province [3, 4]. These retrospective observational studies, with small numbers of patients, allowed us to learn that pregnant women were likely to have severe forms. Similarly, we also learned that non-reassuring fetal heart rate tracings were likely to be associated with maternal COVID-19 infections.

A. J. Vivanti (✉)
Division of Obstetrics and Gynecology, Paris Saclay University Hospitals,
APHP-Paris Saclay University, Clamart, France
e-mail: alexandre.vivanti@aphp.fr

A. Benachi
Obstetrics and Gynecology Department, APHP-University of Paris-Saclay,
Le Kremlin-Bicêtre, France
e-mail: alexandra.benachi@aphp.fr

© The Author(s), under exclusive license to Springer Nature
Switzerland AG 2023
D. De Luca, A. Benachi (eds.), *COVID-19 and Perinatology*,
https://doi.org/10.1007/978-3-031-29136-4_1

The major scientific bodies quickly considered that, in the absence of relevant data, pregnant women should be considered by default as a population at high risk of developing severe forms of COVID-19. Obstetric societies quickly published the first recommendations in March 2020 [5–7]. These recommendations made it possible to lay the foundations for the management of pregnant women in the event of suspected COVID-19 infection: RT-PCR testing of symptomatic patients, clarification of isolation conditions, definitions of severity criteria, etc.

The progressive accumulation of data has made it possible to specify the particularities of the management of COVID-19 infections in pregnant women. This clinical management involves the joint management of both the mother and the fetus. The aim of management is to reduce morbidity and mortality in the mother-fetus dyad.

Any pregnant woman with symptoms suggestive of COVID-19 infection should undergo diagnostic confirmation by nasopharyngeal swab for RT-PCR or, at the very least, an antigenic test (with a minimum sensitivity of 80%). It is now clearly established that pregnant women constitute an independent risk factor for the development of a severe form of COVID-19. In addition, infection with COVID-19 during pregnancy is likely to increase certain obstetrical risks such as premature delivery or preeclampsia [8]. Finally, SARS-CoV-2, via its spike protein, has a particular affinity for the placenta (expression of its ACE2 and TMPRSS receptor) exposing it to an increased risk of non-reassuring fetal heart rate tracings or even of stillbirth. For all these reasons, all symptomatic patients should be offered with clinical, obstetric, and fetal assessment in a gynecology-obstetrics department at symptom onset.

1.2 Initial Clinical Assessment

1.2.1 Search for Risk Factors of Unfavorable Clinical Outcome (Respiratory Distress)

The initial clinical assessment of a patient with a characterized COVID-19 infection should begin by looking for additional risk factors (other than pregnancy), adverse respiratory outcomes such as overweight or obesity, pre-existing chronic disease (diabetes, hypertension, asthma, cancer, cardiovascular disease, immunosuppression, hematological disease), use of toxic substances (tobacco, opioids, alcohol), and lack of vaccination against COVID-19. It is very common for several risk factors to be present.

1.2.2 Search for Signs of Severity and Maternal Complications

The clinical signs of severity in pregnant women are the same as in adults outside pregnancy (Table 1.1). The first signs to look for are severe lung damage such as desaturation, polypnea, and signs of respiratory distress. A search for signs of

1 Clinical Management of COVID-19 During Pregnancy

Table 1.1 COVID-19 infection WHO severity definitions [9]

• Critical COVID-19: Defined by the criteria for acute respiratory distress syndrome (ARDS), sepsis, septic shock, or other conditions that would normally require the provision of life-sustaining therapies such as mechanical ventilation (invasive or noninvasive) or vasopressor therapy
• Severe COVID-19: Defined by any of the following:
– Oxygen saturation <90% in room air
– Respiratory rate >30 breaths/min in adults and children >5 years old, ≥60 breaths/min in children <2 months old, ≥50 in children 2–11 months old, and ≥40 in children 1–5 years old
– Signs of severe respiratory distress (accessory muscle use, inability to complete full sentences, and, in children, very severe chest wall indrawing, grunting, central cyanosis, or presence of any other general danger signs)
• Nonsevere COVID-19: Defined as absence of any criteria for severe or critical COVID-19

sepsis (fever, tachycardia, arterial hypotension) should be performed. It should be remembered that the nadir of symptoms is generally between D7 and D12 from the onset of symptoms. Consequently, a reassuring clinical examination at the onset of the infection must call for vigilance because of the risk of secondary deterioration.

1.2.3 Search for Obstetrical Complications

The state of pregnancy involves the joint assessment of maternal well-being but also of the well-being of the unborn child. The obstetrical assessment time should lead to a search for a situation at risk of preterm delivery [8, 10]. Any state of infection during pregnancy (or simply hyperthermia) can generate uterine contractions and cervical modifications. Similarly, a persistent cough, even in the absence of fever, can stimulate the uterus and cause contractions. The history should indicate the existence of uterine contractions and, where appropriate, cervical changes (by vaginal touch and/or endovaginal ultrasound of the cervix). Uterine contractions should be recorded, especially when the fetus has reached viability.

Because of the increased risk of neonatal acidosis and fetal demise, the patient should be offered an assessment of fetal well-being (Fig. 1.1). It has been shown that a decrease in active fetal movements may be associated with an increased risk of fetal demise [11]. It is therefore important to have the patient specify the existence of active fetal movements. The evaluation of fetal well-being also includes cardiotocography (CTG) for recording of the fetal heart rate when the threshold of viability has been reached (Table 1.2). Obstetrical ultrasound may also be proposed with fetal Doppler evaluation of the exchanges between the mother and her fetus.

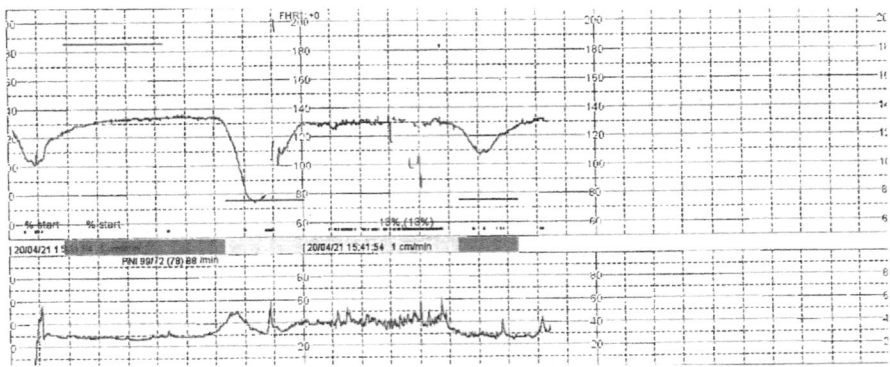

Fig. 1.1 Category III fetal heart rate in a case of mild COVID-19 at 34 weeks. Category III fetal heart rate tracing in a 30-year-old patient with a mild COVID-19 infection (isolated fever) with positive RT-PCR 7 days earlier. The laboratory tests performed on admission showed thrombocytopenia at 53,000 platelets/mm^3 ($N > 150,000$/mm^3), prolonged APTT at 1.36 ($N < 1.20$), D-dimer levels above 20,000 µg/L ($N < 500$ µg/L), liver cytolysis (SGOT = 81 IU/L, SGPT = 47 IU/L), a drop in fibrinogen to 1.3 g/L ($N > 1.5$ g/L), and a rise in C-reactive protein to 101 mg/L ($N < 5$ mg/L). The patient gave birth by emergency cesarean delivery to a 2200 g girl, with a 5-min Apgar score of 2 and severe neonatal acidosis (umbilical artery pH = 6.85; $N > 7.20$). Placental histological analysis showed diffuse lesions of chronic intervillositis and massive fibrin deposits. Placental immunohistochemistry was positive (anti-Covid19N)

Table 1.2 Points of attention for COVID-19 infection during pregnancy in patients with moderate symptoms

COVID-19 infection may cause several types of laboratory abnormalities such as lymphocytopenia, biological inflammatory syndrome (hyperleukocytosis, elevated CRP), prolonged APTT, hepatic cytolysis, thrombocytopenia, fibrinogen consumption, and significant increase in D-dimer. The presence of one or more of these abnormalities should alert the physician managing the patient to the following risks:
1. Maternal respiratory decompensation
If the patient's clinical condition is compatible with outpatient care, it is important to ensure that monitoring is in place to allow regular contact with the patient. Some countries, such as France, have developed remote monitoring tools (COVIDOM platform) that are very useful for remotely assessing the clinical condition of patients (and, if necessary, having them consult in an emergency)
2. Placental damage that can be complicated by acidosis (or even fetal death in utero)
Assessment by cardiotocography (after 24 weeks) should be available for any patient with a symptomatic infection. Some teams propose regular ambulatory heart rate monitoring in order to detect fetal heart rate abnormalities and to limit the risk of neonatal acidosis. Observational data, not yet published, show that in almost 50% of cases of abnormal fetal heart rate tracings (outside of labor), there was maternal thrombocytopenia and hepatic cytolysis

1.3 Management of a Patient with COVID-19 Infection During Pregnancy with Criteria for Hospitalization

1.3.1 Maternal Care

Any patient with one or more of the WHO severity criteria (Table 1.1) should be admitted to hospital for further management. A patient with immediate signs of respiratory distress and/or hypoxemia requiring sustained oxygen therapy (more than 5 L of oxygen per minute) should be managed in an intensive care unit.

If signs of respiratory distress and/or hypoxemia are present, contrasted lung CT-scan can be used to assess the percentage of parenchymal involvement and also to rule out or confirm the existence of an associated pulmonary embolism. Pregnancy is not a contraindication to this examination or to the injection of iodinated contrast. The risk of pulmonary embolism in the context of pregnancy (second and third trimesters) and COVID-19 infection is high [12]. In the presence of a pulmonary embolism, therapeutic anticoagulation with low-molecular-weight heparin should be initiated without delay. If there is no pulmonary embolism on admission, high-level preventive anticoagulation and compression stockings should be provided throughout the management.

The ventilatory management of a pregnant woman should be progressive and adapted. One of the particularities of SARS-CoV-2 infections is the possibility of a sudden worsening of the disease in a "staircase" fashion. Oxygen requirements, initially compensated by low-flow oxygen therapy, can increase significantly and abruptly. Respiratory Critical care of these patients is complex and may require different techniques, both invasive and non-invasive (see chapter 3 in this book). If noninvasive ventilation fails, intubation may be considered during pregnancy but should lead to discussion of the patient's delivery to encourage recruitment of the pulmonary alveoli limited by the reduced ventilatory capacity due to the gravid uterus (see Section 1.2.3). The gravid uterus may also complicate recruitment maneuvers such as the transition to prone position. Finally, in the event of refractory hypoxemia despite all the measures put in place previously, recourse to extracorporeal oxygen therapy is part of the therapeutic arsenal.

The drug management of severe COVID-19 infections has also been greatly improved. The use of systemic corticosteroids (dexamethasone) in severe infections has been shown to improve survival and reduce length of stay in critical care. The use of corticosteroids has had a positive impact on the management of pregnant women in the second and third trimesters [13]. Their use is not contraindicated in pregnancy and should be used in the event of hospitalization of a pregnant woman with severe clinical criteria. Many other drugs are, or have been, the subject of particular attention in the fight against severe infections, such as the use of monoclonal antibodies. Their use during pregnancy should only be considered after evaluation of the benefit-risk balance and should be discussed between intensive care physicians, neonatologists, and obstetricians. National or international scientific bodies can be consulted to assess the impact of the various treatments envisaged on the development of the fetus.

1.3.2 Fetal Management

The risk of adverse short-term maternal clinical outcome should be carefully assessed as delivery may be justified to improve ventilatory management in the event of decompensation. In this sense, it is imperative to take into account the risk of induced prematurity when hospitalizing patients presenting criteria of severity or at risk of decompensation. In utero transfer to a suitable perinatal center with an adult intensive care unit and neonatal intensive care unit is fully justified in the case of severe COVID-19 infection occurring when the viability threshold is reached [14]. Such in utero transfers may be difficult in the pandemic setting because of saturation of intensive care units (adult or neonatal) and should never delay early maternal management.

Because of the risk of spontaneous or induced prematurity in the context of SARS-CoV-2 infection, it seems reasonable to give a course of fetal maturation corticosteroids (betamethasone 12 mg, two intramuscular injections 24 h apart) to any hospitalized patient presenting with criteria of severity between 24 and 33^{+6} weeks of pregnancy, in order to limit complications of prematurity. Dexametasone administered for severe COVID-19 may also have a positive effectonfetallung maturation. Empirically, in cases of severe maternal infection, some teams start with betamethasone for 48 h and follow with dexamethasone. Betamethasone can also be administered in the event of hospitalization for non-reassuring fetal heart tracing between 24 and 33^{+6} weeks if there is a suspicion of placental damage from COVID-19.

The use of magnesium sulfate for fetal neuroprotection is governed by the rules of good practice and may be considered in the event of imminent spontaneous or induced delivery before 31^{+6} weeks of gestation and after a pre-therapeutic check-up (blood creatinine and electrocardiogram). The use of magnesium sulfate should also be discussed between intensive care physicians, neonatologists, and obstetricians because of the possible risk of respiratory depression in the case of overdose in patients with already precarious ventilatory function because of COVID-19 infection.

Finally, the management of a hypoxemic patient (or a patient at high risk of hypoxemia) requires enhanced fetal monitoring by regular CTG when the threshold of viability has been reached. This monitoring can detect possible fetal anoxia due to maternal hypoxemia. Because of the impossibility of monitoring the fetus continuously during the course of the pregnancy in women hospitalized in the intensive care unit, it is advisable to evaluate the medium-term repercussions of maternal hypoxemia on the fetus. This evaluation requires morphological ultrasound scans, or even a fetal brain MRI, remotely from the hospitalization in critical care, if the pregnancy is continued. This evaluation will look for signs of cerebral ischemia (gyration anomalies, ventriculomegaly, porencephaly). The combination of hemodynamic instability with maternal hypoxemia exposes the mother to an increased risk of fetal complications of ischemic/hemorrhagic origin and may lead to termination of pregnancy [15].

1.3.3 Fetal Extraction Criteria

The management of SARS-CoV-2 infection in pregnant women involves the fate of the unborn child. Two settings may involve the decision to induce delivery: management of a patient in respiratory distress and/or the occurrence of non-reassuring fetal heart rate tracing. In both cases, decision-making will take into account the gestational age (the later the term, the easier the birth decision will be because the complications of prematurity will be less important) (Fig. 1.2). In the setting of a patient in respiratory distress, the purpose of performing a maternal rescue cesarean delivery will be to reduce the pressure in the abdominal compartment to facilitate respiratory mechanics. Because of the small uterine volume before 28 weeks, there is little justification for a routine cesarean section in the absence of significant maternal hemodynamic or ventilatory instability. Some teams have successfully used invasive ventilation to overcome the acute stage of acute respiratory distress syndrome during pregnancy [16]. However, after 30 weeks, uterine volume definitely impacts on respiratory capacity. The maternal benefits of fetal extraction after 30 weeks should be considered [17]. It also appears unreasonable to allow a pregnancy to continue in a patient who requires resuscitation after 34 weeks. Each situation and decision should involve the three parties involved, the obstetrician, the pediatrician, and the resuscitator, and the balance of maternal and neonatal risks and benefits should be discussed.

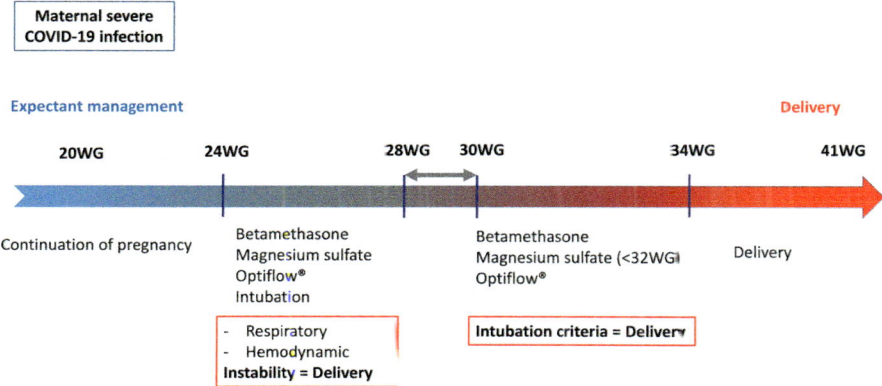

Fig. 1.2 Proposed algorithm for fetal extraction criteria in cases of severe maternal COVID-19 infection. *WG* weeks of gestation

The second situation that may warrant an induced birth is the setting of COVID-19-related placental damage. This rare situation occurs mostly in patients with moderate symptoms and in the absence of pre-established risk factors. Several observations suggest the possibility of an association between laboratory abnormalities and alteration of the fetal heart rate tracing [18–20]. To date, the only alternative to detect possible placental dysfunction is fetal heart rate monitoring. On the other hand, we do not have the necessary hindsight to know whether a policy of systematic and regular fetal heart rate monitoring can reduce neonatal morbidity (acidosis) and mortality.

1.4 Conclusion

The management of pregnant women infected with COVID-19 should be multidisciplinary, involving the skills of obstetricians, neonatologists, and adult intensive care physicians. The aim of management is to reduce maternal and neonatal mortality and morbidity by allowing the pregnancy to continue under the best possible conditions. It will require an assessment of the potential risks associated with the infection, referral of the patient to an appropriate perinatal center if necessary, and the use of drug and ventilatory therapies in line with the severity of the infection and the gestational age.

The management modalities must also consider the spread of new strains of SARS-CoV-2. It is also clear that vaccination against COVID-19 reduces the risk of severe forms during pregnancy and should be widely recommended because of its excellent tolerance and its lack of obstetric adverse outcomes [21–24].

References

1. Mattern J, Vauloup-Fellous C, Zakaria H, Benachi A, Carrara J, Letourneau A, et al. Post lockdown COVID-19 seroprevalence and circulation at the time of delivery, France. MedRxiv. 2020:2020.07.14.20153304. https://doi.org/10.1101/2020.07.14.20153304.
2. Tsatsaris V, Mariaggi A-A, Launay O, Couffignal C, Rousseau J, Ancel PY, et al. SARS-COV-2 IgG antibody response in pregnant women at delivery. J Gynecol Obstet Hum Reprod. 2020;50:102041. https://doi.org/10.1016/j.jogoh.2020.102041.
3. Chen L, Li Q, Zheng D, Jiang H, Wei Y, Zou L, et al. Clinical characteristics of pregnant women with Covid-19 in Wuhan, China. N Engl J Med. 2020;382:e100. https://doi.org/10.1056/NEJMc2009226.
4. Zhu H, Wang L, Fang C, Peng S, Zhang L, Chang G, et al. Clinical analysis of 10 neonates born to mothers with 2019-nCoV pneumonia. Transl Pediatr. 2020;9:51–60. https://doi.org/10.21037/tp.2020.02.06.
5. Peyronnet V, Sibiude J, Deruelle P, Huissoud C, Lescure X, Lucet J-C, et al. SARS-CoV-2 infection during pregnancy. Information and proposal of management care. CNGOF Gynecol Obstet Fertil Senol. 2020;48:436–43. https://doi.org/10.1016/j.gofs.2020.03.014.

6. Poon LC, Yang H, Lee JCS, Copel JA, Leung TY, Zhang Y, et al. ISUOG Interim Guidance on 2019 novel coronavirus infection during pregnancy and puerperium: information for healthcare professionals. Ultrasound Obstet Gynecol. 2020;55:700–8. https://doi.org/10.1002/uog.22013.
7. Royal College of Obstetricians and Gynaecologists. Coronavirus (COVID-19) infection in pregnancy. London: RCOG; 2020. https://www.rcog.org.uk/globalassets/documents/guidelines/2020-03-26-covid19-pregnancy-guidance.pdf.
8. Villar J, Ariff S, Gunier RB, Thiruvengadam R, Rauch S, Kholin A, et al. Maternal and neonatal morbidity and mortality among pregnant women with and without COVID-19 infection: the INTERCOVID multinational cohort study. JAMA Pediatr. 2021;175:817. https://doi.org/10.1001/jamapediatrics.2021.1050.
9. WHO. Living guidance for clinical management of COVID-19. Geneva: WHO; 2020. https://www.who.int/publications-detail-redirect/WHO-2019-nCoV-clinical-2021-2. Accessed 22 Jan 2022.
10. Allotey J, Stallings E, Bonet M, Yap M, Chatterjee S, Kew T, et al. Clinical manifestations, risk factors, and maternal and perinatal outcomes of coronavirus disease 2019 in pregnancy: living systematic review and meta-analysis. BMJ. 2020;370:m3320. https://doi.org/10.1136/bmj.m3320.
11. Favre G, Mazzetti S, Gengler C, Bertelli C, Schneider J, Laubscher B, et al. Decreased fetal movements: a sign of placental SARS-CoV-2 infection with perinatal brain injury. Viruses. 2021;13:2517. https://doi.org/10.3390/v13122517.
12. Servante J, Swallow G, Thornton JG, Myers B, Munireddy S, Malinowski AK, et al. Haemostatic and thrombo-embolic complications in pregnant women with COVID-19: a systematic review and critical analysis. BMC Pregnan Childb. 2021;21:108. https://doi.org/10.1186/s12884-021-03568-0.
13. Magala Ssekandi A, Sserwanja Q, Olal E, Kawuki J, Bashir Adam M. Corticosteroids use in pregnant women with COVID-19: recommendations from available evidence. J Multidiscip Healthc. 2021;14:659–63. https://doi.org/10.2147/JMDH.S301255.
14. ACOG. COVID-19 FAQs for obstetrician-gynecologists, Obstetrics. Washington, DC: ACOG; 2021. https://www.acog.org/en/clinical-information/physician-faqs/covid-19-faqs-for-ob-gyns-obstetrics. Accessed 22 Jan 2022.
15. Düppers AL, Bohnhorst B, Bültmann E, Schulz T, Higgins-Wood L, von Kaisenberg CS. Severe fetal brain damage subsequent to acute maternal hypoxemic deterioration in COVID-19. Ultrasound Obstet Gynecol. 2021;58:490–1. https://doi.org/10.1002/uog.23744.
16. Keita H, James A, Bouvet L, Herrmann E, Le Gouez A, Mazoit J-X, et al. Clinical, obstetrical and anaesthesia outcomes in pregnant women during the first COVID-19 surge in France: a prospective multicentre observational cohort study. Anaesth Crit Care Pain Med. 2021;40:100937. https://doi.org/10.1016/j.accpm.2021.100937.
17. Tolcher MC, McKinney JR, Eppes CS, Muigai D, Shamshirsaz A, Guntupalli KK, et al. Prone positioning for pregnant women with hypoxemia due to coronavirus disease 2019 (COVID-19). Obstet Gynecol. 2020;136:259–61. https://doi.org/10.1097/AOG.0000000000004012.
18. Koumoutsea EV, Vivanti AJ, Shehata N, Benachi A, Le Gouez A, Desconclois C, et al. COVID-19 and acute coagulopathy in pregnancy. J Thromb Haemost. 2020;18:1648. https://doi.org/10.1111/jth.14856.
19. Mongula JE, Frenken MWE, van Lijnschoten G, Arents NLA, de Wit-Zuurendonk LD, Schimmel-de Kok APA, et al. COVID-19 during pregnancy: non-reassuring fetal heart rate, placental pathology and coagulopathy. Ultrasound Obstet Gynecol. 2020;56:773–6. https://doi.org/10.1002/uog.22189.
20. Vivanti AJ, Vauloup-Fellous C, Prevot S, Zupan V, Suffee C, Do Cao J, et al. Transplacental transmission of SARS-CoV-2 infection. Nat Commun. 2020;11:3572. https://doi.org/10.1038/s41467-020-17436-6.

21. Blakeway H, Prasad S, Kalafat E, Heath PT, Ladhani SN, Doare KL, et al. COVID-19 vaccination during pregnancy: coverage and safety. Am J Obstet Gynecol. 2021;226:236.e1. https://doi.org/10.1016/j.ajog.2021.08.007.
22. Magnus MC, Gjessing HK, Eide HN, Wilcox AJ, Fell DB, Håberg SE. Covid-19 vaccination during pregnancy and first-trimester miscarriage. N Engl J Med. 2021;385:2008–10. https://doi.org/10.1056/NEJMc2114466.
23. Zauche LH, Wallace B, Smoots AN, Olson CK, Oduyebo T, Kim SY, et al. Receipt of mRNA Covid-19 vaccines and risk of spontaneous abortion. N Engl J Med. 2021;385:1533–5. https://doi.org/10.1056/NEJMc2113891.
24. Berbece C. COVID-19: latest safety data provide reassurance about use of mRNA vaccines during pregnancy. Amsterdam: European Medicine Agency; 2022. https://www.ema.europa.eu/en/news/covid-19-latest-safety-data-provide-reassurance-about-use-mrna-vaccines-during-pregnancy. Accessed 23 Jan 2022.

Chapter 2
Complications of COVID-19 in Pregnant Women

Charles Egloff and Olivier Picone

SARS-CoV-2 infection during pregnancy is responsible for maternal and obstetric complications.

2.1 Maternal Complications

Many anatomic and physiologic changes occur during pregnancy, beginning in the first trimester. Change in the immune system and cardiac, pulmonary, and other systems results in increased morbidity and mortality with infection during pregnancy [1, 2].

The clinical presentation of COVID-19 ranges from asymptomatic to severe complications, including viral pneumonia and death, especially in patients with comorbidities. The clinical manifestations of SARS-CoV-2 in pregnancy are similar to those in the general population. Main symptoms are fever, cough, dyspnea, and myalgia present in 40% of cases [3, 4]. Other symptoms include headache, dizziness, abdominal pain, diarrhea, nausea, and vomiting.

Current evidence suggests that pregnancy does not increase susceptibility to SARS-CoV-2 infection, but it appears to worsen the clinical course of COVID-19 when compared to nonpregnant females of the same age.

C. Egloff
Department of Gynecology and Obstetrics, Hôpital Louis Mourier, AP-HP, Colombes, France
e-mail: charles.egloff@aphp.fr

O. Picone (✉)
Department of Gynecology and Obstetrics, Hôpital Louis Mourier, AP-HP, Colombes, France

IAME, INSERM, Université Paris Cité, Paris, France

Groupe de Recherche sur les Infections pendant la Grossesse, Paris, France
e-mail: Olviier.picone@aphp.fr

© The Author(s), under exclusive license to Springer Nature Switzerland AG 2023
D. De Luca, A. Benachi (eds.), *COVID-19 and Perinatology*,
https://doi.org/10.1007/978-3-031-29136-4_2

In most cases, disease severity is determined by respiratory failure, as it is the commonest symptom in women with pneumonia. Pregnant COVID-positive patients can also develop moderate cardiac dysfunction and reduced left ventricular ejection fraction (LVEF), but the data is sparse [5]. Other complications include hepatic and renal failure, viral meningitis, cerebrovascular disorder, epilepsy, thrombotic disease, and septic shock in critical patients.

Several studies that have compared pregnant with nonpregnant women of reproductive age have shown that pregnancy is a risk factor for severe disease. A Canadian study analyzed from a national surveillance program for SARS-CoV-2 found that pregnant women with COVID-19 are more likely to be hospitalized for acute respiratory disease (relative risk 2.65 [95% CI, 2.64–2.88]) and to be admitted to an intensive care unit (relative risk 5.46 [95% CI, 4.50–6.53]) among more than 6000 pregnant women with COVID-19 [6]. Meta-analysis and systematic review confirm that COVID-19 during pregnancy is associated with the need for mechanical ventilation (relative risk 2.13 [95% CI, 1.06–4.28]) and death (relative risk 6.09 [95% CI, 1.82–20.38]) compared with the nonpregnant general population [3, 4].

Some data have identified risk factors for more severe illness:

- Like general population: maternal age (relative risk for age >35 years 1.42 [95% CI, 1.13–1.8]), obesity (relative risk for BMI >30 1.89 [95% CI, 1.38–2.58]), or comorbidities such as chronic cardiac or pulmonary disease, preexisting hypertension (relative risk 2.36 [95% CI, 1.54–3.4]), diabetes mellitus (relative risk 2.12 [95% CI, 1.27–3.25]), chronic renal disease, malignancy, and immunosuppression increase the risk of complications from COVID-19 [3, 6].
- The term of pregnancy is the main obstetrical factor associated with the risk of COVID-19 infection. Need for oxygen therapy and need for endotracheal intubation in infected pregnant women are also increased after 20 weeks of gestation [7]. SARS-CoV-2 infection in pregnant women during the late second and early third trimesters increases the risk for adverse obstetric and neonatal outcomes [8].

Studies of COVID-19 suggest that the postpartum period is also one of the increased risks. In a multivariate analysis in Brazil that compared nonpregnant SARS-CoV-2-infected women with those who were pregnant or postpartum (defined as up to 42 days after childbirth), the postpartum period was associated with a highest odds for death [9].

Furthermore, pregnant women have a fourfold higher venous thromboembolism risk compared with age-matched controls owing to hemostatic alterations in preparation for childbirth [10]. Thrombotic events are common complications in COVID-19 patients that include both thrombus formation in large vessels and the microvasculature of the lung and other organs [11]. Thus, particular attention must be paid to a significant risk of thromboembolic complications during pregnancy.

2.2 Obstetrical Complications

Several studies have shown that SARS-CoV-2 infection during pregnancy increases the risk of pregnancy complications. Thus, COVID-19 infection is associated with an increased risk of prematurity, cesarean, stillbirth, preeclampsia, and low birth weight [12, 13]. Differences in the risks of cesarean delivery and preterm birth are primarily related to obstetric intervention practices.

2.2.1 Preeclampsia

One recent meta-analysis shows that women with SARS-CoV-2 infection during pregnancy had a significantly higher odds ratio (1.62; 95% CI, 1.45–1.82) of developing preeclampsia than those without SARS-CoV-2 infection during pregnancy [14]. Moreover, SARS-CoV-2 infection during pregnancy was associated with a significant increase in the odds of preeclampsia with severe features, eclampsia, and HELLP (hemolysis, elevated liver enzymes, and low platelets) syndrome. Both asymptomatic and symptomatic SARS-CoV-2 infections significantly increased the risk for preeclampsia. Nevertheless, the odds of developing preeclampsia were higher among patients with symptomatic illness than among those with asymptomatic illness, which suggests a dose-response gradient effect.

Different mechanisms have been proposed to explain the association between different viral infections during pregnancy and preeclampsia [15–17]:

- Direct effects of infectious agents on trophoblast function and the arterial wall, including endothelial damage or dysfunction
- Acute atherosclerosis
- Local inflammation that may cause relative uteroplacental ischemia
- Indirect effects through an exaggerated maternal systemic inflammatory response

There is evidence that SARS-CoV-2 can infect the syncytiotrophoblast and activate inflammatory responses in placentas of women with a positive RT-PCR test result [18–20]. Entry of SARS-CoV-2 into the placental cell is mediated by the angiotensin-converting enzyme 2 (ACE2) receptor on the cell membrane [21]. The ACE2 receptor is an important component of the renin-angiotensin system (RAS), which converts angiotensin II to angiotensins I–VII [22]. The RAS significantly modulates uteroplacental blood flow, and binding of SARS-CoV-2 to ACE2 receptors would thus promote the vasoconstrictive and proinflammatory effects of angiotensin II. These alterations could play a role in the pathophysiology of preeclampsia in case of SARS-CoV-2 infection.

Therefore, SARS-CoV-2 infection can affect different molecular pathways related to the pathogenesis of preeclampsia such as angiogenesis, hypoxia, inflammatory signaling, thrombin or platelet activation, and imbalance of vasoactive peptides. In summary, multiple mechanisms link SARS-CoV-2 infection to the subsequent development of vascular disease and preeclampsia [14].

2.2.2 Preterm Birth

Numerous studies have shown an increased risk of prematurity. This prematurity is mainly induced by severe maternal respiratory infections requiring fetal extraction for maternal rescue [3, 4, 6]. However, a retrospective analysis of prospectively collected data in France showed that the incidence of spontaneous preterm delivery was also increased [23]. In multivariate analysis, the risk of preterm delivery was significantly increased in the COVID-19 group (OR = 2.5 [2.1–3.5]), including very preterm 28–31SA (OR = 2.6 [1.6–4.2]) and very preterm 22–27SA (OR = 2.9 [1.9–4.5]). The risk was increased for both induced (OR = 3.8 [2.8–5.3]) and spontaneous prematurities (OR = 2.1 [1.7–2.6]) in this French analysis.

2.2.3 Stillbirth

Although maternal-fetal transmission related to SARS-CoV-2-cov-2 is uncommon and of no major consequence for fetal development, placental involvement by the virus during COVID-19 infection is not rare and potentially severe [24–26]. Thus, stillbirth due to SARS-CoV-2 placentitis occurs without evidence of intrauterine transmission to fetus.

Maternal thrombophilia and prenatally diagnosed fetal growth restriction (FGR) were identified as independent predisposing factors for infectious placentitis [24]. Moreover, the severity of the infection does not seem to be related to the severity of the placental damage in these cases. The lesions of SARS-CoV-2 placentitis were rapidly progressive, producing extensive occlusion of the intervillous space and compromising the maternal-fetal exchange.

The main histological lesions found are massive perivillous fibrinoid deposition, severe intervillositis with a mixed inflammatory infiltrate, trophoblast damage, intervillous thrombosis, and chronic histiocytic intervillositis [27].

References

1. Bobrowski RA. Pulmonary physiology in pregnancy. Clin Obstet Gynecol. 2010;53(2):285–300.
2. Abu-Raya B, Michalski C, Sadarangani M, Lavoie PM. Maternal immunological adaptation during normal pregnancy. Front Immunol. 2020;11:575197.
3. Allotey J, Stallings E, Bonet M, Yap M, Chatterjee S, Kew T, et al. Clinical manifestations, risk factors, and maternal and perinatal outcomes of coronavirus disease 2019 in pregnancy: living systematic review and meta-analysis. BMJ. 2020;370:m3320.

4. Wang H, Li N, Sun C, Guo X, Su W, Song Q, et al. The association between pregnancy and COVID-19: a systematic review and meta-analysis. Am J Emerg Med. 2022;56: 188–95.
5. Mercedes BR, Serwat A, Naffaa L, Ramirez N, Khalid F, Steward SB, et al. New-onset myocardial injury in pregnant patients with coronavirus disease 2019: a case series of 15 patients. Am J Obstet Gynecol. 2021;224(4):387.e1–9.
6. McClymont E, Albert AY, Alton GD, Boucoiran I, Castillo E, Fell DB, et al. Association of SARS-CoV-2 infection during pregnancy with maternal and perinatal outcomes. JAMA. 2022;327(20):1983–91.
7. Badr DA, Mattern J, Carlin A, Cordier AG, Maillart E, El Hachem L, et al. Are clinical outcomes worse for pregnant women at ≥20 weeks' gestation infected with coronavirus disease 2019? A multicenter case-control study with propensity score matching. Am J Obstet Gynecol. 2020;223(5):764–8.
8. Badr DA, Picone O, Bevilacqua E, Carlin A, Meli F, Sibiude J, et al. Severe acute respiratory syndrome coronavirus 2 and pregnancy outcomes according to gestational age at time of infection. Emerg Infect Dis. 2021;27(10):2535–43.
9. Knobel R, Takemoto MLS, Nakamura-Pereira M, Menezes MO, Borges VK, Katz L, et al. COVID-19-related deaths among women of reproductive age in Brazil: the burden of postpartum. Int J Gynaecol Obstet. 2021;155(1):101–9.
10. Marik PE, Plante LA. Venous thromboembolic disease and pregnancy. N Engl J Med. 2008;359(19):2025–33.
11. Iba T, Warkentin TE, Thachil J, Levi M, Levy JH. Proposal of the definition for COVID-19-associated coagulopathy. J Clin Med. 2021;10(2):191.
12. Chinn J, Sedighim S, Kirby KA, Hohmann S, Hameed AB, Jolley J, et al. Characteristics and outcomes of women with COVID-19 giving birth at US Academic Centers during the COVID-19 pandemic. JAMA Netw Open. 2021;4(8):e2120456. https://www.ncbi.nlm.nih.gov/pmc/articles/PMC8358731/. Accessed 6 Jun 2022.
13. Wei SQ, Bilodeau-Bertrand M, Liu S, Auger N. The impact of COVID-19 on pregnancy outcomes: a systematic review and meta-analysis. CMAJ. 2021;193(16):E540–8.
14. Conde-Agudelo A, Romero R. SARS-CoV-2 infection during pregnancy and risk of preeclampsia: a systematic review and meta-analysis. Am J Obstet Gynecol. 2022;226(1):68–89.e3.
15. von Dadelszen P, Magee LA. Could an infectious trigger explain the differential maternal response to the shared placental pathology of preeclampsia and normotensive intrauterine growth restriction? Acta Obstet Gynecol Scand. 2002;81(7):642–8.
16. Kwon JY, Romero R, Mor G. New insights into the relationship between viral infection and pregnancy complications. Am J Reprod Immunol. 2014;71(5):387–90.
17. Cardenas I, Means RE, Aldo P, Koga K, Lang SM, Booth CJ, et al. Viral infection of the placenta leads to fetal inflammation and sensitization to bacterial products precisposing to preterm labor. J Immunol. 2010;185(2):1248–57.
18. Vivanti AJ, Vauloup-Fellous C, Prevot S, Zupan V, Suffee C, Do Cao J, et al. Transplacental transmission of SARS-CoV-2 infection. Nat Commun. 2020;11(1):3572.
19. Schwartz DA, Baldewijns M, Benachi A, Bugatti M, Collins RRJ, De Luca D, et al. Chronic histiocytic intervillositis with trophoblast necrosis is a risk factor associated with placental infection from coronavirus disease 2019 (COVID-19) and intrauterine maternal-fetal severe acute respiratory syndrome coronavirus 2 (SARS-CoV-2) transmission in live-born and stillborn infants. Arch Pathol Lab Med. 2021;145(5):517–28.
20. Lu-Culligan A, Chavan AR, Vijayakumar P, Irshaid L, Courchaine EM, Milano KM, et al. SARS-CoV-2 infection in pregnancy is associated with robust inflammatory response at the maternal-fetal interface. medRxiv. 2021:2021.01.25.21250452.
21. Shang J, Ye G, Shi K, Wan Y, Luo C, Aihara H, et al. Structural basis of receptor recognition by SARS-CoV-2. Nature. 2020;581(7807):221–4.
22. Lumbers ER, Delforce SJ, Arthurs AL, Pringle KG. Causes and consequences of the dysregulated maternal renin-angiotensin system in preeclampsia. Front Endocrinol. 2019;10:563.

23. Epelboin S, Labrosse J, Mouzon JD, Fauque P, Gervoise-Boyer MJ, Levy R, et al. Obstetrical outcomes and maternal morbidities associated with COVID-19 in pregnant women in France: a national retrospective cohort study. PLoS Med. 2021;18(11):e1003857.
24. Konstantinidou AE, Angelidou S, Havaki S, Paparizou K, Spanakis N, Chatzakis C, et al. Stillbirth due to SARS-CoV-2 placentitis without evidence of intrauterine transmission to fetus: association with maternal risk factors. Ultrasound Obstet Gynecol. 2022;59(6):813–22.
25. Dubucs C, Groussolles M, Ousselin J, Sartor A, Van Acker N, Vayssière C, et al. Severe placental lesions due to maternal SARS-CoV-2 infection associated to intrauterine fetal death. Hum Pathol. 2022;121:46–55.
26. Schwartz DA, Avvad-Portari E, Babál P, Baldewijns M, Blomberg M, Bouachba A, et al. Placental tissue destruction and insufficiency from COVID-19 causes stillbirth and neonatal death from hypoxic-ischemic injury. Arch Pathol Lab Med. 2022;146(6):660–76.
27. Jaiswal N, Puri M, Agarwal K, Singh S, Yadav R, Tiwary N, Tayal P, Vats B. COVID-19 as an independent risk factor for subclinical placental dysfunction. Eur J Obstet Gynecol Reprod Biol. 2021;259:7. https://pubmed.ncbi.nlm.nih.gov/33556768/. Accessed 7 Jun 2022.

Chapter 3
Peculiarities of ARDS Induced by COVID-19 in Pregnant Patients

Matteo Di Nardo, Francesco Alessandri, Maximilian Fischer, Maria Grazia Frigo, Fabrizia Calabrese, and V. Marco Ranieri

Data on acute respiratory distress syndrome (ARDS) during pregnancy are sparse and consist mainly of case series. However, ARDS represents one of the most common causes of intensive care unit (ICU) admission during pregnancy with a significant mortality and morbidity for both the mother and the fetus [1]. ARDS is a form of respiratory failure characterized by pulmonary edema due to pulmonary inflammation, reduced lung compliance, and acute hypoxemia [2]. Diagnosis of ARDS is

M. Di Nardo
Pediatric Intensive Care Unit, Ospedale Pediatrico Bambino Gesù, IRCCS, Rome, Italy
e-mail: matteo.dinardo@opbg.net

F. Alessandri
Department of Emergency Medicine, Critical Care Medicine and Trauma, Sapienza Università di Roma, Policlinico Umberto I, Rome, Italy
e-mail: francesco.alessandri@uniroma1.it

M. Fischer
Department of Anesthesiology and Critical Care, Azienda Ospedaliero-Universitaria Careggi, Florence, Italy

Department of Health Sciences, Section of Anaesthesiology, Intensive Care and Pain Medicine, University of Florence, Florence, Italy

M. G. Frigo
Obstetric Anesthesia and Intensive Care Unit, Fatebenefratelli Hospital, Rome, Italy

F. Calabrese
Anaesthesia and Intensive Care Unit, Department of Medicine, Padua University Hospital, Padua, Italy

V. M. Ranieri (✉)
Alma Mater Studiorum University of Bologna, Dipartimento di Scienze Mediche e Chirurgiche (DIMEC), Anesthesia and Intensive Care Medicine, Policlinico di Sant'Orsola, IRCCS, Bologna, Italy
e-mail: m.ranieri@unibo.it

© The Author(s), under exclusive license to Springer Nature Switzerland AG 2023
D. De Luca, A. Benachi (eds.), *COVID-19 and Perinatology*,
https://doi.org/10.1007/978-3-031-29136-4_3

Table 3.1 Berlin definition

Timing	Symptoms of worsening respiratory or new respiratory symptoms that occur within one week of known clinical process
Chest imaging	Bilateral infiltrates that cannot be fully explained by atelectasis, lung nodules, or effusions
Origin of edema	Not completely explained by cardiac failure or fluid overload
Oxygenation (PaO_2/FiO_2) with PEEP or CPAP ≥5 cm	Mild = 200 mmHg <PaO_2/FiO_2 ≤300 mmHg
	Moderate = 100 mmHg <PaO_2/FiO_2 ≤200 mmHg
	Severe = PaO_2/FiO_2 <100 mmHg

achieved following the Berlin definition (Table 3.1), and its severity is classified according to three oxygenation criteria [3, 4].

Clinical conditions associated with inflammation and permeability of the alveolar-capillary interface are all potentially responsible for ARDS. Although true for all clinical scenarios, differential diagnosis of the underlying disease responsible for ARDS is particularly important in pregnancy since the high possibility of cardiogenic pulmonary edema is due to peripartum cardiomyopathy and preeclampsia. In the past years, different definitions have been proposed to classify "ARDS during pregnancy," including ARDS during pregnancy or occurring seven days postpartum and ARDS during pregnancy or within one month postpartum [5]. Nevertheless, since the majority of the physiologic changes of pregnancy are maintained till six weeks from delivery, it might be more appropriate to cover a wider postpartum period [5, 6]. Of note, the diagnosis of ARDS according to the Berlin definition includes the presence of bilateral pulmonary infiltrates on chest X-ray or CT scan. Both imaging techniques require ionizing radiation and can produce relevant effects on the fetus depending on the gestation of exposure [7]. These adverse effects include teratogenicity, abnormal neurological development, and an increased risk of childhood leukemia [8]. Fetal teratogenicity risks are greatest during first trimester and are related to the total dose administered (usually requiring >50 mGy). However, the risk of fetal teratogenicity with low radiation exposure (<50 mGy) is minimal. Thus, maternal investigations should not be withheld if they are necessary for management.

The reported incidence of ARDS in the nonpregnant population ranges between 5 and 80 cases per 100,000 population per year [9], while the incidence of ARDS during pregnancy is higher and ranges between 70 and 130 cases per 100,000 deliveries [10, 11] suggesting that pregnancy itself may increase the risk of ARDS. Mortality due to ARDS in the general population is around 40%, while in pregnancy, it is variable and ranges between 25% and 50% [5, 9, 10]. Of note, a significant morbidity may persist even after initial recovery [6]. Data on the effects of maternal ARDS on neonatal outcomes are scarce; however, available case series report high rates of spontaneous preterm labor, fetal heart rate abnormalities, perinatal asphyxia, and fetal death [5].

From an etiological perspective, both changes in physiologic parameters during pregnancy (Table 3.2) and external causes unique to pregnancy (Table 3.3) may

Table 3.2 Physiologic changes during pregnancy (adapted from Carlin A. et al. [12] and Abu-Raya B. et al. [13])

Respiratory changes	Increase in oxygen demand
	Hyperventilation ($\uparrow pO_2$ and $\downarrow pCO_2$)
	Decrease of functional residual capacity due to diaphragmatic elevation
	Reduction of functional residual capacity
Cardiovascular changes	Increase of cardiac output (up to 40%)
	Reduction of systemic vascular resistance due to peripheral vasodilatation (up to 25–30%)
	Reduction of venous return, mainly because of inferior vena cava compression
	Reduction of colloid osmotic pressure/pulmonary capillary wedge pressure gradient, with high risk of pulmonary edema
Hematological changes	Increase of plasma volume (up to 10% above baseline by 7 weeks of gestation, plateaus by 32 weeks at 45–50%), parallel but weaker rise of red blood cell mass (18–25%), determining dilutional anemia
	Increase of white cell count (values as high as 15,000/mm^3 are not uncommon)
	Reduction of platelet count (dilutional effect and/or increased consumption secondary to endothelial-mediated activation)
	Increase of coagulation factors (fibrinogen, factors VII, VIII, IX, X, and XII) and von Willibrand factor circulating levels, maintenance or slight decrease of natural anticoagulant levels (antithrombin III, protein C, protein S), and reduction of fibrinolytic activity (increase of plasminogen activator inhibitors 1 and 2); thus, defining a pro-coagulable state
Immunological changes	Increase of complement system molecules (C3, C4, C5, C9) and regulatory proteins (factor H)
	Increase of neutrophil count, though less active (e.g., lower phagocytosis)
	Reduced NK cell, T helper cell, and T-cytotoxic cell count (increased susceptibility to viral and fungal pneumonias)
	Diversion of Th1/Th2 immunological responses toward a Th2-specific response
	Reduction of B-cell count ("physiological" B-cell lymphopenia), especially innate B-1-cell levels (major source of "innate" IgM antibodies), and function (e.g., loss of responsiveness to mitogens)
	Increase of IgG1 and IgG3 levels (third trimester) and stable IgG2 and IgG4 levels
	Increased proportion of T-regulatory cells (peak in second trimester)
	Increase of CD19+CD24hiCD27+ B-regulatory cell (first trimester, important role in maternal Th1 response suppression)

increase the risk of ARDS [14, 15]. Increase in plasma volume associated with a reduction of the oncotic pressure may predispose to pulmonary edema [5]. Other causes related to pregnancy such as pulmonary edema secondary to preeclampsia, amniotic fluid embolism, tocolytic-associated pulmonary edema, chorioamnionitis, and endometritis may also increase the risk of ARDS [5]. Causes unrelated to pregnancy that may increase the risk of ARDS include sepsis and aspiration that have a

Table 3.3 Causes of ARDS in pregnancy (adapted from Cole DE et al. [5])

Causes related to pregnancy
Tocolytic-induced pulmonary edema
Preeclampsia and eclampsia
Amniotic fluid embolism and trophoblastic embolism
Placental abruption
Obstetric hemorrhage-related causes
Endometritis
Retained placental products
Septic abortion
Increased infections • Viral: varicella and pneumonia • Bacterial: listeria and pyelonephritis • Fungal: blastomycosis and coccidiomycosis • Protozoal: malaria
Causes not related to pregnancy
Sepsis
Pneumonia and pneumonitis
Severe trauma: pulmonary contusion
Multiple transfusions
Aspiration of gastric contents
Acute pancreatitis and pyelonephritis
Fat emboli
Drug overdose
Near drowning

higher incidence in pregnancy report compared to nonpregnant population [14, 15]. Viral pneumonia due to influenza virus is also common in pregnancy due to the alterations in cell-mediated immunity which predispose to pulmonary infections and is associated with increased mortality rates compared with the general population [16].

The management of ARDS during pregnancy includes not only the knowledge of underlying cause of ARDS but also the understanding of the cardiorespiratory physiological changes accompanying pregnancy. Moreover, the maintenance of an adequate perfusion to the uterus and adequate gas exchange ($PaO_2 \geq 70$ mmHg, $PaCO_2 < 45$ mmHg with a pH >7.30) is essential for the fetal well-being [5, 14]. Lung compliance is not altered during pregnancy, but chest wall and total respiratory compliance is reduced in the third trimester. Minute ventilation, instead, is increased; this begins from the first trimester and reaches 20–40% above baseline by term. The major mechanism is an increase in tidal volume of approximately 30–35% mediated by elevated serum progesterone levels. Blood gas measurement in pregnancy reveals a respiratory alkalosis with a compensatory renal excretion of bicarbonate (Table 3.4); consequently, $PaCO_2$ is reduced to 28–32 mmHg and plasma bicarbonate to 18–21 mEq/L [18]. Of note, oxygen consumption and CO_2 production of the mother increase due to both fetal and maternal metabolic

Table 3.4 Arterial blood gas changes in pregnancy (adapted from ACOG Practice Bulletin No. 211 [17])

ABG measurement (sea level)	Nonpregnant state	Pregnancy state	
		First trimester	Third trimester
pH	7.40	7.42–7.46	7.43
PaO_2 (mmHg)	93	105–106	101–106
$PaCO_2$ (mmHg)	37	28–29	26–30
Serum HCO_3-	23	18	17

processes, reaching 20–33% above baseline by the third trimester. This increased oxygen consumption in the presence of a reduced FRC (functional residual capacity) (oxygen reservoir) makes the pregnant patient very susceptible to the rapid development of hypoxia in response to hypoventilation or apnea. Alkalosis (respiratory or metabolic) reduces uterine blood flow and adversely affects fetal oxygenation [5, 18].

Clinically, the signs and symptoms of ARDS reflect the underlying disease process [19]. However, critical patients may exhibit classical generic signs and symptoms of acute hypoxemic respiratory failure, like worsening dyspnea, tachypnea, tachycardia, cyanosis, restlessness, and confusion. Diffuse bilateral crackles or wheezing at lung basis can be appreciated on chest auscultation. Furthermore, clinical, instrumental, and/or laboratory findings of pulmonary hypertension or even of multiple organ dysfunction syndrome could be present.

3.1 SARS-CoV-2 Infection and Pregnancy

The severe acute respiratory syndrome coronavirus 2 (SARS-CoV-2) has spread rapidly across the world in 2020 and was responsible of the coronavirus disease 2019 (COVID-19) pandemic. Early data from China and the United States showed that the risk of severe COVID-19 disease in pregnant women was similar to the general population [20–23]. However, this first enthusiasm was dampened by other data showing that pregnant women with COVID-19 had a higher risk of hospitalization than nonpregnant women [24, 25]. A recent meta-analysis also showed that the prevalence of ICU (intensive care unit) admission and death (2.0–4.2% and 0.1–0.2%, respectively) was similar to that reported in nonpregnant women [26]; however, the risk of ICU admission and adverse maternal and neonatal outcomes has increased with the severity of COVID-19 [27–29]. Several physiologic adaptations to pregnancy may increase maternal susceptibility to infections and in particular to SARS-CoV-2 infection including changes in maternal immune system function, impairment of the respiratory function, and prothrombotic state [30, 31].

Maternal changes of immune function consist of a hormone-mediated shift from a T helper 1 to T helper 2 cell response with a decrease of CD4+ and CD8+ T cells. This asset produces an important immunomodulation associated with an anti-inflammatory cytokine profile to prevent rejection of the fetus [31]. These changes, associated with the reduction of the functional residual capacity, make pregnant women more susceptible to respiratory infections [30, 31]. Moreover, the hypercoagulable state typical of physiological pregnancy is amplified by SARS-CoV-2 infection. SARS-CoV-2 causes a significant activation of both coagulation pathways and fibrinolysis and an endothelial damage (thrombotic microangiopathy) [32]. Thus, pregnant women with COVID-19 may have synergistic factors that may increase the risk for thrombosis and thromboembolic events (pulmonary embolism) and preeclampsia [30, 33].

SARS-CoV-2 infection in pregnant women can be asymptomatic (most of the cases) or symptomatic [30]. Cough, dyspnea, and fever are the most common clinical manifestations, [30] and symptoms do not appear to differ based on gestational age [34]. Symptomatic pregnant women can be classified in mild, moderate, severe, and critical (Table 3.5) according to severity of the respiratory disease and the presence of multiorgan failure and are generally admitted to the hospital in the late second or third trimester [35], and pregnant women with mild COVID-19 reported similar maternal and neonatal outcomes compared with pregnant women without COVID-19 [27]. On the other hand, adverse maternal and neonatal outcomes are reported in pregnant patients with severe or critical COVID-19 [27, 28]. Of note, pregnant women with severe or critical COVID-19 are more likely to be old, Black or Hispanic, or obese, with pre-existing hypertension and diabetes [27, 30]. Differential diagnosis for symptomatic respiratory failure due to COVID-19 in pregnancy is broad and includes pulmonary embolism, cardiomyopathy, preeclampsia, and other etiologies of viral/bacterial pneumonia.

Respiratory failure associated with COVID-19, despite falling in most of the circumstances under the Berlin definition of ARDS, may present distinctive features including a severe hypoxemia often associated with a "near normal" respiratory system compliance. This combination is uncommon in "typical" ARDS and requires a different clinical management at bedside [36, 37]. Recent data suggest that SARS-CoV-2 infection leads to an interstitial pneumonia (ground-glass lesions) associated relatively with small gasless tissue at the beginning of the infection. Thus, loss of hypoxic vasoconstriction may be responsible of hypoxemia [38]. All these features generally cause an increase in respiratory drive which is clinically manifested by an

Table 3.5 Classification of COVID-19 by severity

Classification	Definition
Asymptomatic	Positive SARS-CoV-2 testing, but no symptoms
Mild	Fever and cough, but no shortness of breath, dyspnea, or abnormal imaging on chest X-ray
Moderate	Clinical or radiographic evidence of mild pneumonia (O_2 saturation >93% on room air at sea level)
Severe	Dyspnea, respiratory rate >30/min, O_2 saturation <93%, PaO_2/FiO_2 <300, or >50% lung infiltrates
Critical	Respiratory failure requiring invasive mechanical ventilation, septic shock, and/or multiorgan dysfunction

increase in the respiratory rate rather than an increase tidal volume which is already increased in pregnancy compared with nonpregnant women. A meta-analysis of 42 studies including 247 pregnant women with COVID-19 showed that focal (unilateral or bilateral) ground-glass densities were more frequent in asymptomatic and mild cases, while diffuse ground-glass densities, subpleural lesions, and pleural effusions were more frequent in severe cases [39, 40].

Several key causes may be responsible for the worsening of this form of respiratory failure: (a) the natural evolution of COVID-19 disease in an immunocompromised host [41], (b) the bacterial superinfections [42], and (c) the depth of the negative intrathoracic pressure during spontaneous breathing [38]. All these features may increase lung inflammation, interstitial edema, lung weight, and consequently the amount of atelectasis. The increase of atelectasis, as well as of D-dimer levels, which reflects the endothelial injury caused by COVID-19, contributes to hypoxemia development.

3.2 Maternal and Neonatal Management of COVID-19 ARDS

3.2.1 Respiratory Support

The first and immediate goal in all ARDS pregnant women and thus also in COVID-19 ARDS is to maintain an adequate maternal PaO_2 (>70 mmHg) and $PaCO_2$ (<45 mmHg) [43]. In the early phases of ARDS, these targets may be achieved simply with low flow oxygen administration (e.g. venti-mask); however, when the disease worsens, oxygen supplementation may be delivered by different devices such as high-flow nasal cannula (HFNC), continuous positive airway pressure (CPAP), and noninvasive ventilation (NIV) [44]. Optimal noninvasive respiratory support, time of intubation, and mechanical ventilation settings are still controversial in COVID-19 patients [45]; instead, the indications for invasive mechanical ventilation are the same of non-COVID-19 pregnant women and include an altered mental status, a progressive or refractory hypoxemia, signs of respiratory maternal fatigue, and acidosis [45].

High-flow nasal cannula (HFNC) is the most common technique to provide oxygen supplementation in patients with ARDS. HFNC provides a heated and humidified oxygen flow up to 60 L/min and a FiO_2 up to 100% [46]. This technique may improve the CO_2 washout from the upper airways and may generate a modest positive end-expiratory pressure (PEEP) (2–5 cmH_2O). HFNC may minimize mucosal injury, improve secretion clearance, and reduce transpulmonary driving pressure; HFNC is generally considered comfortable by the patients and reports a higher compliance than other noninvasive devices or techniques such as facial masks, helmet CPAP, or NIV through a ventilator [47]. When HFNC fails, CPAP or NIV through a ventilator can be used. CPAP may be administered with different devices (facial mask or helmet) [48, 49]. There is growing evidence about the use of NIV in pregnancy; however, short trials of NIV should be attempted with caution in pregnant patients before endotracheal intubation [49]. Decreased tone of the lower esophageal sphincter, increased abdominal pressure, and decreased gastric emptying may put pregnant women at risk of aspiration; this risk is further increased during NIV which may lead to gastric distension [45]. Of note, development of high inspiratory efforts during NIV can generate large tidal volumes that are independently associated with NIV failure, barotrauma (i.e., pneumothorax and pneumomediastinum), and self-induced lung injury (SILI) [38].

In pregnant women failing NIV, invasive positive pressure mechanical ventilation is essential to improve gas exchange and reduce the work of breathing [50]. However, since the risk of failed intubation is higher in pregnant women compared to nonpregnant women due to the anatomical changes related to pregnancy (e.g., airway edema), intubation should be performed by experienced staff [5, 29, 51]. Current guidelines suggest that patients should be treated as a classic ARDS with low tidal volume (4–6 mL/kg of PBW) and a plateau pressure (P_{Plat}) limited to 28–30 cmH$_2$O [38]. Of note, since the cause of ventilation-induced lung injury (VILI) is not the pressure applied to the whole respiratory system (Paw), but the one applied to the lung (i.e., the transpulmonary pressure), it follows that the P_{Plat} value of 28–30 cmH$_2$O may be not a good threshold to reduce the risk of VILI [52, 53]. Actually, the relationship between the airway pressure and the transpulmonary pressure in an individual patient is strictly linear and follows the formula: $P_L = Paw*(E_L/E_{tot})$ [52]. The transpulmonary pressure (P_L) equals the applied airway pressure (Paw) times the ratio of lung elastance to total respiratory system elastance (E_L/E_{tot}). In the general population, this ratio averages 0.7; however, in ARDS, it may vary between 0.2 and 0.8 [52]. Thus, the "safe" 30 cmH$_2$O may result in a transpulmonary pressure as low as 6 cmH$_2$O causing hypoxemia or as high as 24 cmH$_2$O causing lung overdistension. In pregnant women, the E_L/E_{tot} is generally low as in obese patients (e.g., 0.2); thus, even a Paw of 28–30 cmH$_2$O may generate a low transpulmonary pressure causing hypoventilation and severe hypoxemia [53]. In these patients, hypoxemia may be easily reversed by safely increasing P_L till 20–21 cmH$_2$O. Further, in patients presenting the H phenotype, PEEP is generally high (>10 cmH$_2$O) and titrated to reach the lower driving pressure with the best respiratory system compliance [52].

3.2.2 Prone Position

Mechanical ventilation with prone position is reserved to severe ARDS with a PaO$_2$/FiO$_2$ <150 mmHg [54]. Repeated cycles of prone position, lasting at least 12–16 h, may improve ventral-dorsal pleural pressure gradient and reduce alveolar shunt. In COVID-19 patients with significant consolidation in the dependent zones, prone position has been recommended [38]. Several reports have described its feasibility and safety also in COVID-19 pregnant patients with ARDS [55, 56]. However, prone position in pregnant women requires appropriate supports to sustain the large

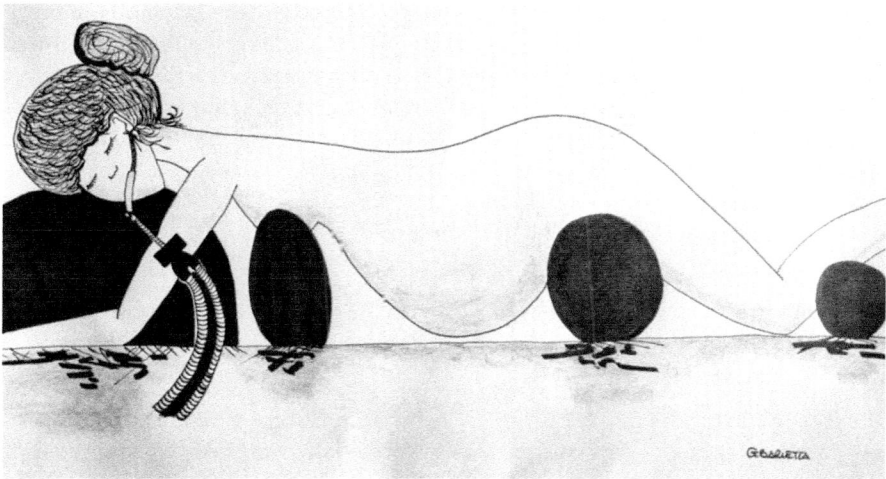

Fig. 3.1 Prone positioning in pregnant patient: the patient is lying down alternating the position of the face. Pillows are placed to support the head, the thorax (above the gravid uterus), the pelvis, and under knees. The bed is in reverse Trendelenburg. Check the gravid abdomen and ensure no pressure

gravid abdomen, and fetal heart rate should be carefully monitored during the procedure to identify any deterioration in clinical status (Fig. 3.1) [55]. The pregnant women should maintain the prone position as long as they can tolerate it. Prone position, instead, should be discontinued if there is no improvement, if fetal or maternal hemodynamic worsen, or if significant improvement is maintained when the patient is returned to the supine position. Furthermore particular attention should be paid to prevent complications associated with prone position, including vascular line and endotracheal tube displacement, facial edema, pressure sores, corneal abrasions, and brachial plexus injury [55, 56]. Though the effect on mortality remains unclear, prone positioning in awake, non-intubated COVID-19 patients improves oxygenation.

3.3 Extracorporeal Membrane Oxygenation (ECMO)

Veno-venous extracorporeal membrane oxygenation (VV-ECMO) is an invasive strategy to support patients with refractory respiratory failure [57]. Indications for VV-ECMO in the general population are PaO_2/FiO_2 <50 mmHg for >3 h or PaO_2/FiO_2 <80 mmHg for >6 h, and pH <7.25 with $PaCO_2$ >60 mmHg for >6 h with a respiratory rate up to 35 breaths/min, along with plateau pressure >30 cmH_2O [57]. Due to the complex management of this technology, patients who meet the ECMO criteria should be treated or referred to experienced, high-volume centers [58]. During the 2009 H1N1 pandemic, ECMO was successfully used to rescue pregnant women with refractory hypoxemia [59]. Positive results were found also during COVID-19 pandemic [60–63]. In a recent retrospective cohort study including 100 COVID-19 pregnant/peripartum patients supported with VV-ECMO, survival to hospital discharge was higher, and ECMO-related complications were lower than that of nonpregnant women supported with VV-ECMO for ARDS [63]. Currently, the guidelines from the Society for Maternal-Fetal Medicine suggest the use of ECMO to rescue COVID-19 ARDS for postpartum and pregnant women <32 weeks gestation to facilitate in utero fetal development [64].

3.4 Delivery

The care of a critically ill COVID-19 pregnant woman requests a multidisciplinary team consisting of obstetricians, intensivists, cardiothoracic surgeons, perfusionists, anesthesiologists, neonatologists, physiotherapists, and nurses. Since few data support the optimal timing and mode of delivery in pregnant women with severe COVID-19, the whole team should carefully evaluate both the fetus gestational age and clinical condition and the maternal health status [5, 29]. Thus, in case of acute changes of maternal respiratory status, continuous fetal monitoring should be promptly initiated. Emergency caesarean section may be considered in case of fetal distress, critical maternal deterioration including septic shock, and multiorgan failure or poor progression in labor [29]. However, before a viable gestational age is reached, delivery is not an option, and any attempt to postpone delivery should be performed [5]. In such cases, the use of VV-ECMO has been advocated to improve maternal gas exchange while awaiting the fetus to reach an adequate gestational age (32–34 weeks) [64]. In late pregnancy instead, an elective delivery has been suggested to improve maternal status (the reduction of the oxygen consumption, the improvement of diaphragmatic excursion, the reduction of intrathoracic pressure, and the resolution of the aortocaval compression) [29, 65]. After delivery, immediate clamping of the umbilical cords and separation of the neonate from the mother are recommended to reduce the risk of vertical infection [29, 43].

References

1. Pollock W, Rose L, Dennis CL. Pregnant and postpartum admissions to the intensive care unit: a systematic review. Intensive Care Med. 2010;36(9):1465–74.
2. Thompson BT, Chambers RC, Liu KD. Acute respiratory distress syndrome. N Engl J Med. 2017;377(6):562–72.
3. Ranieri VM, Rubenfeld GD, Thompson BT, Ferguson ND, Caldwell E, Fan E, et al. Acute respiratory distress syndrome: the Berlin Definition. JAMA. 2012;307(23):2526–33.
4. Ferguson ND, Fan E, Camporota L, Antonelli M, Anzueto A, Beale R, et al. The Berlin definition of ARDS: an expanded rationale, justification, and supplementary material. Intensive Care Med. 2012;38(10):1573–82.

5. Cole DE, Taylor TL, McCullough DM, Shoff CT, Derdak S. Acute respiratory distress syndrome in pregnancy. Crit Care Med. 2005;33(10 Suppl):S269–78.
6. Catanzarite V, Willms D, Wong D, Landers C, Cousins L, Schrimmer D. Acute respiratory distress syndrome in pregnancy and the puerperium: causes, courses, and outcomes. Obstet Gynecol. 2001;97(5 Pt 1):760–4.
7. Guilbaud L, Beghin D, Dhombres F, Blondiaux E, Friszer S, Ducou Le Pointe H, et al. Pregnancy outcome after first trimester exposure to ionizing radiations. Eur J Obstet Gynecol Reprod Biol. 2019;232:18–21.
8. Lowe S. Diagnostic imaging in pregnancy: making informed decisions. Obstet Med. 2019;12(3):116–22.
9. Pham T, Rubenfeld GD. Fifty years of research in ARDS. The epidemiology of acute respiratory distress syndrome. A 50th birthday review. Am J Respir Crit Care Med. 2017;195(7):860–70.
10. Perry KG Jr, Martin RW, Blake PG, Roberts WE, Martin JN Jr. Maternal mortality associated with adult respiratory distress syndrome. South Med J. 1998;91(5):441–4.
11. Vasquez DN, Estenssoro E, Canales HS, Reina R, Saenz MG, Das Neves AV, et al. Clinical characteristics and outcomes of obstetric patients requiring ICU admission. Chest. 2007;131(3):718–24.
12. Carlin A, Alfirevic Z. Physiological changes of pregnancy and monitoring. Best Pract Res Clin Obstet Gynaecol. 2008;22(5):801–23.
13. Abu-Raya B, Michalski C, Sadarangani M, Lavoie PM. Maternal immunological adaptation during normal pregnancy. Front Immunol. 2020;11:575197.
14. Hegewald MJ, Crapo RO. Respiratory physiology in pregnancy. Clin Chest Med. 2011;32(1):1–13.
15. Bandi VD, Munnur U, Matthay MA. Acute lung injury and acute respiratory distress syndrome in pregnancy. Crit Care Clin. 2004;20(4):577–607.
16. Jamieson DJ, Honein MA, Rasmussen SA, Williams JL, Swerdlow DL, Biggerstaff MS, et al. H1N1 2009 influenza virus infection during pregnancy in the USA. Lancet. 2009;374(9688):451–8.
17. ACOG. Practice bulletin no. 211 summary: critical care in pregnancy. Obstet Gynecol. 2019;133(5):1063–6.
18. Lucius H, Gahlenbeck H, Kleine HO, Fabel H, Bartels H. Respiratory functions, buffer system, and electrolyte concentrations of blood during human pregnancy. Respir Physiol. 1970;9(3):311–7.
19. Rush B, Martinka P, Kilb B, McDermid RC, Boyd JH, Celi LA. Acute respiratory distress syndrome in pregnant women. Obstet Gynecol. 2017;129(3):530–5.
20. Chen L, Li Q, Zheng D, Jiang H, Wei Y, Zou L, et al. Clinical characteristics of pregnant women with Covid-19 in Wuhan, China. N Engl J Med. 2020;382(25):e100.
21. Chen L, Zhao Y, Qiao J. More on clinical characteristics of pregnant women with Covid-19 in Wuhan, China. Reply. N Engl J Med. 2020;383(7):697.
22. Breslin N, Baptiste C, Miller R, Fuchs K, Goffman D, Gyamfi-Bannerman C, et al. Coronavirus disease 2019 in pregnancy: early lessons. Am J Obstet Gynecol MFM. 2020;2(2):100111.
23. Lokken EM, Huebner EM, Taylor GG, Hendrickson S, Vanderhoeven J, Kachikis A, et al. Disease severity, pregnancy outcomes, and maternal deaths among pregnant patients with severe acute respiratory syndrome coronavirus 2 infection in Washington State. Am J Obstet Gynecol. 2021;225(1):77.e1–77.e14.
24. Ellington S, Strid P, Tong VT, Woodworth K, Galang RR, Zambrano LD, et al. Characteristics of women of reproductive age with laboratory-confirmed SARS-CoV-2 infection by pregnancy status - United States, January 22-June 7, 2020. MMWR Morb Mortal Wkly Rep. 2020;69(25):769–75.
25. Lokken EM, Taylor GG, Huebner EM, Vanderhoeven J, Hendrickson S, Coler B, et al. Higher severe acute respiratory syndrome coronavirus 2 infection rate in pregnant patients. Am J Obstet Gynecol. 2021;225(1):75.e1–75.e16.
26. Di Toro F, Gjoka M, Di Lorenzo G, De Santo D, De Seta F, Maso G, et al. Impact of COVID-19 on maternal and neonatal outcomes: a systematic review and meta-analysis. Clin Microbiol Infect. 2021;27(1):36–46.

27. Brandt JS, Hill J, Reddy A, Schuster M, Patrick HS, Rosen T, et al. Epidemiology of coronavirus disease 2019 in pregnancy: risk factors and associations with adverse maternal and neonatal outcomes. Am J Obstet Gynecol. 2021;224(4):389.e1–9.
28. Galang RR, Newton SM, Woodworth KR, Griffin I, Oduyebo T, Sancken CL, et al. Risk factors for illness severity among pregnant women with confirmed severe acute respiratory syndrome coronavirus 2 infection-surveillance for emerging threats to mothers and babies network, 22 state, local, and territorial health departments, 29 March 2020-5 March 2021. Clin Infect Dis. 2021;73(Suppl 1):S17–s23.
29. Kumar R, Yeni CM, Utami NA, Masand R, Asrani RK, Patel SK, et al. SARS-CoV-2 infection during pregnancy and pregnancy-related conditions: concerns, challenges, management and mitigation strategies-a narrative review. J Infect Public Health. 2021;14(7):863–75.
30. Boushra MN, Koyfman A, Long B. COVID-19 in pregnancy and the puerperium: a review for emergency physicians. Am J Emerg Med. 2021;40:193–8.
31. Wastnedge EAN, Reynolds RM, van Boeckel SR, Stock SJ, Denison FC, Maybin JA, et al. Pregnancy and COVID-19. Physiol Rev. 2021;101(1):303–18.
32. Bahraini M, Dorgalaleh A. The impact of SARS-CoV-2 infection on blood coagulation and fibrinolytic pathways: a review of prothrombotic changes caused by COVID-19. Semin Thromb Hemost. 2021;48:19.
33. Mendoza M, Garcia-Ruiz I, Maiz N, Rodo C, Garcia-Manau P, Serrano B, et al. Preeclampsia-like syndrome induced by severe COVID-19: a prospective observational study. BJOG. 2020;127(11):1374–80.
34. Liu D, Li L, Wu X, Zheng D, Wang J, Yang L, et al. Pregnancy and perinatal outcomes of women with coronavirus disease (COVID-19) pneumonia: a preliminary analysis. AJR Am J Roentgenol. 2020;215(1):127–32.
35. Knight M, Bunch K, Vousden N, Morris E, Simpson N, Gale C, et al. Characteristics and outcomes of pregnant women admitted to hospital with confirmed SARS-CoV-2 infection in UK: national population based cohort study. BMJ. 2020;369:m2107.
36. Camporota L, Chiumello D, Busana M, Gattinoni L, Marini JJ. Pathophysiology of COVID-19-associated acute respiratory distress syndrome. Lancet Respir Med. 2021;9(1):e1.
37. Fan E, Beitler JR, Brochard L, Calfee CS, Ferguson ND, Slutsky AS, et al. COVID-19-associated acute respiratory distress syndrome: is a different approach to management warranted? Lancet Respir Med. 2020;8(8):816–21.
38. Gattinoni L, Chiumello D, Caironi P, Busana M, Romitti F, Brazzi L, et al. COVID-19 pneumonia: different respiratory treatments for different phenotypes? Intensive Care Med. 2020;46(6):1099–102.
39. Galang RR, Chang K, Strid P, Snead MC, Woodworth KR, House LD, et al. Severe coronavirus infections in pregnancy: a systematic review. Obstet Gynecol. 2020;136(2):262–72.
40. Moradi B, Kazemi MA, Gity M. CT findings of pregnant women with coronavirus disease (COVID-19) pneumonia. AJR Am J Roentgenol. 2020;215(1):W9.
41. Gattinoni L, Busana M, Camporota L, Marini JJ, Chiumello D. COVID-19 and ARDS: the baby lung size matters. Intensive Care Med. 2021;47(1):133–4.
42. Cataño-Correa JC, Cardona-Arias JA, Porras Mancilla JP, García MT. Bacterial superinfection in adults with COVID-19 hospitalized in two clinics in Medellín-Colombia, 2020. PLoS One. 2021;16(7):e0254671.
43. Lapinsky SE. Acute respiratory failure in pregnancy. Obstet Med. 2015;8(3):126–32.
44. Navas-Blanco JR, Dudaryk R. Management of respiratory distress syndrome due to COVID-19 infection. BMC Anesthesiol. 2020;20(1):177.
45. Bhatia PK, Biyani G, Mohammed S, Sethi P, Bihani P. Acute respiratory failure and mechanical ventilation in pregnant patient: a narrative review of literature. J Anaesthesiol Clin Pharmacol. 2016;32(4):431–9.
46. Nishimura M. High-flow nasal cannula oxygen therapy in adults: physiological benefits, indication, clinical benefits, and adverse effects. Respir Care. 2016;61(4):529–41.
47. Coppadoro A, Zago E, Pavan F, Foti G, Bellani G. The use of head helmets to deliver noninvasive ventilatory support: a comprehensive review of technical aspects and clinical findings. Crit Care. 2021;25(1):327.

48. Raoof S, Nava S, Carpati C, Hill NS. High-flow, noninvasive ventilation and awake (nonintubation) proning in patients with coronavirus disease 2019 with respiratory failure. Chest. 2020;158(5):1992–2002.
49. Al-Ansari MA, Hameed AA, Al-jawder SE, Saeed HM. Use of noninvasive positive pressure ventilation during pregnancy: case series. Ann Thorac Med. 2007;2(1):23–5.
50. Russotto V, Bellani G, Foti G. Respiratory mechanics in patients with acute respiratory distress syndrome. Ann Transl Med. 2018;6(19):382.
51. Munnur U, de Boisblanc B, Suresh MS. Airway problems in pregnancy. Crit Care Med. 2005;33(10 Suppl):S259–68.
52. Gattinoni L, Marini JJ, Collino F, Maiolo G, Rapetti F, Tonetti T, et al. The future of mechanical ventilation: lessons from the present and the past. Crit Care. 2017;21(1):183.
53. Tonetti T, Vasques F, Rapetti F, Maiolo G, Collino F, Romitti F, et al. Driving pressure and mechanical power: new targets for VILI prevention. Ann Transl Med. 2017;5(14):286.
54. Guérin C, Albert RK, Beitler J, Gattinoni L, Jaber S, Marini JJ, et al. Prone position in ARDS patients: why, when, how and for whom. Intensive Care Med. 2020;46(12):2385–96.
55. Cavalcante FML, Fernandes CDS, Rocha LDS, Galindo-Neto NM, Caetano J, Barros LM. Use of the prone position in pregnant women with COVID-19 or other health conditions. Rev Lat Am Enfermagem. 2021;29:e3494.
56. Tolcher MC, McKinney JR, Eppes CS, Muigai D, Shamshirsaz A, Guntupalli KK, et al. Prone positioning for pregnant women with hypoxemia due to coronavirus disease 2019 (COVID-19). Obstet Gynecol. 2020;136(2):259–61.
57. Combes A, Peek GJ, Hajage D, Hardy P, Abrams D, Schmidt M, et al. ECMO for severe ARDS: systematic review and individual patient data meta-analysis. Intensive Care Med. 2020;46(11):2048–57.
58. Barbaro RP, Odetola FO, Kidwell KM, Paden ML, Bartlett RH, Davis MM, et al. Association of hospital-level volume of extracorporeal membrane oxygenation cases and mortality. Analysis of the extracorporeal life support organization registry. Am J Respir Crit Care Med. 2015;191(8):894–901.
59. Jamieson DJ, Rasmussen SA. An update on COVID-19 and pregnancy. Am J Obstet Gynecol. 2021;226:177.
60. Khalil M, Butt A, Kseibi E, Althenayan E, Alhazza M, Sallam H. COVID-19-related acute respiratory distress syndrome in a pregnant woman supported on ECMO: the juxtaposition of bleeding in a hypercoagulable state. Membranes. 2021;11(7):544.
61. Barrantes JH, Ortoleva J, O'Neil ER, Suarez EE, Beth Larson S, Rali AS, et al. Successful treatment of pregnant and postpartum women with severe COVID-19 associated acute respiratory distress syndrome with extracorporeal membrane oxygenation. ASAIO J. 2021;67(2):132–6.
62. Rushakoff JA, Polyak A, Caren J, Parrinella K, Salabat R, Wong M, et al. A case of a pregnant patient with COVID-19 infection treated with emergency c-section and extracorporeal membrane oxygenation. J Card Surg. 2021;36(8):2982–5.
63. O'Neil ER, Lin H, Shamshirsaz AA, Naoum EE, Rycus PR, Alexander PM, et al. Pregnant/peripartum women with COVID-19 high survival with ECMO: an ELSO registry analysis. Am J Respir Crit Care Med. 2021;205:248.
64. Society for Maternal-Fetal Medicine (SFMF). Management considerations for pregnant patients with COVID-19. Washington, DC: SFMF; 2021. https://s3.amazonaws.com/cdn.smfm.org/media/2734/SMFM_COVID_Management_of_COVID_pos_preg_patients_2-2-21_(final).pdf. Accessed 1 Jun 2022.
65. Tomlinson MW, Caruthers TJ, Whitty JE, Gonik B. Does delivery improve maternal condition in the respiratory-compromised gravida? Obstet Gynecol. 1998;91(1):108–11.

Chapter 4
Miscarriage and Fetal Death

Baptiste Tarasi and David Baud

4.1 Introduction

The SARS-CoV-2 pandemic has been the subject of extensive research resulting in multiple publications associated with pregnancy. This research has been much more voluminous than the ones devoted to other viral diseases. The discoveries continue, and it is important to keep in mind that what we think and understand today may be wrong tomorrow [1]. At the beginning of the pandemic, data on past coronavirus epidemics were briefly summarized in a literature review. The SARS-CoV-1 and the MERS-CoV were known to cause severe complications during pregnancy, resulting in numerous maternal and fetal adverse outcomes [2]. Fortunately, the first studies published afterward were reassuring, both in terms of maternal and fetal outcomes [3–5]. Shortly after, during the early part of the pandemic, our team discovered a case of fetal death in a SARS-CoV-2-positive woman during the second trimester of her pregnancy. The placental swabs were positive for this virus, and placental histological analysis showed a mixed inflammatory infiltrate. No other cause of fetal death was identified [6]. Information about the risk of miscarriage and fetal death in patients during the Covid-19 pandemic was not available at that time and many questions followed. What do we know today? This subject will be discussed in this chapter, in the form of a narrative review.

B. Tarasi · D. Baud (✉)
Materno-Fetal and Obstetric Research Unit, Obstetric service, Woman-Mother-Child Department, University Hospital of Lausanne, Lausanne, Switzerland
e-mail: baptiste.tarasi@chuv.ch; david.baud@chuv.ch

4.2 Definitions

According to the International Classification of Diseases, 10th revision (ICD 10) definitions, a miscarriage is defined as a loss of pregnancy before 22 completed weeks of gestational age. If a pregnancy loss occurs after 22 weeks, it will be defined as fetal death. This can be differentiated into "early fetal death" if it occurs before 28 weeks of gestational age and "late fetal death" if it occurs after [7]. Before the Covid-19 pandemic, the risk of miscarriage in a recognized pregnancy was estimated to be 15.3% [8]. Much less frequent, fetal death was estimated to occur in 5.7 per 1000 births in the European region in 2019 [9]. The causes are multifactorial and will not be explained in detail in this chapter, but it is important to mention that some systemic infections may be one of them [7, 10].

4.3 Miscarriages

At the beginning of the pandemic, a Canadian cross-sectional study compared the reason of consultations in the emergency department during the early part of the pandemic with a control group from a past period. Curiously, a decrease in the number of miscarriages was reported. However, the number of emergency department visits also decreased, raising an important point that could potentially explain the lower number of diagnosed miscarriages [11]. The publication of other studies followed with reassuring results. For example, the case-control study by Cosma et al. on 225 patients demonstrated that a SARS-CoV-2 infection in the first trimester of pregnancy does not appear to be associated with a higher risk of miscarriage (odds ratio, 1.28; 95% CI, 0.53–3.08) [5]. Other studies, including the one of Rotshenker-Olshinka et al., a retrospective study comparing first-trimester pregnancy outcomes in early 2020 with early 2019, or the one of Jacoby et al., a prospective study in which data on miscarriage during the pandemic were comparable to the national pre-pandemic miscarriage rate, reinforced the previously published findings [12, 13]. Moreover, the meta-analysis by Cavalcante et al. estimated the miscarriage rates during the pandemic to be 15.3% (95% CI, 10.94–20.59) [14], corresponding to the pre-pandemic data [8].

A prospective study published in early 2022 focuses, in addition to clinical features, on biomarkers of pregnancy and inflammatory markers between weeks 8 and 14 of pregnancy. In addition to a more marked lymphopenia and increased IL-6 levels, this study found that PAPP-A (pregnancy-associated plasma protein-A) levels were higher in symptomatic women than in the asymptomatic and the negative ones.

The higher expression of PAPP-A in symptomatic women suggests that it may be involved in the inflammatory response to SARS-CoV-2. However, its role in the Covid-19 disease needs to be further investigated [15].

In summary, the outcomes of the first trimester of pregnancy in SARS-CoV-2-infected pregnant women are comparable to those noninfected, as are the outcomes comparing pregnant women in the first trimester during the SARS-CoV-2 pandemic in general with those during the pre-pandemic period.

4.4 Fetal Death

Regarding fetal death, the phenomenon could be different. The study by Khalil et al., which took place in the United Kingdom during the early part of the pandemic, identified an increase in the fetal death rates compared to the pre-pandemic period, from 2.38 per 1000 to 9.31 per 1000 births (difference, 6.93; 95% CI, 1.83–12.0). Although no cases involved women with Covid-19, the question of a direct consequence of SARS-CoV-2 infections arose. In parallel, the author also reported a significant decrease in the number of medical consultations during the pandemic, which could also be linked to the indirect increased rate in fetal death rates [16]. Thereafter, Gurol-Urganci et al. confirmed this hypothesis. Their study included more than 340,000 pregnant women, of whom 3527 had a confirmed SARS-CoV-2 infection. Fetal death was more frequent in women infected with SARS-CoV-2 than in those not infected (adjusted odds ratio, 2.21; 95% CI, 1.58–3.11) [17]. Other articles have subsequently reinforced this hypothesis, such as the study by Cruz Melguizo et al. reporting a higher rate of fetal death in patients with SARS-CoV-2 infection (0 2% vs. 0.7%; p-value 0.023) [18].

In addition, Chmielewska et al. assessed the collective evidence of the effects of the pandemic on maternal, fetal, and neonatal outcomes in their meta-analysis. Out of a total of 40 studies, 12 concerned fetal death. The result was a significant increase in it (odds ratio, 1.28; 95% CI, 1.07–1.54) [19]. Other meta-analyses followed, including the one of Allotey et al. with 9 studies and resulting in an increased risk of fetal death (odds ratio, 2.84; 95% CI, 1.25–6.45) [20] as well as the one of Wei et al. in which 6 of the 42 studies included data concerning the same subject, resulting in a significantly increased risk (odds ratio, 2.11; 95% CI, 1.14–3.90) [21].

It may also be worth mentioning the study conducted by Kc et al., focusing on the rate of fetal death right before and during Nepal's lockdown. The rate increased from 14 per 1000 before to 21 per 1000 births during the lockdown in Nepal (95% CI, 12–16, respectively, 18–25). This study raised one more time the suspicion that the decrease in medical consultations from pregnant women may also lead to an increased rate of fetal death [22].

In summary, the increase in fetal death rates is likely due to direct effects caused by maternal SARS-CoV-2 infection as well as indirect effects such as a change in access to the health-care system [23].

Although many studies reported an increase in fetal death, the evidence remains controversial. Some data, mostly from smaller studies, do not confirm this trend [24–28]. The period during which the study was conducted could be a potential explanation. Indeed, DeSisto et al. demonstrated that variants could have an influence. Documented SARS-CoV-2 infections were associated with an increased risk of fetal death, with a stronger association during the period of Delta variant predominance. The adjusted relative risk of fetal death was higher for women with Covid-19 than for women without Covid-19 between March 2020 and September 2021 (adjusted relative risk, 1.90; 95% CI, 1.69–2.15), including during the pre-Delta period (adjusted relative risk, 1.47; 95% CI, 1.27–1.71) and the Delta period (adjusted relative risk, 4.04; 95% CI, 3.28–4.97) [29]. In the latter, 2.7% of all pregnancies infected with SARS-CoV-2 were complicated by a fetal death, a rate much higher than the 0.6% in noninfected pregnant women.

4.5 Conclusion

The number of studies investigating Covid-19 and its effects on pregnancy continues to grow [1]. Currently, the available data indicate that a SARS-CoV-2 infection does not appear to be associated with pregnancy loss during the first trimester [5, 11–13]. Regarding fetal death, the literature describes that a SARS-CoV-2 infection is likely to increase its risk [16–21]. This one probably varies depending on the variants [29]. Being the subject of another chapter in this book, the vertical transmission was not discussed in detail here. However, a decrease in fetal movements following the week of a SARS-CoV-2 infection should be carefully monitored [30, 31]. It is also important to remember that medical follow-up of pregnant women should not be hampered by the pandemic. Indeed, studies reported that the number of consultations was decreasing during the pandemic compared to the pre-pandemic period. This could have an impact on fetal deaths as well [11, 22]. Pregnant women should therefore take special precautions against Covid-19. Compliance with barrier measures and vaccination are important means of prevention, the latter being, according to published data, without risk for pregnancy [32–34].

Bibliography

1. Lambelet V, Vouga M, Pomar L, Favre G, Gerbier E, Panchaud A, et al. SARS-CoV-2 in the context of past coronaviruses epidemics: consideration for prenatal care. Prenat Diagn. 2020;40(13):1641–54.
2. Favre G, Pomar L, Musso D, Baud D. 2019-nCoV epidemic: what about pregnancies? Lancet. 2020;395(10224):e40.
3. Chen H, Guo J, Wang C, Luo F, Yu X, Zhang W, et al. Clinical characteristics and intrauterine vertical transmission potential of COVID-19 infection in nine pregnant women: a retrospective review of medical records. Lancet. 2020;395(10226):809–15.
4. Chen L, Li Q, Zheng D, Jiang H, Wei Y, Zou L, et al. Clinical characteristics of pregnant women with Covid-19 in Wuhan, China. N Engl J Med. 2020;382(25):e100.
5. Cosma S, Carosso AR, Cusato J, Borella F, Carosso M, Bovetti M, et al. Coronavirus disease 2019 and first-trimester spontaneous abortion: a case-control study of 225 pregnant patients. Am J Obstet Gynecol. 2021;224(4):391.e1–7.

6. Baud D, Greub G, Favre G, Gengler C, Jaton K, Dubruc E, et al. Second-trimester miscarriage in a pregnant woman with SARS-CoV-2 infection. JAMA. 2020;323(21):2198–200.
7. Lawn JE, Blencowe H, Waiswa P, Amouzou A, Mathers C, Hogan D, et al. Stillbirths: rates, risk factors, and acceleration towards 2030. Lancet. 2016;387(10018):587–603.
8. Quenby S, Gallos ID, Dhillon-Smith RK, Podesek M, Stephenson MD, Fisher J, et al. Miscarriage matters: the epidemiological, physical, psychological, and economic costs of early pregnancy loss. Lancet. 2021;397(10285):1658–67.
9. WHO European health information at your fingertips. [Internet]. [cited 2022 Mar 15]. https://gateway.euro.who.int/en/indicators/hfa_82-1160-fetal-deaths-per-1000-births/.
10. Giakoumelou S, Wheelhouse N, Cuschieri K, Entrican G, Howie SEM, Horne AW. The role of infection in miscarriage. Hum Reprod Update. 2016;22(1):116–33.
11. Gomez D, Simpson AN, Sue-Chue-Lam C, de Mestral C, Dossa F, Nantais J, et al. A population-based analysis of the impact of the COVID-19 pandemic on common abdominal and gynecological emergency department visits. CMAJ. 2021;193(21):E753–60.
12. Rotshenker-Olshinka K, Volodarsky-Perel A, Steiner N, Rubenfeld E, Dahan MH. COVID-19 pandemic effect on early pregnancy: are miscarriage rates altered, in asymptomatic women? Arch Gynecol Obstet. 2021;303(3):839–45.
13. Jacoby VL, Murtha A, Afshar Y, Gaw SL, Asiodu I, Tolosa J, et al. Risk of pregnancy loss before 20 weeks' gestation in study participants with COVID-19. Am J Obstet Gynecol. 2021;225(4):456–7.
14. Cavalcante MB, de Melo Bezerra Cavalcante CT, Cavalcante ANM, Sarno M, Barini R, Kwak-Kim J. COVID-19 and miscarriage: from immunopathological mechanisms to actual clinical evidence. J Reprod Immunol. 2021;148:103382.
15. Trilla C, Mora J, Crovetto F, Crispi F, Gratacós E, Llurba E, et al. First-trimester SARS-CoV-2 infection: clinical presentation, inflammatory markers and obstetric outcomes. Fetal Diagn Ther. 2022;49:67.
16. Khalil A, von Dadelszen P, Draycott T, Ugwumadu A, O'Brien P, Magee L. Change in the incidence of stillbirth and preterm delivery during the COVID-19 pandemic. JAMA. 2020;324:705.
17. Gurol-Urganci I, Jardine JE, Carroll F, Draycott T, Dunn G, Fremeaux A, et al. Maternal and perinatal outcomes of pregnant women with SARS-CoV-2 infection at the time of birth in England: national cohort study. Am J Obstet Gynecol. 2021;225(5):522.e1–522.e11.
18. Cruz Melguizo S, de la Cruz Conty ML, Carmona Payán P, Abascal-Saiz A, Pintando Recarte P, González Rodríguez L, et al. Pregnancy outcomes and SARS-CoV-2 infection: The Spanish Obstetric Emergency Group Study. Viruses. 2021;13(5):853.
19. Chmielewska B, Barratt I, Townsend R, Kalafat E, van der Meulen J, Gurol-Urganci I, et al. Effects of the COVID-19 pandemic on maternal and perinatal outcomes: a systematic review and meta-analysis. Lancet Glob Health. 2021;9(6):e759–72.
20. Allotey J, Stallings E, Bonet M, Yap M, Chatterjee S, Kew T, et al. Clinical manifestations, risk factors, and maternal and perinatal outcomes of coronavirus disease 2019 in pregnancy: living systematic review and meta-analysis. BMJ. 2020;370:m3320.
21. Wei SQ, Bilodeau-Bertrand M, Lu S, Auger N. The impact of COVID-19 on pregnancy outcomes: a systematic review and meta-analysis. CMAJ. 2021;193(16):E540–8.
22. Kc A, Gurung R, Kinney MV, Sunry AK, Moinuddin M, Basnet O, et al. Effect of the COVID-19 pandemic response on intrapartum care, stillbirth, and neonatal mortality outcomes in Nepal: a prospective observational study. Lancet Glob Health. 2020;8(10):e1273–81.
23. Khalil A, Blakeway H, Samara A, O'Brien P. COVID-19 and stillbirth: direct vs indirect effect of the pandemic. Ultrasound Obstet Gynecol. 2022;59(3):288–95
24. Arnaez J, Ochoa-Sangrador C, Caserío S, Gutiérrez EP, Jiménez MDP, Castañón L, et al. Lack of changes in preterm delivery and stillbirths during COVID-19 lockdown in a European region. Eur J Pediatr. 2021;180(6):1997–2002.
25. Bunnell ME, Koenigs KJ, Roberts DJ, Quade BJ, Hornick JL, Goldfarb IT. Third trimester stillbirth during the first wave of the SARS-CoV-2 pandemic: similar rates with increase in placental vasculopathic pathology. Placenta. 2021;109:72–4.

26. Simon E, Cottenet J, Mariet A-S, Bechraoui-Quantin S, Rozenberg P, Gouyon J-B, et al. Impact of the COVID-19 pandemic on preterm birth and stillbirth: a nationwide, population-based retrospective cohort study. Am J Obstet Gynecol. 2021;225(3):347–8.
27. Yang J, D'Souza R, Kharrat A, Fell DB, Snelgrove JW, Murphy KE, et al. COVID-19 pandemic and population-level pregnancy and neonatal outcomes: a living systematic review and meta-analysis. Acta Obstet Gynecol Scand. 2021;100(10):1756–70.
28. Stowe J, Smith H, Thurland K, Ramsay ME, Andrews N, Ladhani SN. Stillbirths during the COVID-19 pandemic in England, April-June 2020. JAMA. 2021;325(1):86–7.
29. DeSisto CL, Wallace B, Simeone RM, Polen K, Ko JY, Meaney-Delman D, et al. Risk for stillbirth among women with and without COVID-19 at delivery hospitalization - United States, March 2020-September 2021. MMWR Morb Mortal Wkly Rep. 2021;70(47):1640–5.
30. Schoenmakers S, Snijder P, Verdijk RM, Kuiken T, Kamphuis SSM, Koopman LP, et al. Severe acute respiratory syndrome Coronavirus 2 placental infection and inflammation leading to fetal distress and neonatal multi-organ failure in an asymptomatic woman. J Pediatr Infect Dis Soc. 2021;10(5):556–61.
31. Linehan L, O'Donoghue K, Dineen S, White J, Higgins JR, Fitzgerald B. SARS-CoV-2 placentitis: an uncommon complication of maternal COVID-19. Placenta. 2021;104:261–6.
32. Male V. Are COVID-19 vaccines safe in pregnancy? Nat Rev Immunol. 2021;21(4):200–1.
33. Shimabukuro TT, Kim SY, Myers TR, Moro PL, Oduyebo T, Panagiotakopoulos L, et al. Preliminary findings of mRNA Covid-19 vaccine safety in pregnant persons. N Engl J Med. 2021;384(24):2273–82.
34. Blakeway H, Prasad S, Kalafat E, Heath PT, Ladhani SN, Le Doare K, et al. COVID-19 vaccination during pregnancy: coverage and safety. Am J Obstet Gynecol. 2022;226(2):236.e1–236.e14.

Chapter 5
COVID-19 in Perinatology: Obstetrical Counseling to Pregnant Women During Pandemics

Inês Martins and Diogo Ayres-de-Campos

5.1 Clinical Implications of COVID-19 Infection During Pregnancy

Changes during pregnancy occur in women's immune, respiratory, and cardiovascular physiology, causing a well-known increased vulnerability to infectious pathogens. Previous public healthcare emergencies, such as human immunodeficiency virus (HIV), H1N1 pandemic influenza, and Ebola and Zika virus outbreaks, demonstrated that pregnant women are particularly affected by emerging infectious pathogens, and the COVID-19 pandemic is no exception. Particularly during the third trimester of pregnancy and when associated comorbidities exist, pregnant women are at increased risk of severe illness from SARS-CoV-2 infection [1–3], when compared to nonpregnant women of the same age. Intensive care unit admission and need for invasive mechanical ventilation or extracorporeal membrane oxygenation is *circa* three times higher in pregnant women, and the overall risk of death from COVID-19 is about 70% higher in this population [4–6]. COVID-19 is also associated with an increased risk of adverse obstetric outcomes [1, 3]. Preterm birth occurs about three times more often, mainly due to iatrogenic preterm delivery, and the risk of stillbirth is *circa* two times higher [2, 4, 5, 7]. There is also evidence suggesting that COVID-19 is associated with an increased risk of preeclampsia or preeclampsia-like syndromes [2, 8].

I. Martins
Department of Obstetrics and Gynecology, Santa Maria University Hospital, Lisbon, Portugal

D. Ayres-de-Campos (✉)
Department of Obstetrics and Gynecology, Santa Maria University Hospital, Lisbon, Portugal

Department of Obstetrics and Gynecology, Medical School, University of Lisbon, Lisbon, Portugal

© The Author(s), under exclusive license to Springer Nature Switzerland AG 2023
D. De Luca, A. Benachi (eds.), *COVID-19 and Perinatology*,
https://doi.org/10.1007/978-3-031-29136-4_5

In many countries around the world, obstetric and perinatal outcomes worsened during the pandemic, namely, those related to maternal and perinatal mortality. This is likely to have occurred, not only from COVID-19 disease directly affecting pregnant women but also from reduced access of this population to healthcare facilities, a phenomenon that occurred at various stages of the pandemic. Several reports also document a weakened maternal mental health status, likely due to reduced social interactions, and this could also have impacted obstetric indicators [9].

5.2 Changes to Obstetric Healthcare During the Pandemic

Several leading scientific societies and healthcare institutions, such as the World Health Organization (WHO), Centers for Disease Control (CDC), and the International Federation of Gynecology and Obstetrics (FIGO), released recommendations on the provision of obstetric care in SARS-CoV-2-infected pregnant patients and also on the adaptations of obstetric care to the general population during the pandemic. Initial guidelines were based on little more than case series and expert opinion, but the real impact of COVID-19 on pregnancy soon became much clearer [10]. Guidelines were updated as more robust data became accessible, and the major points are summarized below and in Table 5.1 [11].

Table 5.1 Summary of changes to obstetric healthcare during the pandemic

	General obstetric population	SARS-Cov-2-positive women
Prenatal care	Screen for COVID-19 symptoms and high-risk exposure	Postpone prenatal visits, laboratory analyses, and obstetric ultrasounds, if these are not time-sensitive, or schedule them at the end of the working day
	Substitution of some in-presence prenatal appointments by video appointments, with self-evaluation of maternal weight and blood pressure	
	Schedule laboratory analyses and obstetric ultrasounds on the same day	
Intrapartum care	Screen for COVID-19 symptoms and high-risk exposure	Individual labor and delivery rooms
	Nasopharyngeal swab for SARS-CoV-2 infection, prior to or on the day of admission	Consider cesarean delivery only in severe maternal disease with compromised fetal oxygenation
	Maintain the presence of an asymptomatic accompanying person	
Postnatal care	Maintain mothers together with their newborns. Continue to encourage breastfeeding	

5.2.1 Prenatal Care

Substitution of some in-presence prenatal appointments by video appointments, after self-evaluation of maternal weight and blood pressure, should be considered, in both infected and noninfected women. Efforts should be made to have laboratory analyses and obstetric ultrasounds scheduled on the same day. Postponing prenatal visits, laboratory analyses, and obstetric ultrasounds should be considered in infected patients, if the former are not time-sensitive. All pregnant women attending outpatient clinics should be screened for COVID-19 symptoms and high-risk exposure to infected individuals. Appropriate cleaning of clinical equipment needs to be performed.

5.2.2 Intrapartum Care

Screening for COVID-19 symptoms and high-risk exposure to infected individuals should be performed, as well as a nasopharyngeal swab for SARS-CoV-2 infection, on the previous day or on admission to the labor ward. Individual labor and delivery rooms should be used for infected patients, but women should continue to be accompanied by one asymptomatic person during their stay in the labor ward. Staff need to use appropriate personnel protective equipment, specifically face masks, when providing support to infected patients. Appropriate cleaning of clinical equipment needs to be performed. Timing and mode of delivery do not need to be altered in infected individuals, except in severe disease affecting fetal oxygenation, when consideration must be given to performing a life-saving cesarean delivery.

5.2.3 Postnatal Care

Separation of infected mothers from their babies is unnecessary, if they are both in stable condition. Breastfeeding should continue to be encouraged in these situations, reinforcing the need for maternal hand hygiene and use of face masks. Consideration should be given to shortening the length of hospital stay if adequate home support is available.

5.3 Use of COVID-19-Specific Medication During Pregnancy

The vast majority of studies evaluating the effect of medication used for the treatment of COVID-19 (remdesivir, lopinavir-ritonavir, interferon beta, corticosteroids, chloroquine, hydroxychloroquine, and ivermectin) excluded pregnant women at enrolment. This occurred even with medication known to have low or absent safety concerns during pregnancy [12]. The COVID-19 pandemic again exposed the increased vulnerability of pregnant women in infectious disease situations, exacerbated by their exclusion from clinical trials, thus limiting their access to potentially beneficial interventions [13].

Although pharmaceutical companies producing *m*RNA vaccines for COVID-19 have announced the conduction of clinical trials involving pregnant women, evidence for their use in pregnancy is currently still of very limited quality [14–16]. The strongest evidence regarding safety and effectiveness derives mainly from self-reported effects of vaccination in online registries. In the "COVID-19 Vaccine Pregnancy Registry" platform launched by the CDC, as of 21 March 2022, a total of 210,896 pregnant women had reported their experience, with similar incidence of side effects and effectiveness as in the nonpregnant population [17].

Despite the limited quality of evidence and the short-term follow-up of individuals, medications and vaccines have been recommended in pregnant women by leading scientific institutions and healthcare authorities [10, 12–15], based mainly on the counterbalancing concerns of the greater risk of severe disease in this population.

5.4 Pregnancy and Pandemics: Lessons for the Future

COVID-19 is not the first pandemic to affect pregnant women and is unlikely to be the last. Several reflections on how society, science, and healthcare systems should prepare for emerging infectious diseases, particularly when affecting pregnant women and their infants, have been proposed by leading individuals and institutions [10, 18–20]. Some of the major points requiring consideration are summarized below and in Table 5.2.

Table 5.2 Summary of lessons learnt from the pandemic (for society, science, and healthcare systems)

Prediction	Investment in microbiological and epidemiological research:
	• Identification of zoonotic pathogens
	• Improving knowledge on the transmission of infections in pregnant women
	• Establishing the moment and mode of intervention before a pathogen reaches the human population
Preparedness	Strengthening and modernizing existing healthcare and public health systems:
	• Upgrading healthcare infrastructures to provide more individual and isolation rooms
	• Reinforcing public health systems, and their capacity to prevent, detect, and respond to future outbreaks, with adequate support from epidemiologists, infectiologists, and obstetricians
	• Assuring adequate coordination between public health agencies
	• Promoting a science-based approach to public health policy and decision-making
	• Preestablishing networks for local and international research collaborations in infectious diseases, with preprepared study designs for public health emergencies
	• Pre-implementation of databases including linked mother and infant data
	• Inclusion of pregnant women in clinical trials evaluating medications and vaccines for emergent infectious agents

5.4.1 Prediction

Recent pandemics were caused by zoonotic viruses originated in wildlife, developing through changes in the ecological environment, but also in socioeconomic behaviors. Prediction of upcoming potential emergent infectious agents requires investment in microbiological and epidemiological research. Identification of zoonotic pathogens has been substantially improved by advances in molecular diagnostics, but establishing the conditions (moment, time, mode) for researchers to intervene before a pathogen reaches the human population is still a major challenge [19]. Improving knowledge on the transmission of infections in pregnant women is particularly needed, in order to offer more protection to this vulnerable population [10].

5.4.2 Preparedness

Existing infrastructural and organizational conditions present in individual countries made an enormous difference to the impact of the pandemic on mortality rates. Strengthening and modernizing existing health and public health systems need therefore to be a priority in the future. Upgrading infrastructures to provide more individual or isolation rooms will avoid many of the major hospital adaptations that were required during the pandemic [10, 20].

Reinforcing public health systems may also be required in many countries, to develop their capacity to prevent, detect, and respond to future outbreaks [10, 20]. Adequate coordination between public health agencies is essential to address future challenges, ensuring that a response strategy is in place before the next pandemic occurs [10, 20]. Input from obstetric healthcare professionals is required to tackle issues related to pregnancy. Further input from epidemiologists and infectious disease and public health specialists is also necessary for aspects related to prevention of transmission, interpretation of surveillance and research results, and the development of clinical management guidelines [10]. A science-based approach to public health policy and decision-making needs to be actively promoted and engaged at all levels (government, public health agencies, academia, media, and civil society) [20].

The capacity to conduct clinical studies early in public health emergencies, particularly with the extra challenge of involving pregnant women, may quickly affect management decisions and have an impact on health outcomes. This can be greatly facilitated when research networks are preestablished and study designs are prepared in advance. Ensuring funding for international networks of research collaboration is a key element for this purpose. These collaborations need to include researchers, infectiologists, epidemiologists, obstetricians, and pediatricians and to possess the adequate know-how for developing research protocols, constructing robust databases, and producing scientific publications. Linked maternal and infant data need to be implemented in advance, and adaptable research protocols need to be created [18].

Lastly, inclusion of pregnant women in clinical trials evaluating medication and vaccines for emergent infectious agents needs to be considered, as soon as evidence of safety is established, ensuring an ethically responsible and socially just inclusion of this population [15].

References

1. Vouga M, Favre G, Martinez-Perez O, et al. Maternal outcomes and risk factors for COVID-19 severity among pregnant women. Sci Rep. 2021;11(1):13898.
2. Villar J, Ariff S, Gunier RB, et al. Maternal and neonatal morbidity and mortality among pregnant women with and without COVID-19 infection: the INTERCOVID Multinational Cohort Study. JAMA Pediatr. 2021;175(8):817–26.
3. Jamieson DJ, Rasmussen SA. An update on COVID-19 and pregnancy. Am J Obstet Gynecol. 2022;226(2):177–86.
4. Zambrano LD, Ellington S, Strid P, et al. Update: characteristics of symptomatic women of reproductive age with laboratory-confirmed SARS-CoV-2 infection by pregnancy status - United States, January 22-October 3, 2020. MMWR Morb Mortal Wkly Rep. 2020;69(44):1641–7.
5. Allotey J, Stallings E, Bonet M, et al. Clinical manifestations, risk factors, and maternal and perinatal outcomes of coronavirus disease 2019 in pregnancy: living systematic review and meta-analysis. BMJ. 2020;370:3320.
6. Delahoy MJ, Whitaker M, O'Halloran A, et al. Characteristics and maternal and birth outcomes of hospitalized pregnant women with laboratory-confirmed COVID-19 - COVID-NET, 13 States, March 1-August 22, 2020. MMWR Morb Mortal Wkly Rep. 2020;69(38):1347–54.
7. DeSisto CL, Wallace B, Simeone RM, et al. Risk for stillbirth among women with and without COVID-19 at delivery hospitalization - United States, March 2020-September 2021. MMWR Morb Mortal Wkly Rep. 2021;70(47):1640–5.
8. Mendoza M, Garcia-Ruiz I, Maiz N, et al. Pre-eclampsia-like syndrome induced by severe COVID-19: a prospective observational study. BJOG. 2020;127(11):1374–80.
9. Chmielewska B, Barratt I, Townsend R, et al. Effects of the COVID-19 pandemic on maternal and perinatal outcomes: a systematic review and meta-analysis. Lancet Glob Health. 2021;9(6):e759–72.
10. Rasmussen SA, Jamieson DJ. Coronavirus disease 2019 and pregnancy is deja vu all over again. BJOG. 2022;129(2):188–91.
11. Narang K, Ibirogba ER, Elrefaei A, et al. SARS-CoV-2 in pregnancy: a comprehensive summary of current guidelines. J Clin Med. 2020;9(5):1521.
12. Taylor MM, Kobeissi L, Kim C, et al. Inclusion of pregnant women in COVID-19 treatment trials: a review and global call to action. Lancet Glob Health. 2021;9(3):e366–71.
13. Modi N, Ayres-de-Campos D, Bancalari E, et al. Equity in Covid-19 vaccine development and deployment. Am J Obstet Gynecol. 2021;224(5):423–7.
14. Heath PT, Le-Doare K, Khalil A. Inclusion of pregnant women in COVID-19 vaccine development. Lancet Infect Dis. 2020;20(9):1007–8.
15. Krubiner CB, Faden RR, Karron RA, et al. Pregnant women & vaccines against emerging epidemic threats: ethics guidance for preparedness, research, and response. Vaccine. 2021;39(1):85–120.
16. Garg I, Shekhar R, Sheikh AB, Pal S. COVID-19 vaccine in pregnant and lactating women: a review of existing evidence and practice guidelines. Infect Dis Rep. 2021;13(3):685–99.
17. CDC. V-safe COVID-19 Vaccine Pregnancy Registry. Updated 21 March 2022. https://www.cdc.gov/coronavirus/2019-ncov/vaccines/safety/vsafepregnancyregistry.html.

18. Faherty LJ, Rasmussen SA, Lurie N. A call for science preparedness for pregnant women during public health emergencies. Am J Obstet Gynecol. 2017;216(1):34.e1–5.
19. Morse SS, Mazet JA, Woolhouse M, et al. Prediction and prevention of the next pandemic zoonosis. Lancet. 2012;380(9857):1956–65.
20. Daszak P, Keusch GT, Phelan AL, et al. Infectious disease threats: a rebound to resilience. Health Aff. 2021;40(2):204–11.

Part II
Perinatal Medicine

Chapter 6
Biological Mechanisms of Transplacental SARS-COV-2 Transmission

Serena Pirola and Luisa Patanè

6.1 The Maternal–Fetal Interface

Most viruses that infect the placenta do so via hematogenous spread leading to infection of the villi [1, 2].

Infection of the placenta, and subsequently of the fetus, typically occurs by direct villous trophoblastic infection or by "paracellular route" via damage to the villous trophoblastic barrier. The virus must be transported across the villous stroma and through the vascular endothelium to enter the fetal bloodstream and cause congenital (vertical) infection [3]. Alternatively, the virus can enter the placental/fetal bloodstream more directly via villous vasculosyncytial membrane infection, where the villous syncytiotrophoblast (ST) and the villous capillary endothelium are apposed, essentially functioning as a single unit [4].

Viruses gain access to the cells within the decidua and placenta by ascending from the lower reproductive tract [5, 6]. Following access to the upper reproductive tract, viral tropism for the decidua and/or placenta is then dependent on both viral entry receptor expression by the cellular component of these tissues and the specific maternal immune response to the virus. These factors vary by cell type and gestational age and can be affected by changes to the in utero environment and maternal immunity. Some viruses can directly infect the fetus at specific times during gestation, while some only infect the placenta.

Systemic maternal viral infections can also affect the pregnancy, and these can be very dangerous, because pregnant women suffer higher virus-associated morbidity and mortality than do nonpregnant counterparts. Therefore, the virus-host interaction during pregnancy is complex and highly variable.

S. Pirola (✉) · L. Patanè
Department of Gynecology and Obstetrics, ASST Papa Giovanni XXIII, Bergamo, Italy
e-mail: spirola@asst-pg23.it; lpatane@asst-pg23.it

© The Author(s), under exclusive license to Springer Nature Switzerland AG 2023
D. De Luca, A. Benachi (eds.), *COVID-19 and Perinatology*, https://doi.org/10.1007/978-3-031-29136-4_6

The human placenta is a chimeric organ composed of maternal and fetal structures [7]. During the first trimester of pregnancy, fetal-derived trophoblast progenitor cells differentiate into several cell subpopulations, including cytotrophoblasts (CTBs) which retain a proliferative capacity and the syncytiotrophoblast (ST) terminally differentiated multi-nucleated cells, together forming the placental villi [8, 9].

The floating and anchoring placental villi facilitate maternal–fetal exchange of gases, nutrients, and waste products. The fetal-derived floating villi, containing CTBs that are covered by syncytiotrophoblast (ST) cell layer, bath in maternal blood flowing into the intervillous space. The anchoring villi are attached to the basal plate by CTBs that form cell columns. CTBs differentiate into invasive extravillous CTBs at the distal ends of the cell column and invade the maternal decidua, anchoring the placenta to the uterus. A subset of these cells remodels the uterine vasculature in the decidua at the maternal–fetal interface. This process is controlled through the coordinated actions of multiple interrelated invasion and angiogenesis-promoting factors [8, 10–14].

The maternal–fetal interface includes multiple cell types that contribute to the development of the fetus, regulation of the maternal immune system, and protection against microorganisms. The maternal side is made from the stroma of the uterus, or decidual cells, and a wide range of immune cells including natural killer cells (NK), macrophages, dendritic cells (DCs), and regulatory T cells (Tregs).

The fetal side consists of the placental villus, which contains fetal blood vessels surrounded by fibroblasts and fetal macrophages (known as Hofbauer cells), cytotrophoblasts (CTBs), and, finally, the multinucleated syncytiotrophoblast (ST), an epithelial covering that is in direct contact with maternal blood.

While this creates a barrier for the controlled movement and transport of molecules, the placenta is not an impermeable barrier. There is evidence for the bidirectional movement of maternal and fetal cells [15]. This may be explained, in part, by the presence of gaps in the syncytiotrophoblast (ST), particularly later in gestation [16]. In addition, the extravillous trophoblast is in direct contact with cells from the decidua, including maternal immune cells, endothelial cells, and microorganisms present in the uterus (Fig. 6.1). Importantly, malfunction and impaired invasion capacity of CTBs have been associated with major pregnancy complications such as repeated miscarriages, IUGR (intrauterine growth restriction), and preeclampsia [17–25].

Innate immune cells, including natural killer cells (NK), dendritic cells (DCs), and macrophages, and the maternal humoral response play a critical role in regulating and controlling the infection and, consequently, determining its severity. Innate cells phagocytize virus complexes and can kill infected cells, while antibodies facilitate viral clearance. Contrary to nonpregnant women, during pregnancy, the function of the innate immune system is influenced and regulated by the fetal/placenta unit.

In summary, the route of viral transmission, abundance of permissive cell types (which changes with gestational age), and maternal immune function, all influence viral infections at the maternal–fetal interface.

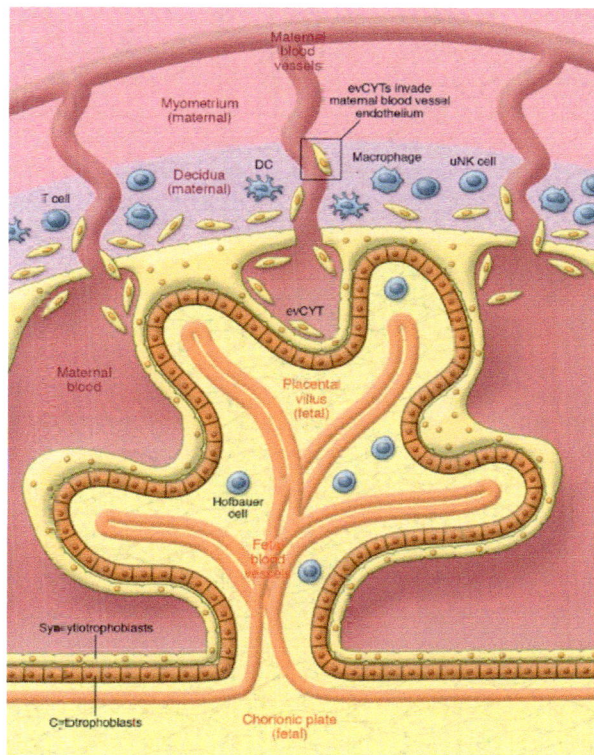

Fig. 6.1 The maternal–fetal interface

The critical function of the placenta in protecting the fetus against invading pathogens during gestation must be balanced with awareness and tolerance of the semi-allogeneic fetus [26–31].

In pregnant females, local adaptation of the maternal immune system allows for successful coexistence between the mother and the semi-allograft that is the fetus/placenta unit expressing both maternal (self) and paternal (non-self) genes [32–35]. Cytotoxic adaptive immune responses are diminished, bypassed, or even abrogated, while regulatory adaptive immunity is enhanced [36, 37]. By contrast, innate (natural) immunity remains intact, serving two purposes: one, to continue to provide host defense against infection, and two, to interact with fetal tissues to promote successful placentation and pregnancy [35, 38–41]. Altered infection-based placental innate defenses and breach of placental integrity may lead to pregnancy complications.

The defense mechanisms used by the placenta against diverse microbial infections have remained largely unknown, despite intense research efforts and studies in animal models.

A certain level of protection is provided by the continuous layer of the syncytiotrophoblast (ST), located at the placental villous surface and in direct contact with maternal blood [31]. Moreover, it is increasingly recognized that CTBs have strong innate defense mechanisms against intracellular pathogens [30, 31]. It is suggested that the invasive role of CTBs and their active breakdown of extracellular matrix may involve degradative pathways that can also interfere with the life cycle of intracellular pathogens [30, 31]. In addition to their antimicrobial defense function, CTBs play an important role in the maternal tolerance toward the semi-allogeneic fetus [27–30, 42–44].

The maternal decidua (the specialized endometrium of pregnancy, constituting the uterine implantation site) is a multicell-type structure consisting of maternal cells as well as fetal interstitially invading CTBs. In addition to solid tissue cells, it is composed of ~40% immune cells (of which 70% are unique decidual natural killer cells (dNK), 20–25% are macrophages, and 3–10% are T cells) [45–49].

During normal placentation, a highly specialized environment is created in the decidua, in order to allow immunological tolerance of the semi-allogeneic fetal origin CTBs, which lie in proximity to maternal cells [26, 32, 50, 51]. Among the central mechanisms maintaining the decidual immune function is the decidual immune cell composition, characterized by limited lymphocyte access. This special composition has been shown to be governed by the controlled expression of local chemokines [50, 51] and is further maintained by adaptation of both fetal and maternal cells [26–29].

The level of immunity may vary during pregnancy, with a highly regulated pro-inflammatory state early in pregnancy, which is subsequently attenuated until late in pregnancy, when inflammation is associated with labor [28]. Alterations in this tightly controlled environment can adversely impact the outcome of pregnancy.

6.2 SARS-COV-2 Infection: Virus Characteristics (Genomic and Taxonomy)

Coronaviruses (CoVs) of the family Coronaviridae are enveloped, positive-sense single-stranded RNA viruses [52]. All of the highly pathogenic CoVs, including SARS-CoV-2, belong to the *Betacoronavirus* genus, group 2 [52].

As a novel betacoronavirus, SARS-CoV-2 shares 79% genome sequence identity with SARS-CoV and 50% with MERS-CoV [53]. Its genome comprises 14 open reading frames (ORFs), two-thirds of which encode 16 nonstructural proteins that make up the replicase complex [53, 54]. The remaining one-third encodes nine accessory proteins (ORFs) and four structural proteins, spike (S), envelope (E), membrane (M), and nucleocapsid (N), of which spike mediates SARS-CoV entry into host cells [55]. The six functional open reading frames (ORFs) are arranged in

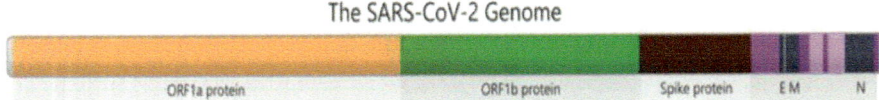

Fig. 6.2 SARS-CoV-2 genome

Human Coronavirus Structure

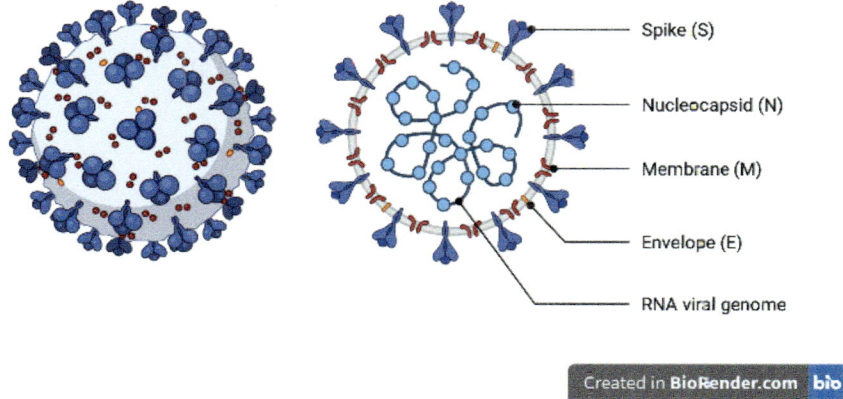

Fig. 6.3 Human coranavirus structure

order from replicase (ORF1a/ORF1b), spike (S), envelope (E), membrane (M), and nucleocapsid (N) (Figs. 6.2 and 6.3).

The SARS-CoV-2 S protein has a full size of 1273 amino acids, and the S gene of SARS-CoV-2 is highly variable from SARS-CoV. Spike has a receptor-binding domain (RBD) that mediates direct contact with a cellular receptor, angiotensin-converting enzyme 2 (ACE2), and an S1/S2 polybasic cleavage site that is proteolytically cleaved by cellular cathepsin-L and transmembrane protease serine 2 (TMPRSS2) [56–58].

The S1 subunit of the coronavirus is further divided into two functional domains, an N-terminal domain and a C-terminal domain.

Structural and biochemical analyses identified a 211-amino acid region (amino acids 319–529) at the S1 C-terminal domain of SARS-CoV-2 as the RBD (receptor-binding domain of S protein) which has a key role in virus entry and is the target of neutralizing antibodies [59, 60].

6.3 SARS-COV-2 and Cell Entry: Mechanism and Receptors

The RBM (receptor-binding motif) mediates contact with the ACE2 receptor.

SARS-CoV-2 needs proteolytic processing of the S protein to activate the endocytic route (Fig. 6.4).

It has been shown that host proteases participate in the cleavage of the S protein and activate the entry of SARS-CoV-2, including transmembrane protease serine 2 (TMPRSS2), cathepsin-L, and furin [58, 61, 62].

Single-cell RNA sequencing data showed that TMPRSS2 (transmembrane protease serine 2) is highly expressed in several tissues and body sites and is co-expressed

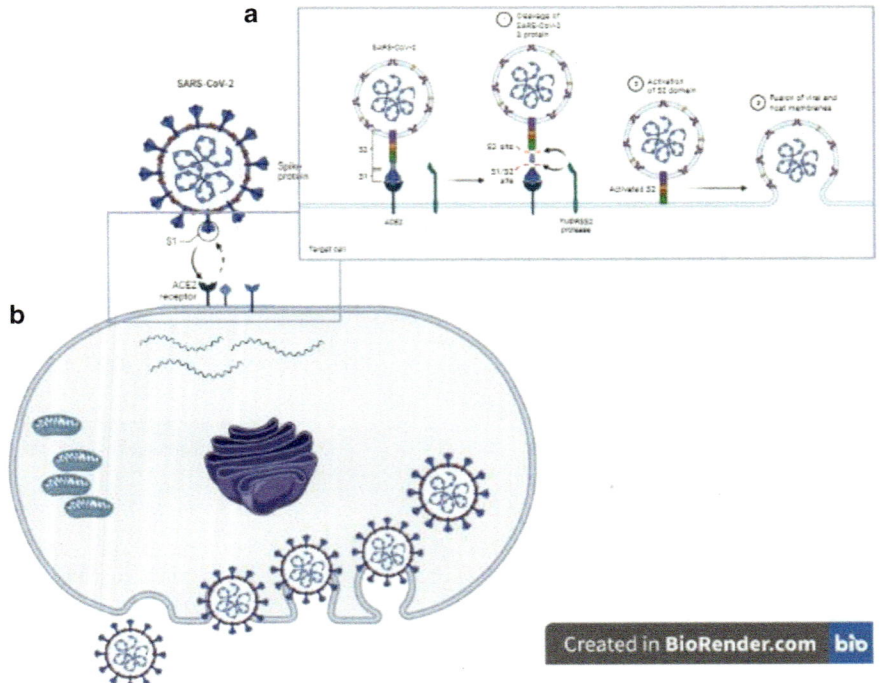

Fig. 6.4 SARS-CoV-2 virus and proposed mechanisms of placental cell entry. (**a**) ACE2 receptors mediated endocytosis. (**b**) Proteases mediated membrane fusion

with ACE2 (angiotensin-converting enzyme 2) in nasal epithelial cells, lungs, and bronchial branches, which explains some of the tissue tropism of SARS-CoV-2 [63, 64]. SARS-CoV-2 pseudovirus entry assays revealed that TMPRSS2 and cathepsin-L have cumulative effects with furin on activating virus entry [62].

A structural study suggested that the furin cleavage site can reduce the stability of SARS-CoV-2 S protein and facilitate the conformational adaption that is required for the binding of the RBD (receptor-binding domain) to its receptor [65].

TMPRSS2 (transmembrane protease serine 2) facilitates viral entry at the plasma membrane surface, whereas cathepsin-L activates SARS-CoV-2 spike in endosomes and can compensate for entry into cells that lack TMPRSS2 [58].

Once the genome is released into the host cytosol, ORF1a and ORF1b (opening reading frames) are translated into viral replicase proteins, which are cleaved into individual (nsps) nonstructural proteins [55]. Here, the replicase components rearrange the endoplasmic reticulum (ER) into double-membrane vesicles (DMVs) that facilitate viral replication of genomic and subgenomic RNAs (sgRNA); the latter are translated into accessory and viral structural proteins that facilitate virus particle formation [66, 67] (Fig. 6.5).

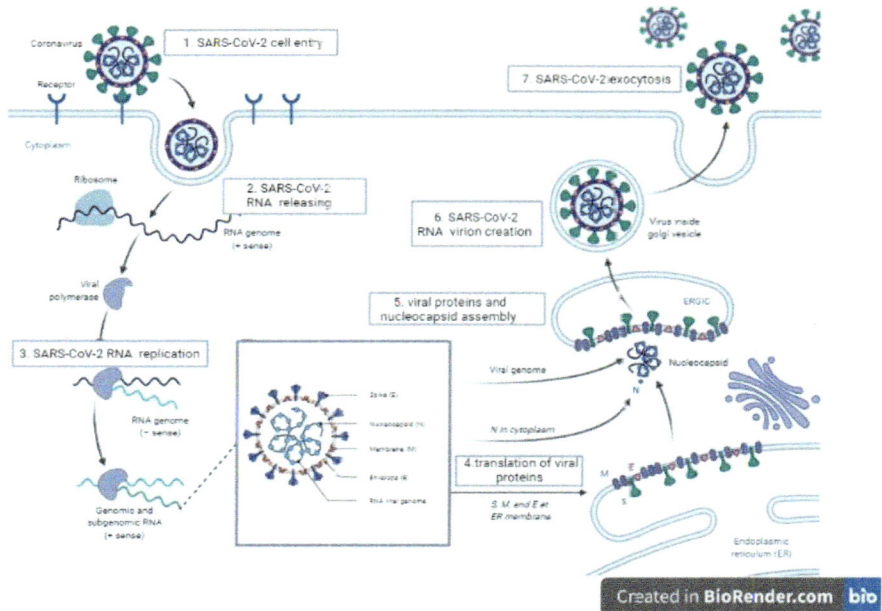

Fig. 6.5 Proposed mechanisms of cell entry, replication, and structure of SARS-CoV-2

6.4 ACE2 and TMPRSS2: Role in the Placental Transmission

It is already said that to enter and infect cells, SARS-CoV-2 requires a receptor, most commonly ACE2, and a serine protease, usually TMPRSS2 receptor, and protease must be co-expressed in cells for SARS-CoV-2 infection to occur [68].

In previous works, it has been shown that ACE2 is expressed in the syncytiotrophoblast (ST), extravillous trophoblast (EVT), and cytotrophoblasts (CTBs) and that TMPRSS2 was usually not detected by immunohistochemistry in any late-gestation placental cells [69, 70]. The function of ACE2 in the placenta is thought to activate the renin–angiotensin system in chorionic villi and extravillous trophoblast (EVT). ACE2 may play a role in trophoblast invasion and changes in vascular flow [71–74]. When present, TMPRSS2 was rarely and very weakly detected in the placental (fetal) endothelium and syncytiotrophoblasts [69, 70]. The role of TMPRSS2 expression in the placenta is largely unknown.

ACE2 receptor needed for cellular SARS-CoV-2 placental infection is expressed in the placental syncytiotrophoblasts (ST), extravillous trophoblasts (EVT), and cytotrophoblasts (CTBs) across all three pregnancy trimesters While in third trimester pregnancies exposed to SARS-CoV-2 [69, 70] was find rare, weak expression of the serine protease TMPRSS2 in the placental endothelium is very rare in the syncytiotrophoblasts (ST). TMPRSS2 is not detectable or weakly expressed in the placental villous tissues throughout pregnancy.

In addition, recent studies demonstrated that ACE2 expression is polarized, such that the apical syncytiotrophoblast (ST) surface directly exposed to maternal blood usually does not express the protein, but rather ACE2 expression is biased to the syncytiotrophoblast (ST) stromal (basal) side. This expression pattern could offer some barrier to placental cellular SARS-CoV-2 infection when spread hematogenously (apparent low prevalence of SARS-CoV-2 viremia in pregnancy) [69] while reported rates of viremia in nonpregnant populations range widely, from 1 to 27% [75, 76].

However, in early gestation, ACE2 is expressed more frequently circumferentially in the ST. Relatively higher ACE2 expression on the apical ST surface in early gestation suggests a weakness of the syncytiotrophoblast (ST) barrier function which could result in higher placental infection rates and vertical SARS-CoV-2 transmission in the setting of early pregnancy exposures, although this has not been reported to date.

The presence of ACE2 (angiotensin-converting enzyme 2), the main receptor for SARS-CoV-2, in human placentas indicates that this organ can be vulnerable for viral infection during pregnancy.

Recently, it has been found that the placental expression of ACE2 receptor and TMPRSS2 is similar between the women affected by COVID-19 or not and between those with or without transplacental transmission [77].

Nowadays, we know that a minority of cases of SARS-CoV-2 transplacental infection may occur through placental macrophages (Hofbauer cells) and circulating fetal monocytes [78, 79].

Even if SARS-CoV-2 transplacental transmission is a rare event, it can lead to negative consequences for the offspring. Many factors influencing transplacental transmission are still unclear such as placental expression of viral receptors, viral load, and inflammation status.

A recent study [77] shows that transplacental transmission of SARS-CoV-2 is not related to the placental expression of ACE2 (angiotensin-converting enzyme 2) and TMPRSS2 (transmembrane protease serine 2) receptors (the existence of alternative receptors has recently been hypothesized and should be studied further [80]), viral load, or any common clinical perinatal characteristics.

On the other hand, it was associated with placental inflammation and particularly with intervillositis with peculiar pathological signs as massive fibrin deposition, diffuse chronic intervillositis with necrosis, and positive viral staining in the intervillositis lesions. This may damage the placental barrier and is associated with fetal distress, acidosis at the birth, and need for neonatal intensive care (NCU). So when placental inflammatory damage is sufficient to determine fetal distress and acidosis at birth, placental transmission of SARS-CoV-2 seems to be possible.

6.5 Latest News

Viruses are constantly changing, and this includes SARS-CoV-2, the virus that causes COVID-19. These genetic variations occur over time and can lead to the emergence of new variants that may have different characteristics. Some variant viruses are of particular concern because they spread more easily, cause more severe disease, or may escape the body's immune response.

Mutations are changes in the genetic code of a virus that naturally occur over time when an animal or person is infected. It is important to monitor circulating viruses for key mutation(s) that happen in important regions of the genome. Many mutations, fortunately, do not affect the virus' ability to spread or cause disease because they do not alter the major proteins involved in infection; eventually these are outcompeted by variants with mutations that are more beneficial for the virus.

On November 2021, South Africa reported the identification of a new SARS-CoV-2 variant, B.1.1.529, to the World Health Organization (WHO). B.1.1.529 was first detected in specimens collected in Botswana and South Africa.

Then this variant was designated by WHO and the European Center for Disease Prevention and Control as a variant of concern (VOC) due to concerns regarding immune escape and potentially increased transmissibility compared to previous known variants [81].

WHO designated B.1.1.529 as a VOC named omicron [82].

The spike glycoprotein (S), which promotes viral entry into cells [83, 84] of the omicron variant, is characterized by at least 30 amino acid substitutions, 3 small deletions, and 1 small insertion. Notably, 15 of the 30 amino acid substitutions are in the receptor-binding domain (RBD). Although the omicron RBD harbors 15 residue mutations, it binds to the human ACE2 (angiotensin-converting enzyme 2) entry receptor with high affinity and can efficiently recognize ACE2 [85].

These mutations have a net enhancing effect on binding of the omicron RBD to human ACE2 relative to the original Wuhan virus, which suggests that structural epistasis enables immune evasion while retaining efficient receptor engagement [86].

Analysis of the changes in the spike protein indicates that the omicron variant is likely to have increased transmission compared to the original SARS-CoV-2 virus. Some detected mutations can increase binding to the ACE2 (angiotensin-converting enzyme 2) receptor, which could increase transmission, and the combination of some of them may increase binding affinity even more; however, other substitutions in the omicron spike protein are expected to decrease binding to ACE2. As such, receptor-binding affinity needs to be assessed [87] using the full spectrum of spike protein substitutions found in the omicron variant. Another mutation is proximal to the furin cleavage site and may increase spike cleavage, which could aid transmission. Moreover, omicron variant shares some mutations showing the enhancement of spike cleavage, which could aid transmission, with other variants.

It is known that previous different viral strains (such as Alpha or Delta variant) are more environmentally transmittable, the same can be said about the omicron variant, but how this can impact transplacental transmission deserves more specific studies.

6.6 Conclusions

COVID-19 seems to be a challenging disease in terms of transplacental transmission, whose mechanisms seem complex and mainly represented by inflammatory placental damage, which is associated with a strong local immune response at the maternal–fetal interface and increased levels of circulating cytokines in the fetal circulation [88, 89]. This situation is similar to the so-called cytokine storm observed during severe pulmonary SARS-CoV-2 infection: it is likely that this excessive local response might eventually lead to placental insufficiency and allow transplacental viral passage and may cause other organ dysfunctions [90].

Conflict of Interest The authors report no conflict of interest.

References

1. Kaplan C. The placenta and viral infections. Semin Diagn Pathol. 1993;10:232–50.
2. Koi H, Zhang J, Parry S. The mechanisms of placental viral infection. Ann N Y Acad Sci. 2001;943:148–56.
3. Mahyuddin AP, Kanneganti A, Wong J, et al. Mechanisms and evidence of vertical transmission of infections in pregnancy including SARS-CoV-2. Prenat Diagn. 2020;40:1655.
4. Benirschke K, Burton GJ, Baergen RN. Pathology of the human placenta. 6th ed. Berlin: Springer; 2012.
5. Salzberger B, Myerson D, Boeckh M. Circulating cytomegalovirus (CMV)-infected endothelial cells in marrow transplant patients with CMV disease and CMV infection. J Infect Dis. 1997;176(3):778–81.
6. Fisher S, Genbacev O, Maidji E, Pereira L. Human cytomegalovirus infection of placental cytotrophoblasts in vitro and in utero: implications for transmission and pathogenesis. J Virol. 2000;74(15):6808–20.
7. Weisblum Y, Panet A, Zakay-Rones Z, Haimov-Kochman R, Goldman-Wohl D, Ariel I, et al. Modeling of human cytomegalovirus maternal-fetal transmission in a novel decidual organ culture. J Virol. 2011;85:13204–13.
8. Cross JC, Werb Z, Fisher SJ. Implantation and the placenta: key pieces of the development puzzle. Science. 1994;266:1508–18.
9. Hamilton WJ, Boyd JD. Development of the human placenta in the first three months of gestation. J Anat. 1960;94:297–328.
10. Rossant J, Cross JC. Placental development: lessons from mouse mutants. Nat Rev Genet. 2001;2:538–48.
11. Adler SP, Nigro G, Pereira L. Recent advances in the prevention and treatment of congenital cytomegalovirus infections. Semin Perinatol. 2007;31:10–8.
12. Knofler M. Critical growth factors and signalling pathways controlling human trophoblast invasion. Int J Dev Biol. 2010;54:269–80.
13. Pereira L, Maidji E, McDonagh S, Tabata T. Insights into viral transmission at the uterine-placental interface. Trends Microbiol. 2005;13:164–74.
14. Red-Horse K, Zhou Y, Genbacev O, Prakobphol A, Foulk R, McMaster M, et al. Trophoblast differentiation during embryo implantation and formation of the maternal-fetal interface. J Clin Invest. 2004;114:744–54.
15. Gammill HS, Nelson JL. Naturally acquired microchimerism. Int J Dev Biol. 2010;54:531.
16. Frank HG. Placental development. In: Polin RA, Abman SH, Rowitch D, Benitz WE, editors. Fetal and neonatal physiology, vol. 1. 5th ed. Amsterdam: Elsevier; 2017. p. 103.
17. Lyall F, Robson SC, Bulmer JN. Spiral artery remodeling and trophoblast invasion in preeclampsia and fetal growth restriction: relationship to clinical outcome. Hypertension. 2013;62:1046–54.
18. Zhou Y, Gormley MJ, Hunkapiller NM, Kapidzic M, Stolyarov Y, Feng V, et al. Reversal of gene dysregulation in cultured cytotrophoblasts reveals possible causes of preeclampsia. J Clin Invest. 2013;123:2862–72.

19. Burton GJ, Jauniaux E, Charnock-Jones DS. The influence of the intrauterine environment on human placental development. Int J Dev Biol. 2010;54:303–12.
20. Hustin J, Gillerot Y, Collette J, Franchimont P. Placental alkaline phosphatase in developing normal and abnormal gonads and in germ-cell tumours. Virchows Arch A Pathol Anat Histopathol. 1990;417:67–72.
21. Jauniaux E, Van Oppenraaij RH, Burton GJ. Obstetric outcome after early placental complications. Curr Opin Obstet Gynecol 2010;22:452–7.
22. John R, Hemberger M. A placenta for life. Reprod Biomed Online. 2012;25:5–11.
23. Norwitz ER. Defective implantation and placentation: laying the blueprint for pregnancy complications. Reprod Biomed Online. 2006;13:591–9.
24. Pijnenborg R, Anthony J, Davey DA, Rees A, Tiltman A, Vercruysse L, et al. Placental bed spiral arteries in the hypertensive disorders of pregnancy. Br J Obstet Gynaecol. 1991;98:648–55.
25. Pijnenborg R, Ball E, Bulmer JN, Hanssens M, Robson SC, Vercruysse L. In vivo analysis of trophoblast cell invasion in the human. Methods Mol Med. 2006; 22:11–44.
26. Arck PC, Hecher K. Fetomaternal immune cross-talk and its consequences for maternal and offspring's health. Nat Med. 2013;19:548–56.
27. Erlebacher A. Immunology of the maternal-fetal interface. Annu Rev Immunol. 2013;31:387–411.
28. Mor G, Cardenas I. The immune system in pregnancy: a unique complexity. Am J Reprod Immunol. 2010;63:425–33.
29. Zenclussen AC. Adaptive immune responses during pregnancy. Am J Reprod Immunol. 2013;69:291–303.
30. Mouillet JF, Ouyang Y, Bayer A, Coyne CB, Sadovsky Y. The role of trophoblastic microRNAs in placental viral infection. Int J Dev Biol. 2014;58:281–9.
31. Zeldovich VB, Bakardjiev AI. Host defense and tolerance: unique challenges in the placenta. PLoS Pathog. 2012;8:e1002804.
32. Hunt JS. Stranger in a strange land. Immunol Rev. 2006;213:36.
33. Robertson SA. Immune regulation of conception and embryo implantation-all about quality control? J Reprod Immunol. 2010;85:51.
34. Stoller M, Traupe T, Khattab AA, et al. Effects of coronary sinus occlusion on myocardial ischaemia in humans: role of coronary collateral function. Heart. 2013;99:548.
35. Mor G, Abrahams VM. The immunology of pregnancy. In: Creasy RK, Resnik R, Iams JD, et al., editors. Creasy and Resnik's maternal-fetal medicine: principles and practice. 7th ed. Philadelphia: Elsevier; 2014. p. 80.
36. Guerin LR, Prins JR, Robertson SA. Regulatory T-cells and immune tolerance in pregnancy: a new target for infertility treatment? Hum Reprod Update. 2009;15:517.
37. Leber A, Teles A, Zenclussen AC. Regulatory T cells and their role in pregnancy. Am J Reprod Immunol. 2010;63:445.
38. Barrientos G, Tirado-González I, Klapp BF, et al. The impact of dendritic cells on angiogenic responses at the fetal-maternal interface. J Reprod Immunol. 2009;83:35.
39. Dekel N, Gnainsky Y, Granot I, Mor G. Inflammation and implantation. Am J Reprod Immunol. 2010;63:17.
40. Nagamatsu T, Schust DJ. The contribution of macrophages to normal and pathological pregnancies. Am J Reprod Immunol. 2010;63:460.
41. Zhang J, Chen Z, Smith GN, Croy BA. Natural killer cell-triggered vascular transformation: maternal care before birth? Cell Mol Immunol. 2011;8:1.
42. Bainbridge DR. Evolution of mammalian pregnancy in the presence of the maternal immune system. Rev Reprod. 2000;5:67–74.
43. Ishitani A, Sageshima N, Lee N, Dorofeeva N, Hatake K, Marquardt H, et al. Protein expression and peptide binding suggest unique and interacting functional roles for HLA-E, F, and G in maternal- placental immune recognition. J Immunol. 2003;171:1376–84.
44. Rapacz-Leonard A, Dabrowska M, Janowski T. Major histocompatibility complex I mediates immunological tolerance of the trophoblast during pregnancy and may mediate rejection during parturition. Mediators Inflamm. 2014;2014:579279.

45. Bulmer JN, Pace D, Ritson A. Immunoregulatory cells in human decidua: morphology, immunohistochemistry and function. Reprod Nutr Dev. 1988;28:1599–613.
46. King A, Loke YW, Chaouat G. NK cells and reproduction. Immunol Today. 1997;18:64–6.
47. Mor G, Straszewski-Chavez SL, Abrahams VM. Macrophage-trophoblast interactions. Methods Mol Med. 2006;122:149–63.
48. Wicherek L, Basta P, Pitynski K, Marianowski P, Kijowski J, Wiatr J, et al. The characterization of the subpopulation of suppressive B7H4(+) macrophages and the subpopulation of CD25(+) CD4(+) and FOXP3(+) regulatory T-cells in decidua during the secretory cycle phase, Arias Stella reaction, and spontaneous abortion - a preliminary report. Am J Reprod Immunol. 2009;61:303–12.
49. Manaster I, Mandelboim O. The unique properties of uterine NK cells. Am J Reprod Immunol. 2010;63:434–44.
50. Red-Horse K, Drake PM, Fisher SJ. Human pregnancy: the role of chemokine networks at the fetal-maternal interface. Expert Rev Mol Med. 2004;6:1–14.
51. Nancy P, Tagliani E, Tay CS, Asp P, Levy DE, Erlebacher A. Chemokine gene silencing in decidual stromal cells limits T cell access to the maternal-fetal interface. Science. 2012;336:1317–21.
52. Gorbalenya AE, et al. The species severe acute respiratory syndrome-related coronavirus: classifying 2019-nCoV and naming it SARS-CoV-2. Nat Microbiol. 2020;5:536–44.
53. Lu R, et al. Genomic characterisation and epidemiology of 2019 novel coronavirus: implications for virus origins and receptor binding. Lancet. 2020;395:565–74.
54. Zhang YZ, Holmes EC. A genomic perspective on the origin and emergence of SARS-CoV-2. Cell. 2020;181:223–7.
55. Perlman S, Netland J. Coronaviruses post-SARS: update on replication and pathogenesis. Nat Rev Microbiol. 2009;7:439–50.
56. Zhou P, et al. A pneumonia outbreak associated with a new coronavirus of probable bat origin. Nature. 2020;579:270–3.
57. Wu F, et al. A new coronavirus associated with human respiratory disease in China. Nature. 2020;579:265–9.
58. Hoffmann M, et al. SARS-CoV-2 cell entry depends on ACE2 and TMPRSS2 and is blocked by a clinically proven protease inhibitor. Cell. 2020;181:271–80.
59. Shang J, et al. Structural basis of receptor recognition by SARS-CoV-2. Nature. 2020;581:221–4.
60. Walls AC, et al. Structure, function, and antigenicity of the SARS-CoV-2 spike glycoprotein. Cell. 2020;181:281–92.
61. Ou X, et al. Characterization of spike glycoprotein of SARS-CoV-2 on virus entry and its immune cross- reactivity with SARS-CoV. Nat Commun. 2020;11:1620.
62. Shang J, et al. Cell entry mechanisms of SARS-CoV-2. Proc Natl Acad Sci U S A. 2020;117:11727–34.
63. Sungnak W, et al. SARS-CoV-2 entry factors are highly expressed in nasal epithelial cells together with innate immune genes. Nat Med. 2020;26:681–7.
64. Lukassen S, et al. SARS-CoV-2 receptor ACE2 and TMPRSS2 are primarily expressed in bronchial transient secretory cells. EMBO J. 2020;39:e105114.
65. Wrobel AG, et al. SARS-CoV-2 and bat RaTG13 spike glycoprotein structures inform on virus evolution and furin-cleavage effects. Nat Struct Mol Biol. 2020;27:763–7.
66. Snijder EJ, et al. Ultrastructure and origin of membrane vesicles associated with the severe acute respiratory syndrome coronavirus replication complex. J Virol. 2006;80:5927–40.
67. Wu H-Y, Brian DA. Subgenomic messenger RNA amplification in coronaviruses. Proc Natl Acad Sci U S A. 2010;107:12257–62.
68. Hoffmann M, Kleine-Weber H, Schroeder S, et al. SARS-CoV-2 cell entry depends on ACE2 and TMPRSS2 and is blocked by a clinically proven protease inhibitor. Cell. 2020; 181(271-80):e8.
69. Edlow AG, Li JZ, Collier AY, et al. Assessment of maternal and neonatal SARS-CoV-2 viral load, transplacental antibody transfer, and placental pathology in pregnancies during the COVID-19 pandemic. JAMA Netw Open. 2020;3:e2030455.

70. Hecht JL, Quade B, Deshpande V, et al. SARS-CoV-2 can infect the placenta and is not associated with specific placental histopathology: a series of 19 placentas from COVID-19- positive mothers. Mod Pathol. 2020;33:2092–103.
71. Anton L, Merrill DC, Neves LA, et al. Activation of local chorionic villi angiotensin II levels but not angiotensin (1-7) in preeclampsia. Hypertension. 2008;51:1066–72.
72. Pique-Regi R, Romero R, Tarca AL, et al. Does the human placenta express the canonical cell entry mediators for SARS-CoV-2? Elife. 2020;9:e58716.
73. Valdes G, Corthorn J, Bharadwaj MS, Joyner J, Schneider D, Brosnihan KB. Utero-placental expression of angiotensin-(1-7) and ACE2 in the pregnant guinea-pig. Reprod Biol Endocrinol. 2013;11:5.
74. Valdes G, Neves LA, Anton L, et al. Distribution of angiotensin-(1-7) and ACE2 in human placentas of normal and pathological pregnancies. Placenta. 2006;27:200–7.
75. Wang W, Xu Y, Gao R, et al. Detection of SARS-CoV-2 in different types of clinical specimens. JAMA. 2020;323:1843–4.
76. Fajnzylber J, Regan J, Coxen K et al. SARS-CoV-2 viral load is associated with increased disease severity and mortality. Nat Commun. 2020;11:5493.
77. Vivanti AJ, et al. Factors influencing SARS-CoV-2 transplacental transmission. Preprint 2022. https://ssrn.com/abstract=3989785.
78. Schwartz DA, Baldewijns M, Benachi A, Bugatti M, Bulfamante G, Cheng K, et al. 542 Hofbauer cells and coronavirus disease 2019 (COVID-19) in pregnancy: molecular pathology analysis of villous macrophages, endothelial cells, and placental findings from 22 placentas infected by severe acute respiratory syndrome coronavirus 2 (SARS-CoV-2) with and without fetal transmission. Arch Pathol Lab Med. 2021;145(11):1328–40.
79. Facchetti F, Bugatti M, Drera E, Tripodo C, Sartori E, Cancila V, et al. SARS-CoV2 547 vertical transmission with adverse effects on the newborn revealed through integrated immunohistochemical, electron microscopy and molecular analyses of placenta. EBioMedicine. 2020;59:102951.
80. Argueta LB, Lacko LA, Bram Y, Tada T, Carrau L, Zhang T, et al. SARS-CoV-2 infects syncytiotrophoblast and activates inflammatory responses in the placenta. bioRxiv. 2021:2021.06.01.446676. https://doi.org/10.1101/2021.06.01.446676.
81. https://www.ecdc.europa.eu/en/publications-data/threat-assessment-brief-emergence-sars-cov-2-variant-b.1.1.529.
82. https://www.who.int/news/item/26-11-2021-classification-of-omicron-(b.1.1.529)-sars-cov-2-variant-of-concern.
83. Walls AC, et al. Structure, function, and antigenicity of the SARS-CoV-2 spike glycoprotein. Cell. 2020;181:281–92.e6
84. Wrapp D, et al. Cryo-EM structure of the 2019-ncoV spike in the prefusion conformation. Science. 2020;367:1260–3.
85. Cameroni E, et al. Lectins enhance SARS-CoV-2 infection and influence neutralizing antibodies. Nature. 2021; https://doi.org/10.1038/s41586-021-03925-1.
86. Starr TN, et al. SARS-CoV-2 RBD antibodies that maximize breadth and resistance to escape. Nature. 2021;597:97–102.
87. McCallum, et al. Structural basis of SARS-CoV-2 Omicron immune evasion and receptor engagement. Science. 2022;375:864–8.
88. Garcia-Flores V, Romero R, Xu Y, Theis K, Arenas-Hernandez M, Miller D, et al. Maternal-fetal immune responses in pregnant women infected with SARS-CoV-2. Res Sq [Preprint] 2021:rs.3.rs-362886. https://doi.org/10.21203/rs.3.rs-362886/v1.
89. Lu-Culligan A, Chavan AR, Vijayakumar P, Irshaid L, Courchaine EM, Milano KM, et al. Maternal respiratory SARS-CoV-2 infection in pregnancy is associated with a robust inflammatory response at the maternal-fetal interface. Med (N Y). 2021;2(5):591–610.e10.
90. Fajgenbaum DC, June CH. Cytokine storm. N Engl J Med. 2020;383:2255–73.
91. Ben H, et al. Characteristics of SARS-CoV-2 and COVID-19. Nat Rev Microbiol. 2021;19:141–54. https://doi.org/10.1038/s41579-020-00459-7.

92. Cui J, Li F, Shi ZL. Origin and evolution of pathogenic coronaviruses. Nat Rev Microbiol. 2019;17:181–92.
93. Wu JT, Leung K, Leung GM. Nowcasting and forecasting the potential domestic and international spread of the 2019-nCoV outbreak originating in Wuhan, China: a modelling study. Lancet. 2020;395:689–97.
94. Hui DS, et al. The continuing 2019-nCoV epidemic threat of novel coronaviruses to global health - the latest 2019 novel coronavirus outbreak in Wuhan, China. Intl J Infect Dis. 2020;91:264–6.
95. www.who.int/publications/i/item/WHO-2019-nCoV-mother-to-child-transmission5382021.1. Accessed 15 Dec 2021.
96. Celik E, et al. Placental deficiency during maternal SARS-CoV-2 infection. Placenta. 2022;117:47–56. https://doi.org/10.1016/j.placenta.2021.10.012.
97. Gulersen M, Prasannan L, Tam H, Metz CN, Rochelson B, Meirowitz N, Shan W, Edelman M, Millington KA. Histopathologic evaluation of placentas after diagnosis of maternal severe acute respiratory syndrome coronavirus 2 infection. Am J Obstet Gynecol MFM. 2020;2:100211. https://doi.org/10.1016/j.ajogmf.2020.100211.

Chapter 7
Placental Pathology During COVID-19

David A. Schwartz

7.1 Introduction

Following the identification of an outbreak of respiratory tract disease caused by a novel coronavirus infection, later termed coronavirus disease 2019 (COVID-19), in Wuhan, China, in December 2019 [1, 2], there was consternation for the potential effects of the illness on pregnant women and their infants [3–7]. At that time, it was unknown whether this newly recognized coronavirus, termed the severe acute respiratory syndrome coronavirus 2 (SARS-CoV-2), would adversely affect pregnant mothers. In particular, there was widespread concern that SARS-CoV-2 could be transmitted from an infected mother to her fetus or neonate, a process termed vertical infection [6, 8, 9]. During previous outbreaks of two different but highly pathogenic coronavirus infections, Middle East respiratory syndrome coronavirus (MERS-CoV) and severe acute respiratory syndrome coronavirus (SARS-CoV), there had been both maternal and infant morbidity and mortality, but no confirmed cases of vertical transmission had been identified [3, 4]. Analysis of other respiratory RNA viruses infecting pregnant women demonstrated that they were rarely, if ever, transmitted to the fetus [4]. Based upon the initial reports of pregnant women developing COVID-19 in Wuhan and surrounding areas in China during the early stage of the pandemic, no confirmed cases of vertical transmission were identified [6, 9–12], although there were some suspicious cases [13, 14]. As COVID-19 continued to spread throughout China and subsequently extend to other countries, increasing numbers of neonates testing positive for the virus were reported [15–20]. As a result, it became even more important to understand whether vertical transmission was occurring [12, 21, 22]. Among the three mechanisms for vertical transmission—intrauterine, intrapartum, and postpartum—the possibility that intrauterine

---

D. A. Schwartz (✉)
Perinatal Pathology Consulting, Atlanta, GA, USA

© The Author(s), under exclusive license to Springer Nature Switzerland AG 2023
D. De Luca, A. Benachi (eds.), *COVID-19 and Perinatology*,
https://doi.org/10.1007/978-3-031-29136-4_7

transplacental transmission with SARS-CoV-2 was occurring in some cases became of particular interest. In order to evaluate this mechanism of transmission, studies of the placenta from infected mothers became necessary.

7.2 Role of Placental Pathology in Emerging Infections

Placental pathology has been shown to be a highly valuable method for delineating the mechanisms and risk factors for maternal-fetal infection associated with emerging viral diseases. Expert pathology analysis can identify the maternal and fetal components of the cellular and immunological response to the infectious agent; the nature and extent of the inflammatory response; the occurrence, localization, and nature of cytopathic damage; and other associated pathology abnormalities and can exclude the presence of other microbial agents. Nucleic acid and antibody-based pathology techniques can be performed to supplement standard histopathological methods, with the benefit of obtaining additional significant information including the specific identification of the virus, estimating the viral burden, and determining the placental cell tropism and distribution of the virus in infected tissues [23–26]. These methods can include techniques such as immunohistochemical or immunofluorescent analysis using antibodies to viral antigens as well as nucleic acid techniques such as nucleic acid in situ hybridization that identify target RNA or DNA molecules within intact cells. Immunohistochemical and nucleic acid methodologies are capable of identifying the location of virus within specific cell types in defined anatomic compartments of the placenta, and many of these techniques can be used in placental tissues that have been formalin fixed and paraffin embedded. The performance of these specialized pathologic methods used together with routine histopathological methods has been successful in previous outbreaks of emerging viral infections such as the Zika and Ebola virus, where immunohistochemistry and molecular pathology have demonstrated the spectrum of placental cells susceptible for viral infection and confirmed intrauterine transplacental maternal-fetal transmission [23–25]. In addition, molecular pathology analysis of the placenta can be useful in delineating the spectrum and immunophenotype of inflammatory cells of both maternal and fetal origins, helping to understand the nature of the immunologic response to placental infection. The use of double-staining techniques can analyze placental cells for two different markers, permitting the simultaneous identification of the virus and specific cell types. Additionally, immunohistochemistry and immunofluorescence can identify specific cytoskeletal components, proteins, and markers of cell activation that can characterize responses at the maternal-fetal interface to viral infection. Placental pathology has also contributed to understanding the mechanisms of fetal morbidity and mortality from such TORCH agents as herpes virus, toxoplasmosis, *Trypanosoma cruzi*, cytomegalovirus, listeriosis, parvovirus, and many others.

7.3 Placental Pathology and COVID-19

In a few studies performed during the early phases of the COVID-19 pandemic, placentas were collected and analyzed to determine the potential for SARS-CoV-2 to cause placental damage and infect the fetus. However, the initial results from examining placentas from mothers with COVID-19 were variable and differed significantly between reports. These results included finding fetal vascular malperfusion or maternal vascular malperfusion [27, 28], both processes [29–31], as well as a spectrum of different inflammatory lesions that included chronic histiocytic intervillositis, villitis, funisitis, and chorioamnionitis [29–31]. In contrast, other reports described a lack of specific findings of COVID-19 in placentas from infected women [32, 33] including one article with the title "SARS-CoV-2 can infect the placenta and is not associated with specific placental histopathology." These reports added to the variability and confusion regarding the effects of SARS-CoV-2 on the placenta. A caveat of these disparate results was that the large majority of placentas evaluated had not been infected with SARS-CoV-2 and were from infants that tested negative for the virus.

In order to provide standardized guidelines to evaluate the occurrence of maternal-fetal transmission of SARS-CoV-2, in 2020, Schwartz and colleagues proposed diagnostic criteria for determining intrauterine transmission by examining placentas from maternal-neonatal dyads that were infected with COVID-19 [34]. These criteria included identifying the presence of SARS-CoV-2 in the placenta using molecular pathology and/or immunohistochemical methods from mother-neonatal dyads that both tested positive for SARS-CoV-2. However, these proposed criteria for intrauterine transmission did not address specific microscopic abnormalities occurring in placentas from cases of suspected transplacental transmission.

Eventually, placental pathology analysis from several investigators confirmed that maternal-fetal transmission from infected mothers was occurring in a small percentage of infants [35–39], making SARS-CoV-2 the newest congenitally transmissible agent to be described [40]. The first description of pregnant women and their neonates testing positive for COVID-19 in which the fetal tissues of the placenta were found to be infected using molecular methods was from Patanè and colleagues at the Papa Giovanni XXIII Hospital in Bergamo, Italy [35]. The placentas from two infected infants were abnormal and demonstrated chronic histiocytic intervillositis in which the intervillous spaces contained numerous CD68-positive macrophages. Both RNA in situ hybridization for the spike protein mRNA of SARS-CoV-2 and immunohistochemistry for SARS-CoV-2 antigens showed extensive positive staining in the syncytiotrophoblast of both placentas. Vivanti et al. [36] described an infected and symptomatic pregnant primigravida who at 35^{+2} weeks gestation had SARS-CoV-2 in the amniotic fluid and in her blood, nasopharynx, and vagina. The neonate was also infected, having nasopharyngeal and rectal swabs, blood, and non-bronchoscopic bronchoalveolar lavage fluid positive for SARS-CoV-2. Placental tissue was found to be positive for SARS-CoV-2 by RT-PCR at levels higher than in maternal and fetal blood and the amniotic fluid. Microscopic examination of the placenta revealed diffuse perivillous fibrin deposition, infarction, trophoblast necrosis, and acute and chronic histiocytic intervillositis. The inflammatory infiltrate in the intervillous space consisted of histiocytes and neutrophils—the histiocytes stained positively with the anti-CD68 antibody. The syncytiotrophoblast stained intensely positive using immunohistochemistry and an antibody to SARS-CoV-2 N-protein. Sisman et al. [37] reported a pregnant woman who developed COVID-19 at 34 weeks gestation and delivered an infected neonate that developed respiratory distress. The neonate's placenta was large for gestational age and had abnormal microscopic findings including chronic histiocytic intervillositis, chronic villitis, villous necrosis, and karyorrhexis and infarction. Immunohistochemistry for SARS-CoV-2 nucleocapsid protein was positive in the cytoplasm of the syncytiotrophoblastic cells, and ultrastructural analysis showed structures consistent with viral particles clustered within membrane-bound cisternal spaces in syncytiotrophoblastic cells. Fachetti et al. [38] reported a 29-year-old woman hospitalized at 37^5 weeks with COVID-19 and idiopathic thrombocytopenia who delivered a neonate testing positive for SARS-CoV-2 and developed pneumonia requiring intubation. Placental pathology included histiocytic-neutrophilic intervillositis and syncytiotrophoblast thinning and necrosis. Prominent perivillous fibrin deposition was present, together with fetal vascular malperfusion consisting of avascular and fibrotic villi and stroma-vascular karyorrhexis. Accelerated villous maturation and chorangiosis were also present. Hofbauer cells were increased and expressed programmed death ligand-1 (PD-L1). Scattered neutrophil extracellular traps (NETs) were identified by immunofluorescence. Analysis of the placenta using RNA in situ hybridization for SARS-CoV-2 demonstrated strong positivity in the syncytiotrophoblast and also within scattered CD14+ mononuclear cells in the intervillous space. Immunohistochemistry for SARS-CoV-2 spike and nucleocapsid proteins demonstrated positivity in syncytiotrophoblast for both proteins. Electron microscopy revealed coronavirus-like particles in the cytoplasm of syncytiotrophoblast cells and also in the endothelium of fetal capillaries and fibroblasts. Particles consistent with the appearance of coronaviruses were seen within the cytoplasm of cells within the capillary lumina, which were probably monocytes.

The placental pathology effects of SARS-CoV-2 became clearer following a report from Schwartz and Morotti that examined pathology differences between placentas based upon the infection status of their babies [41]. This study found that maternal-fetal dyads infected with COVID-19 in which the placentas were positive for SARS-CoV-2 using immunohistochemistry or RNA in situ hybridization had a unique and highly repetitive pattern of pathological findings compared with the variable pathology findings in uninfected cases. In addition to positive staining of the syncytiotrophoblast for SARS-CoV-2, the pathology findings included villous trophoblast necrosis and chronic histiocytic intervillositis, with some cases also having increased fibrin deposition. Based on this report and others, it appeared that a determining factor of the spectrum of placental pathology with COVID-19 was based on the occurrence of SARS-CoV-2 infection of the pregnant mother, placenta, and the baby. Additional cases were reported in which placentas that tested positive for SARS-CoV-2 contained a spectrum of pathological findings including villous trophoblast necrosis, chronic histiocytic intervillositis, and increased fibrin up to the level of massive perivillous fibrin deposition (Figs. 7.1 and 7.2) [42–45].

In 2021, an investigation by Schwartz and colleagues of 11 still- and live-born babies having placentas infected with SARS-CoV-2 confirmed that these placental findings were pathology risk factors for intrauterine viral transmission and perinatal morbidity and mortality [46]. In all 11 placentas, the syncytiotrophoblast stained positively for SARS-CoV-2 using immunohistochemistry (Fig. 7.3), RNA in situ hybridization, or both. Following examination of additional placentas, the

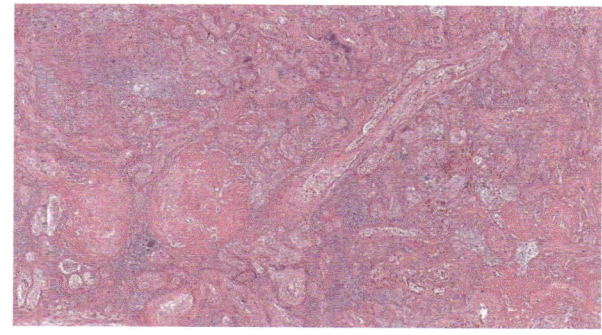

Fig. 7.1 Typical appearance of massive perivillous fibrin deposition in a placenta infected with SARS-CoV-2. Hematoxylin and eosin, ×10

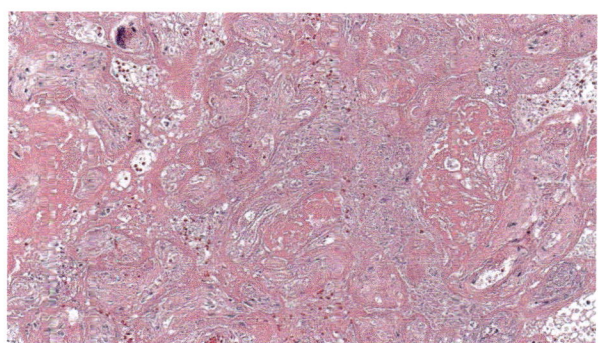

Fig. 7.2 Massive perivillous fibrin deposition demonstrating ischemic necrosis of chorionic villi with trophoblast necrosis and residual inflammatory cells in the intervillous space. Hematoxylin and eosin, ×20

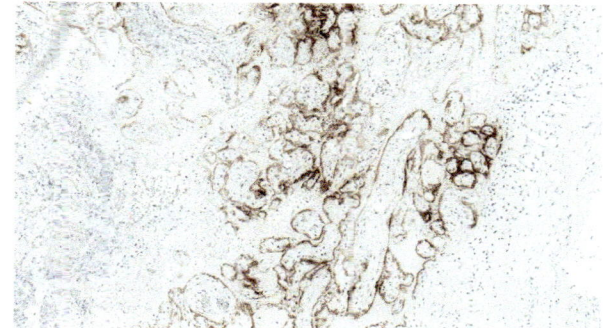

Fig. 7.3 Typical staining pattern of a placenta infected with SARS-CoV-2 illustrating confluent syncytiotrophoblast positivity (brown staining) using immunohistochemistry. Antibody to SARS-CoV-2 spike protein, ×10

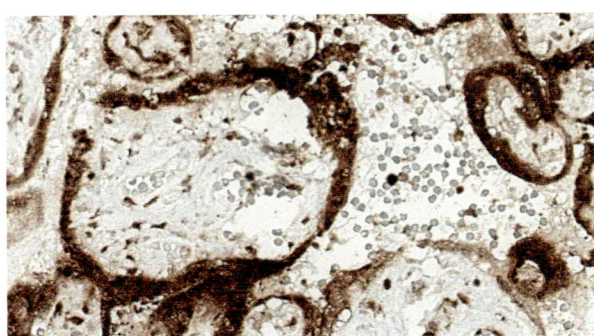

Fig. 7.4 In this infected placenta from a stillborn fetus, the syncytiotrophoblast stains intensely positive for SARS-CoV-2 using immunohistochemistry. Also present are positive-staining cells in the villous stroma and maternal inflammatory cells in the intervillous space. Antibody to SARS-CoV-2 spike protein, ×40

term SARS-CoV-2 placentitis was used by Watkins et al. [47] to refer to the triad of findings of chronic histiocytic intervillositis, perivillous fibrin deposition (typically reaching the level of massive perivillous fibrin deposition), and villous trophoblast necrosis occurring in placentas from mothers having COVID-19. In their study of six infected placentas from live-born neonates and one stillborn fetus, they found evidence that placental damage was mediated by complement activation as there was C4d expression present along the villous borders in six of the seven cases.

Although these and other reports indicate that among placentas infected with SARS-CoV-2, the syncytiotrophoblast is the most frequent cell type involved, there are other villous cells that also stain positive for the virus. These include the cytotrophoblast, Hofbauer cells (the resident population of chorionic villous macrophages), and villous stromal and endothelial cells (Fig. 7.4), as well as maternal inflammatory cells in the intervillous space [40, 48, 49]. Although Hofbauer cells have previously been found to be infected with other viruses and microbial agents [50] and can stain positive for SARS-CoV-2 in a minority of infected placentas, there has been no evidence that this positivity was associated with transplacental transmission in COVID-19 [40, 51].

In studying the prevalence of COVID-19 among pregnant women and the number of neonates with confirmed infection, it appears that both SARS-CoV-2 placentitis and maternal-fetal viral transmission are at least uncommon and possibly rare. In order to determine the frequency of intrauterine transmission, Raschetti and colleagues [52] performed a meta-analysis in which 74 published reports were analyzed that included a total of 176 neonates testing positive for SARS-CoV-2. The authors estimated that among all reported cases of neonates testing positive for SARS-CoV-2, approximately 70% acquired their infection through postpartum transmission (i.e., environmental exposure) and 30% likely became infected either through intrauterine or intrapartum mechanisms. Among all, 5.7% were stated to have confirmed congenital (i.e., prepartum) infection.

7.4 SARS-CoV-2 Placentitis

SARS-CoV-2 placentitis has emerged as the characteristic finding in placentas infected with SARS-CoV-2. This diagnostic entity consists of three discrete pathological findings occurring together in the same placenta—increased fibrin deposition which typically reaches the level of massive perivillous fibrin deposition, chronic histiocytic intervillositis, and villous trophoblast necrosis.

Increased perivillous fibrin (or fibrinoid) deposition is a pathological finding that was described long before the recognition of COVID-19, as a single entity has been associated with poor obstetric outcomes including neurological injury [53]. Its significance as a potential risk factor for poor perinatal outcome is associated with several factors that include its extent and chronicity and its quantity, placental size (small placentas may be compromised with a smaller volume of fibrin), and the occurrence of other placental risk factors such as findings of maternal or fetal malperfusion [54]. Increased perivillous fibrin is believed by some authors to result from turbulence and decreased blood flow, particularly at the placental margins or immediately under the chorionic plate. In addition, abnormally increased perivillous fibrin may be a reaction to trophoblastic damage and necrosis resulting in villous stromal exposure to the maternal space stimulating the clotting cascade [54, 55]. Massive perivillous fibrin deposition (Figs. 7.1 and 7.2) is another lesion characterized by increased intervillous fibrin but is a more severe pathological abnormality that can involve a significant proportion of the placental tissues. Massive perivillous fibrin deposition, sometimes referred to as massive fibrin deposition, is a rare lesion, reported in less than 1% of all pregnancies. The gross and microscopic features of this abnormality are typically striking, with greater than 25% of the placenta involved by contiguous areas of fibrin/fibrinoid within the intervillous space associated with ischemic degeneration of the entrapped chorionic villi. It is often accompanied by necrosis of the syncytiotrophoblast and proliferation of septal/chorionic extravillous trophoblast [54] Transmural involvement of the placental parenchyma by dense fibrin within the intervillous space is a characteristic finding. Partially because massive perivillous fibrin deposition obstructs both maternal and fetal blood flows within the affected regions of the placenta, it is associated with a variety of poor perinatal outcomes including intrauterine growth restriction, preterm birth, neurological injury, pregnancy loss including stillbirth, and recurrence in subsequent pregnancies [54, 56]. There is evidence that the severity of the neonatal outcomes is directly associated with the extent of fibrin deposition [56]. Prior to the COVID-19 pandemic, massive perivillous fibrin deposition was occasionally reported to occur together with intervillositis or villitis.

Chronic histiocytic intervillositis is a rare inflammatory placental abnormality that was first identified by Labarre and Mullen in 1987, who termed it massive chronic intervillositis [57], and has since then been referred to by a variety of terms in the medical literature. Chronic histiocytic intervillositis is a condition of unknown etiology that has a high rate of recurrence and an association with poor obstetric outcomes—these include pregnancy loss and stillbirth, intrauterine growth restriction, and preterm delivery [41, 54]. It is an unusual placental abnormality, and although its exact prevalence is unknown, prior to the COVID-19 pandemic, it had been estimated to occur in approximately 6 of 10,000 (0.6%) second- and third-trimester placentas. The microscopic features consist of the accumulation of mononuclear inflammatory cells that are predominantly histiocytes within the intervillous space which stain positive anti-CD68 and other immunohistochemical markers of histiocytes and macrophages. Although the histiocytes usually compose greater than 80% of the inflammatory cell population in the intervillous space, lymphocytes and occasionally neutrophils can also be present [41]. The risk for recurrence of chronic histiocytic intervillositis in cases prior to the COVID-19 pandemic was very high, with ranges varying from almost 70% to 100%, although lower rates have been reported [54].

7.5 Determining Placental Infection with SARS-CoV-2

Unlike some viruses which can infect the fetus in the absence of infecting the placenta, in the case of SARS-CoV-2, placental infection appears to be a necessary step for intrauterine mother-to-fetal transmission. In order to arrive at a working definition of SARS-CoV-2 placental infection, in December 2021, Roberts and colleagues proposed a consensus-driven set of diagnostic criteria that were based upon the collected published experience of reported cases of placental involvement with the virus [58]. These proposed criteria were based on the rigor of diagnostic testing. Definite infection indicated documentation of the presence, location, and replication of the virus using either an RNA probe to the antisense strand, showing a positive signal in placental tissues with appropriate positive and negative controls, or positive staining by RNA in situ hybridization for double-stranded RNA, produced as replication intermediate for positive-sense RNA virus in placental tissues with appropriate positive and negative controls. Probable placental infection includes the documentation of viral RNA or proteins within placental tissues, without evidence of active replication, through an RNA probe to the positive-sense strand, showing a positive signal in placental tissues with appropriate positive and negative controls, or positive staining by immunohistochemistry in placental tissues with antibodies to SARS-CoV-2 proteins, with appropriate positive and negative controls. Possible placental infection is a less specific diagnostic entity for detection of virus which could be used for detecting viral particles engulfed by macrophages rather than actively replicating virus. RT-PCR of placental homogenates theoretically may have a positive result owing to maternal viremia (although this is a rare entity), rather than placental involvement. This utilizes RT-PCR detection or quantification of viral RNA in PBS (phosphate-buffered saline)-rinsed placental homogenates with no tissue localization or electron microscopic detection of viral-like particles in placental tissues. Unlikely placental infection includes negative results from any of the above tests.

7.6 Placental Pathology and Stillbirth from COVID-19

During the early phases of the global COVID-19 pandemic, the relationship between SARS-CoV-2 infection in pregnancy and stillbirth remained indeterminate, with some studies showing an increase in fetal loss, others showing a decrease, and some demonstrating no effect [59]. However, in November 2021 the causal association of SARS-CoV-2 infection with stillbirth was confirmed when the US Centers for Disease Control and Prevention described a population-based study of 1,249,634 delivery hospitalizations demonstrating that pregnant women with COVID-19 had an increased risk for stillbirth compared with uninfected women and that the strength of this association was greatest during the period of the SARS-CoV-2 B.1.617.2 (Delta) variant predominance [60].

Placental analysis using routine, immunohistochemical, and molecular methods has been instrumental in the understanding of the mechanism(s) for intrauterine fetal demise from COVID-19. Schwartz et al. in 2020 [46] described the pathology findings in placentas infected with SARS-CoV-2 from five stillborn fetuses which were not only remarkably consistent with one another but also with the infected placentas of 6 live-born neonates. The findings included chronic histiocytic intervillositis, necrosis of villous trophoblast, and positivity of syncytiotrophoblast for SARS-CoV-2 using immunohistochemistry or RNA in situ hybridization. Extensive intervillous fibrin deposition, which involved 70% or more of the placental tissues in one case, was identified in the placentas from all five stillborns. Additional reports of the placental pathology from stillborn fetuses delivered to mothers with COVID-19 showed that placentas were significantly abnormal with extensive involvement from increased or massive intervillous fibrin deposition, chronic histiocytic intervillositis, and villous trophoblast necrosis [59, 61, 62].

The largest study of the role of the placenta in COVID-19-related stillbirth was performed by Schwartz and colleagues [63] who analyzed 64 stillborn fetuses and 4 early neonatal deaths from 12 countries that were delivered to unvaccinated mothers. All 68 babies in this cohort of perinatal deaths had placentas that tested positive for SARS-CoV-2, ensuring that there was intimate exposure to the virus. Delivery of the 64 stillbirths varied from 15 weeks to 39.2 weeks of gestation, with 8 (13%) stillbirth cases delivered at full term. Stillbirths occurred at an average gestational age of 30 weeks, and the neonatal death cases had a mean gestational age of 30.8 weeks and survived an average of 3.5 days following delivery. Every placenta from this cohort demonstrated severe pathology findings from 2 or more of the lesions composing SARS-CoV-2 placentitis and associated findings. Increased fibrin deposition was present together with chronic histiocytic intervillositis and trophoblast necrosis in 65/68 (97%) of placentas. Two of the three placentas that did not have all three of the constituents of SARS-CoV-2 placentitis did have both massive perivillous fibrin deposition and trophoblast necrosis. There was increased fibrin deposition present in all 68 placentas which reached the level of massive perivillous fibrin deposition in 63 (93%) cases. Trophoblast necrosis was also present in all 68 placentas and chronic histiocytic intervillositis was present in 66/68 (97%). In addition to SARS-CoV-2 placentitis, other abnormalities included intervillous thrombi/hemorrhages in 25 (37%) placentas, villitis in 22 (32%), maternal vascular malperfusion in 12 (18%), fetal vascular malperfusion in 7 (10%), and acute chorioamnionitis in 9 (13%) of cases. There were 23 placentas that measured below the tenth percentile of weight stratified for gestational age. An important aspect of this study was the estimation of placental involvement with the destructive lesions of SARS-CoV-2 placentitis. This metric was calculated for each of 68 placentas to understand the impact of the pathology findings on placental function. The results were striking—the average placenta had 77.7% involvement from SARS-CoV-2 placentitis, a degree of placental damage and resulting malperfusion that greatly exceeded the extent of placental destruction typically present with infections with other TORCH agents. This high level of placental damage severely impeded the delivery of sufficient oxygen and nutrients to the fetus, rendering the placenta incapable of sustaining life. Results of autopsy examination performed on 30 babies showed no evidence that the stillbirth or neonatal death was the result of SARS-CoV-2 causing direct fetal somatic organ damage following placental infection and transplacental transmission. The results of this study, including not only the presence of the destructive placental abnormalities of SARS-CoV-2 placentitis but also the presence of additional placental pathology findings that included intervillous thrombi, villitis, and maternal vascular malperfusion, demonstrated that placental insufficiency had resulted in fetal hypoxia, causing a hypoxic-ischemic fetal or neonatal demise. In a 2023 article Schwartz et al. [64] addressed the protective role of maternal COVID-19 vaccination in reducing or preventing SARS-CoV- 2 placentitis and stillbirth, as the reported cases of perinatal demise have occurred in unvaccinated mothers. Schwartz and colleagues also proposed that SARS-CoV-2 placentitis is associated with maternal viremia and has an underlying immunological basis that may be the result of failure of maternal-fetal tolerance and rejection of fetal-derived tissues such as the placenta, analogous to the rejection syndromes occurring in allogeneic solid organ transplantation.

References

1. Zhu N, Zhang D, Wang W, Li X, Yang B, Song J, et al. A novel coronavirus from patients with pneumonia in China, 2019. N Engl J Med. 2020;382:727–33. https://doi.org/10.1056/NEJMoa2001017.
2. Li Q, Guan X, Wu P, Wang X, Zhou L, Tong Y, et al. Early transmission dynamics in Wuhan, China, of novel coronavirus-infected pneumonia. N Engl J Med. 2020;382:1199–207. https://doi.org/10.1056/NEJMoa2001316.
3. Schwartz DA, Graham AL. Potential maternal and infant outcomes from coronavirus 2019-nCoV (SARS-CoV-2) infecting pregnant women: lessons from SARS, MERS, and other human coronavirus infections. Viruses. 2020;12:194. https://doi.org/10.3390/v12020194.
4. Schwartz DA, Dhaliwal A. Infections in pregnancy with COVID-19 and other respiratory RNA virus diseases are rarely, if ever, transmitted to the fetus: experiences with coronaviruses, parainfluenza, metapneumovirus respiratory syncytial virus, and influenza. Arch Pathol Lab Med. 2020;144:920–8. https://doi.org/10.5858/arpa.2020-0211-SA.

5. Schwartz DA, Dhaliwal A. Coronavirus diseases in pregnant women, the placenta, fetus, and neonate. Adv Exp Med Biol. 2021;1318:223–41. https://doi.org/10 1007/978-3-030-63761-3_14.
6. Chen H, Guo J, Wang C, Luo F, Yu X, et al. Clinical characteristics and intrauterine vertical transmission potential of COVID-19 infection in nine pregnant women: a retrospective review of medical records. Lancet. 2020;395:809–15. https://doi.org/10.1016/S0140-6736(20)30360-3.
7. Schwartz DA. The effects of pregnancy on women with COVID-19: maternal and infant outcomes. Clin Infect Dis. 2020;71:2042–4. https://doi.org/10.1093/cid/ciaa559.
8. Qiancheng X, Jian S, Lingling P, Lei H, Xiaogan J, Weihua L, et al. Coronavirus disease 2019 in pregnancy. Int J Infect Dis. 2020 95:376–83. https://doi.org/10.1016/j.ijid.2020.04.065.
9. Schwartz DA. An analysis of 38 pregnant women with COVID-19, their newborn infants, and maternal-fetal transmission of SARS-CoV-2: maternal coronavirus infections and pregnancy outcomes. Arch Pathol Lab Med. 2020;144:799–805. https://doi.org/10.5858/arpa.2020-0901-SA.
10. Chen Y, Peng H, Wang L, Zhao Y, Zeng L, Gao H, Liu Y. Infants born to mothers with a new coronavirus (COVID-19). Front Pediatr. 2020;8:104. https://doi.org/10.3389/fped.2020.00104.
11. Zhu H, Wang L, Fang C, Peng S, Zhang L, Chang G, et al. Clinical analysis of 10 neonates born to mothers with 2019-nCoV pneumonia. Transl Pediatr. 2020;9:51–60. https://doi.org/10.21037/tp.2020.02.06.
12. Simões E, Silva AC, Leal CRV. Is SARS-CoV-2 vertically transmitted? Front Pediatr. 2020;8:276. https://doi.org/10.3389/fped.2020.00276.
13. Zeng L, Xia S, Yuan W, Yan K, Xiao F, Shao J, et al. Neonatal early-onset infection with SARS-CoV-2 in 33 neonates born to mothers with COVID-19 in Wuhan, China. JAMA Pediatr. 2020;174:722–5. https://doi.org/10.1001/jamapediatrics.2020.0878.
14. Wang S, Guo L, Chen L, Liu W, Cao Y, Zhang J, et al. A case report of neonatal 2019 coronavirus disease in China. Clin Infect Dis. 2020;71:853–7. https://doi.org/10.1093/cid/ciaa225.
15. Knight M, Bunch K, Vousden N, Morris E, Simpson N, Gale C, et al. Characteristics and outcomes of pregnant women admitted to hospital with confirmed SARS-CoV-2 infection in UK: national population based cohort study. BMJ. 2020;369:m2107. https://doi.org/10.1136/bmj.m2107.
16. Schwartz DA, Mohagheghi P, Beigi B, Zafaranloo N, Moshfegh F, Yazdani A. Spectrum of neonatal COVID-19 in Iran: 19 infants with SARS-CoV-2 perinatal infections with varying test results, clinical findings and outcomes. J Matern Fetal Neonatal Med. 2022;35:2731–40. https://doi.org/10.1080/14767058.2020.1797672.
17. Meslin P, Guiomard C, Chouakria M, Porcher J, Duquesne F, Tiprez C, et al. Coronavirus disease 2019 in newborns and very young infants: a series of six patients in France. Pediatr Infect Dis J. 2020;39(7):e145–7. https://doi.org/10.1097/INF.0000000000002743.
18. Oncel MY, Akın IM, Kanburoglu MK, Tayman C, Coskun S, Narter F, et al. A multicenter study on epidemiological and clinical characteristics of 125 newborns born to women infected with COVID-19 by Turkish Neonatal Society. Eur J Pediatr. 2021 180:733–42. https://doi.org/10.1007/s00431-020-03767-5.
19. Lamouroux A, Attie-Bitach T, Martinovic J, Leruez-Ville M, Ville Y. Evidence for and against vertical transmission for severe acute respiratory syndrome coronavirus 2. Am J Obstet Gynecol. 2020;223(1):91.e1–4. https://doi.org/10.1016/j.ajog.2020.04.039.
20. Gordon M, Kagalwala T, Rezk K, Rawlingson C, Ahmed MI, Guleri A. Rapid systematic review of neonatal COVID-19 including a case of presumed vertical transmission. BMJ Paediatr Open. 2020;4:e000718. https://doi.org/10.1136/bmjpo-2020-000718.
21. Auriti C, De Rose DU, Tzialla C, Caforio L, Ciccia M, Manzoni P, et al. Vertical transmission of SARS-CoV-2 (COVID-19): are hypotheses more than evidences? Am J Perinatol. 2020;37(Suppl 02):S31–8. https://doi.org/10.1055/s-0040-1714346.
22. Hijona Elósegui JJ, Carballo García AL, Fernández Risquez AC, Bermúdez Quintana M, Expósito Montes JF. Does the maternal-fetal transmission of SARS-CoV-2 occur during pregnancy? [Existe transmission materno-fetal del SARS-CoV-2 durante la gestación?]. Rev Clin Esp. 2020;221:93–6. https://doi.org/10.1016/j.rce.2020.06.001.

23. Muehlenbachs A, de la Rosa VO, Bausch DG, Schafer IJ, Paddock CD, Nyakio JP, et al. Ebola virus disease in pregnancy: clinical, histopathologic, and immunohistochemical findings. J Infect Dis. 2017;215:64–9. https://doi.org/10.1093/infdis/jiw206.
24. Schwartz DA. Viral infection, proliferation, and hyperplasia of Hofbauer cells and absence of inflammation characterize the placental pathology of fetuses with congenital Zika virus infection. Arch Gynecol Obstet. 2017;295:1361–8. https://doi.org/10.1007/s00404-017-4361-5.
25. Ritter JM, Martines RB, Zaki SR. Zika virus: pathology from the pandemic. Arch Pathol Lab Med. 2017;141:49–59. https://doi.org/10.5858/arpa.2016-0397-SA.
26. Schwartz DA, Thomas KM. Characterizing COVID-19 maternal-fetal transmission and placental infection using comprehensive molecular pathology. EBioMedicine. 2020;60:102983. https://doi.org/10.1016/j.ebiom.2020.102983.
27. Gao L, Ren J, Xu L, Ke X, Xiong L, Tian X, et al. Placental pathology of the third trimester pregnant women from COVID-19. Diagn Pathol. 2021;16:8. https://doi.org/10.1186/s13000-021-01067-6.
28. Prabhu M, Cagino K, Matthews KC, Friedlander RL, Glynn SM, Kubiak JM, et al. Pregnancy and postpartum outcomes in a universally tested population for SARS-CoV-2 in New York City: a prospective cohort study. BJOG. 2020;127:1548–56. https://doi.org/10.1111/1471-0528.16403.
29. Shanes ED, Mithal LB, Otero S, Azad HA, Miller ES, Goldstein JA. Placental pathology in COVID-19. Am J Clin Pathol. 2020;154:23–32. https://doi.org/10.1093/ajcp/aqaa089.
30. Sharps MC, Hayes DJL, Lee S, Zou Z, Brady CA, Almoghrabi Y, et al. A structured review of placental morphology and histopathological lesions associated with SARS-CoV-2 infection. Placenta. 2020;101:13–29. https://doi.org/10.1016/j.placenta.2020.08.018.
31. Baergen RN, Heller DS. Placental pathology in Covid-19 positive mothers: preliminary findings. Pediatr Dev Pathol. 2020;23:177–80. https://doi.org/10.1177/1093526620925569.
32. Gulersen M, Prasannan L, Tam Tam H, Metz CN, Rochelson B, Meirowitz N, et al. Histopathologic evaluation of placentas after diagnosis of maternal severe acute respiratory syndrome coronavirus 2 infection. Am J Obstet Gynecol MFM. 2020;2:100211. https://doi.org/10.1016/j.ajogmf.2020.100211.
33. Hecht JL, Quade B, Deshpande V, Mino-Kenudson M, Ting DT, Desai N, et al. SARS-CoV-2 can infect the placenta and is not associated with specific placental histopathology: a series of 19 placentas from COVID-19-positive mothers. Mod Pathol. 2020;33:2092–103. https://doi.org/10.1038/s41379-020-0639-4.
34. Schwartz DA, Morotti D, Beigi B, Moshfegh F, Zafaranloo N, Patanè L. Confirming vertical fetal infection with COVID-19: neonatal and pathology criteria for early onset and transplacental transmission of SARS-CoV-2 from infected pregnant mothers. Arch Pathol Lab Med. 2020;144:1451–6. https://doi.org/10.5858/arpa.2020-0442-SA.
35. Patanè L, Morotti D, Giunta MR, Sigismondi C, Piccoli MG, et al. Vertical transmission of coronavirus disease 2019: severe acute respiratory syndrome coronavirus 2 RNA on the fetal side of the placenta in pregnancies with coronavirus disease 2019-positive mothers and neonates at birth. Am J Obstet Gynecol MFM. 2020;2:100145. https://doi.org/10.1016/j.ajogmf.2020.100145.
36. Vivanti AJ, Vauloup-Fellous C, Prevot S, Zupan V, Suffee C, et al. Transplacental transmission of SARS-CoV-2 infection. Nat Commun. 2020;11:3572. https://doi.org/10.1038/s41467-020-17436-6.
37. Sisman J, Jaleel MA, Moreno W, Rajaram V, Collins RRJ, et al. Intrauterine transmission of SARS-COV-2 infection in a preterm infant. Pediatr Infect Dis J. 2020;39:e265–7. https://doi.org/10.1097/INF.0000000000002815.
38. Facchetti F, Bugatti M, Drera E, Tripodo C, Sartori E, et al. SARS-CoV2 vertical transmission with adverse effects on the newborn revealed through integrated immunohistochemical, electron microscopy and molecular analyses of placenta. EBioMedicine. 2020;59:102951. https://www.sciencedirect.com/science/article/pii/S2352396420303273\.

39. Kirtsman M, Diambomba Y, Poutanen SM, Malinowski AK, Vlachodimitropoulou E, et al. Probable congenital SARS-CoV-2 infection in a neonate born to a woman with active SARS-CoV-2 infection. CMAJ. 2020;192:E647–50. https://doi.org/10.1503/cmaj.200821.
40. Schwartz DA, Baldewijns M, Benachi A, Bugatti M, Bulfamante G, et al. Hofbauer cells and COVID-19 in pregnancy. Molecular pathology analysis of villous macrophages, endothelial cells, and placental findings from 22 placentas infected by SARS-CoV-2 with and without fetal transmission. Arch Pathol Lab Med. 2021;145(11):1328–40. https://doi.org/10.5858/arpa.2021-0296-SA.
41. Schwartz DA, Morotti D. Placental pathology of COVID-19 with and without fetal and neonatal infection: Trophoblast necrosis and chronic histiocytic intervillositis as risk factors for transplacental transmission of SARS-CoV-2. Viruses. 2020;12:1308. https://doi.org/10.3390/v12111308.
42. Hosier H, Farhadian SF, Morotti RA, Deshmukh U, Lu-Culligan A, et al. SARS-CoV-2 infection of the placenta. J Clin Invest. 2020;130(9):4947–53. https://doi.org/10.1172/JCI139569.
43. Pulinx B, Kieffer D, Michiels I, Petermans S, Strybol D, et al. Vertical transmission of SARS-CoV-2 infection and preterm birth. Eur J Clin Microbiol Infect Dis. 2020;39:2441–5. https://doi.org/10.1007/s10096-020-03964-y.
44. Debelenko L, Katsyv I, Chong AM, Peruyero L, Szabolcs M, Uhlemann AC. Trophoblast damage with acute and chronic intervillositis: disruption of the placental barrier by severe acute respiratory syndrome coronavirus 2. Hum Pathol. 2020;109:69–79. https://doi.org/10.1016/j.humpath.2020.12.004.
45. Schoenmakers S, Snijder P, Verdijk RM, Kuiken T, Kamphuis SSM, et al. Severe acute respiratory syndrome coronavirus 2 placental infection and inflammation leading to fetal distress and neonatal multiorgan failure in an asymptomatic woman. J Pediatr Infect Dis Soc. 2020;10:556–61. https://doi.org/10.1093/jpids/piaa153.
46. Schwartz DA, Baldewijns M, Benachi A, Bugatti M, Collins RRJ, et al. Chronic histiocytic intervillositis with trophoblast necrosis is a risk factor associated with placental infection from coronavirus disease 2019 (COVID-19) and intrauterine maternal-fetal severe acute respiratory syndrome coronavirus 2 (SARS-CoV-2) transmission in live-born and stillborn infants. Arch Pathol Lab Med. 2021;145:517–28. https://doi.org/10.5858/arpa.2020-0771-SA.
47. Watkins JC, Torous VF, Roberts DJ. Defining severe acute respiratory syndrome coronavirus 2 (SARS-CoV-2) placentitis. Arch Pathol Lab Med. 2021;145:1341–9. https://doi.org/10.5858/arpa.2021-0246-SA.
48. Schwartz DA, Levitan D. Severe acute respiratory syndrome coronavirus 2 (SARS-CoV-2) infecting pregnant women and the fetus, intrauterine transmission, and placental pathology during the coronavirus disease 2019 (COVID-19) pandemic: it's complicated. Arch Pathol Lab Med. 2021;145:925–8. https://doi.org/10.5858/arpa.2021-0164-ED.
49. Schwartz DA, Bugatti M, Santoro A, Facchetti F. Molecular pathology demonstration of SARS-CoV-2 in cytotrophoblast from placental tissue with chronic histiocytic intervillositis, trophoblast necrosis and COVID-19. J Dev Biol. 2021;9:33. https://doi.org/10.3390/jdb9030033.
50. Fakonti G, Pantazi P, Bokun V, Holder B. Placental macrophage (Hofbauer Cell) responses to infection during pregnancy: a systematic scoping review. Front Immunol. 2022;12:756035. https://doi.org/10.3389/fimmu.2021.756035.
51. Morotti D, Cadamuro M, Rigoli E, Sonzogni A, Gianatti A, et al. Molecular pathology analysis of SARS-CoV-2 in syncytiotrophoblast and Hofbauer cells in placenta from a pregnant woman and fetus with COVID-19. Pathogens. 2021;10:479. https://doi.org/10.3390/pathogens10040479.
52. Raschetti R, Vivanti AJ, Vauloup-Fellous C, Loi B, Benachi A, et al. Synthesis and systematic review of reported neonatal SARS-CoV-2 infections. Nat Commun. 2020;11:5164. https://doi.org/10.1038/s41467-020-18982-9.

53. Redline RW, O'Riordan MA. Placental lesions associated with cerebral palsy and neurologic impairment following term birth. Arch Pathol Lab Med. 2000;124:1785–91. https://doi.org/10.5858/2000-124-1785-PLAWCP.
54. Chen A, Roberts DJ. Placental pathologic lesions with a significant recurrence risk – what not to miss! APMIS. 2018;126:589–601. https://doi.org/10.1111/apm.12796.
55. Benirschke K, Burton GJ, Baergen RN. Pathology of the human placenta. 6th ed. New York: Springer; 2012.
56. Lampi K, Papadogiannakis N, Sirotkina M, Pettersson K, Ajne G. Massive perivillous fibrin deposition of the placenta and pregnancy outcome: a retrospective observational study. Placenta. 2022;117:213–8. https://doi.org/10.1016/j.placenta.2021.12.013.
57. Labarrere C, Mullen E. Fibrinoid and trophoblastic necrosis with massive chronic intervillositis: an extreme variant of villitis of unknown etiology. Am J Reprod Immunol Microbiol. 1987;15:85–91. https://doi.org/10.1111/j.1600-0897.1987.tb00162.x.
58. Roberts DJ, Edlow AG, Romero RJ, Coyne CB, Ting DT, et al. A standardized definition of placental infection by SARS-CoV-2, a consensus statement from the National Institutes of Health/Eunice Kennedy Shriver National Institute of Child Health and Human Development SARS-CoV-2 placental infection workshop. Am J Obstet Gynecol. 2021;225:593.e1–9. https://doi.org/10.1016/j.ajog.2021.07.029.
59. Schwartz DA. Stillbirth after COVID-19 in unvaccinated mothers can result from SARS-CoV-2 placentitis, placental insufficiency, and hypoxic ischemic fetal demise, not direct fetal infection: potential role of maternal vaccination in pregnancy. Viruses. 2022;14:458. https://doi.org/10.3390/v14030458.
60. DeSisto CL, Wallace B, Simeone RM, Polen K, Ko JY, Meaney-Delman D, et al. Risk for stillbirth among women with and without COVID-19 at delivery hospitalization—United States, March 2020–September 2021. MMWR Morb Mortal Wkly Rep. 2021;70:1640–5. https://doi.org/10.15585/mmwr.mm7047e1.
61. Zaigham M, Gisselsson D, Sand A, Wikström AK, von Wowern E, et al. Clinical-pathological features in placentas of pregnancies with SARS-CoV-2 infection and adverse outcome: case-series with and without congenital transmission. BJOG. 2022;129:1361. https://doi.org/10.1111/1471-0528.17132.
62. Fitzgerald B, O'Donoghue K, McEntagart N, Gillan JE, Kelehan P, et al. Fetal deaths in Ireland due to SARS-CoV-2 placentitis caused by SARS-CoV-2 alpha. Arch Pathol Lab Med. 2022;146:529. https://doi.org/10.5858/arpa.2021-0586-SA.
63. Schwartz DA, Avvad-Portari E, Babál P, Baldewijns M, Blomberg M, et al. Placental tissue destruction and insufficiency from COVID-19 causes stillbirth and neonatal death from hypoxic-ischemic injury: a study of 68 cases with SARS-CoV-2 placentitis from 12 countries. Arch Pathol Lab Med. 2022;146:660. https://doi.org/10.5858/arpa.2022-0029-SA.
64. Schwartz DA, Mulkey SB, Roberts D. SARS-CoV-2 placentitis stillbirth and maternal COVID-19 vaccination: clinical–pathologic correlations. Am J Obstet Gynecol. 2023;228:261–69. https://doi.org/10.1016/j.ajog.2022.10.001.

Chapter 8
Perinatal Diagnostic of SARS-CoV-2 Infection

Christelle Vauloup-Fellous

Laboratory diagnostic tests play a central role in identifying individuals with an active SARS-CoV-2 infection, in order to ensure that infected patients get appropriate management and to enable rapid isolation of infected individuals to prevent further spread of infection. Tests are also performed to identify if a person has been infected with the SARS-CoV-2 virus in the past or has been vaccinated. This chapter currently focuses on giving an overview of performances and interpretation of diagnostic tests that may be used in pregnant women and neonates to assess SARS-CoV-2 infection as recommended by WHO (World Health Organization) [1].

Conventionally, there are two main types of diagnostic tests for infectious viral diseases. The first type is by detecting the presence of the virus itself establishing current infection status (by detection of viral RNA by RT-PCR/LAMP or antigen tests). The second is by detecting the presence of specific antibodies of the virus (by serology). Each approach has its own advantages and shortcoming. Thus, diagnostic methods present different performances depending on the type of assay, the specimen tested, and the stage of the disease. Various diagnostic methods have been developed, each of them having a different degree of sensibility/specificity and based on different SARS-CoV-2 target molecules (Table 8.1) [2, 3].

C. Vauloup-Fellous (✉)
Division of Virology, Department of Biology Genetics and PUI, APHP-Paris Saclay University, Villejuif, France

INSERM U1193, Université Paris Saclay, Villejuif, France
e-mail: christelle.vauloup-fellous@aphp.fr

© The Author(s), under exclusive license to Springer Nature Switzerland AG 2023
D. De Luca, A. Benachi (eds.), *COVID-19 and Perinatology*,
https://doi.org/10.1007/978-3-031-29136-4_3

Table 8.1 Main types of viral/serological methods used for detection of COVID-19

Type of diagnostic test	Technology	Molecule tested	Processing place	Delay for result	Sample site	Number of sample/batch	Sensibility
Detection of SARS-CoV-2 virus	RT-PCR	Viral RNA	Laboratory	2–6 h	Any[a]	Up to 96	++++
	LAMP	Viral RNA	Laboratory or PoC	1–2 h	NP swab, sputum	1–4	+++ (for high viral loads)
	Lateral flow	Viral antigen	PoC	15–20 min	NP swab, sputum	1	++
	ELISA	Viral antigen	Laboratory	1–2 h	NP swab, sputum	Up to 96	++
	Sequencing	Viral RNA	Laboratory	1–2 days	Any[a]	12–48	++
Detection of SARS-CoV-2 antibodies	ELISA	IgG/IgM	Laboratory	1–3 h	Serum	Up to 96	++++
	Lateral flow	IgG/IgM	PoC	15–30 min	Finger prick blood drop	1	++
	VNA	Neutralizing antibodies	Laboratory	3–5 days	Serum	1–12	+++
	sVNA	Neutralizing antibodies	Laboratory	1–2 h	Serum	12–48	+++

PoC point of care device, *NP* nasopharyngeal, *VNA* virus neutralization assay, *sVNA* surrogate virus neutralization assay

[a]Samples' sites are NP, oropharyngeal, nasal, saliva, sputum, lower respiratory tract secretions, blood, urine, stool, vaginal swab, amniotic fluid, placenta, and biopsies

8.1 Samples Suitable for Testing

As per the Centers for Disease Control and Prevention (CDC) recommendations, in order to diagnose COVID-19, upper respiratory specimen, especially nasopharyngeal (NP), is the best choice for methods detecting the presence of the virus itself. CDC also suggests other specimens such as oropharyngeal, nasal mid-turbinate, anterior nares (nasal swab), nasopharyngeal wash/aspirate, or nasal aspirate as alternatives whenever NP specimens could not be obtained [4]. Additionally, a various range of specimens, such as saliva, sputum, lower respiratory tract secretions, blood, urine, stool, vaginal swab, amniotic fluid, placenta, and biopsies, can be used to detect SARS-CoV-2 [5, 6]. After collection, specimens are transported to laboratories in a suitable viral transport medium. Additionally, minimum essential medium, sterile phosphate buffer, and 0.9% saline solutions were all found to be good alternatives to viral transport media.

Blood sample for serological assay should be collected as usual.

All necessary personal protective equipment and strict adherence to infection control and prevention guidelines as stated by WHO should be followed and monitored by all healthcare professionals involved [7].

8.2 Detecting the Presence of SARS-CoV-2 Virus

Currently, diagnostic techniques based on **reverse transcriptase real-time PCR (RT-PCR)** are the gold standard diagnostic methods for COVID-19 especially because of its high specificity ($\approx$100%). It is the first-line screening method of choice for SARS-CoV-2 detection and recommended by different health agencies [8]. Additionally, RT-PCR techniques are suitable, as they allow viral detection and quantification in specimens collected from symptomatic and asymptomatic patients and provide a relatively rapid result (average 2–6 h). However, RT-PCR for SARS-CoV-2 virus has some pitfalls that all healthcare workers should be aware of.

Numerous RT-PCR tests were rapidly developed and are now currently widely available on several platforms [9]. Sensitivity, stability, accuracy, and assay time depends on the assay. In general, these tests involve three main steps: (1) extraction of viral RNA from the collected specimens, (2) reverse transcription of viral RNA to a single-stranded DNA (cDNA) using the enzyme reverse transcriptase, and (3) amplification of the cDNA coupled with fluorescent detection [9]. An ideal nucleic acid test design should include a conserved region and a specific region of the viral genome in order to minimize against the effects of SARS-CoV-2 genetic drift [10]. E and RdRp genes are the most commonly used as both have high analytical sensitivity (technical limit of detection < 100 copies/mL) [11–13]. Unlike OFR1b and N, the E and RdRp genes are more conserved in the SARS-CoV-2 genome, which leads to a high performance of the test and, consequently, a lower probability of cross-reactivity with other homologous viruses [3, 13, 14]. Overall, specificity of RT-PCR assays is usually 100%, but evidence has shown that sensibility of many of the available commercial RT-PCR assays for detecting SARS-CoV-2 may be lower than optimal (70–100%) [14–16]. The accuracy of the test depends on specimen quality and quantity, time of collection during the course of the disease, and the inherent quality of the test kit.

Swab specimens are not possible from bedridden patients with severe respiratory involvement or those undergoing mechanical ventilation. Invasive procedures to obtain endotracheal aspirates, sputum, and bronchial lavage are possible ways to obtain specimens from such patients. Throat swabs were found to result in false-negative results as viral RNA was recovered from sputum samples of patients after viral load in the throat had decreased to undetectable levels [17]. As course of illness progresses, lower respiratory tract specimens become the best choice [18]. However, collection of specimens from the lower respiratory tract may increase infection risk to healthcare workers owing to aerosol generation during collection procedures [19]. Saliva and nasal wash specimens have been found to be good alternatives [20–22]. Stool specimens were found to contain SARS-CoV-2 and viral

RNA has been successfully detected from such specimens by RT-PCR (Fig. 8.1); however, their diagnostic value has not been studied thoroughly [23].

One of the main reasons of the false-negative rate in RT-PCR results in COVID-19 is the time of sampling after the onset of symptoms. Indeed, it was shown that the false-negative rate of the test varies over time [24]. Another explanation could be related to the variation of the viral load among different specimens and patients. The highest viral loads are usually found in the lower respiratory tracts of COVID-19 patients compared to the upper respiratory tract [25]. Finally, it seems that different variant may be detected differently depending on specimens. For example, it has been recently shown that RT-PCR happens to be more sensitive in saliva containing the omicron variant than in NP swabs [26]. Another important point is that the timeline of RT-PCR positivity is different depending on the type of specimen used. It has been shown that RT-PCR positivity decreases more slowly in sputum and can still be positive even after NP swabs are negative (Fig. 8.1) [27]. Therefore, it is recommended that the molecular tests should be performed soon after the onset of symptoms from respiratory tract specimens, especially those obtained from the lower respiratory tract, to minimize the chances of false-negative results. Despite the recommendation to perform the RT-PCR test on samples collected from the appearance of symptoms, since the viral load is higher, some studies indicate that the Ct (cycle threshold) value between symptomatic and asymptomatic patients is similar [28–31].

It is important to note that PCR positivity does not always correlate with the clinical severity of the disease [32]. The viral load of SARS-CoV-2 is normally defined through the cycle threshold (Ct), and in a practical application, it is considered that a Ct value less than 40 is clinically reported as PCR positive [33]. Ct value is defined as the number of replication cycles in which the fluorescence of the sample exceeds a chosen threshold above the calculated background fluorescence. In other words, the lower the Ct value obtained, the more the gene exists in the sample, which can reflect a higher viral load. However, detectable SARS-CoV-2 RNA does

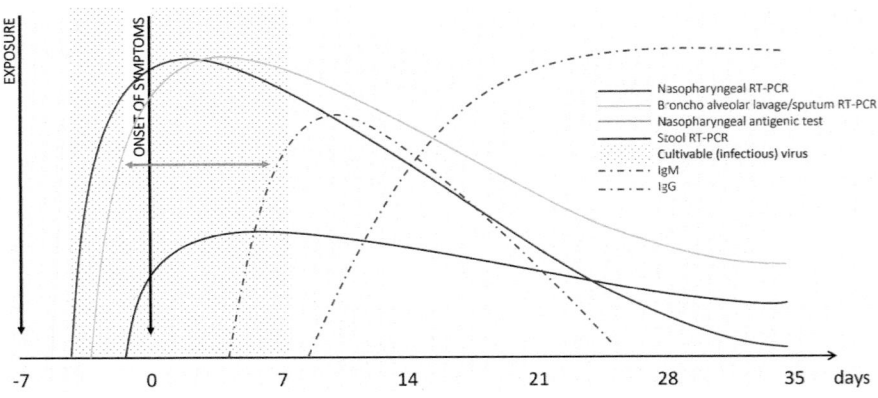

Fig. 8.1 Estimated variation over time of SARS-CoV-2 diagnostic tests

not necessarily mean infectious virus is excreted by the patients. Indeed, although RT-PCR may stay positive for several weeks (usually 2–5 weeks) whatever the clinical presentation, median duration of infectious virus shedding is 4–8 days (range 1–20 days) (Fig. 8.1). Moreover, RT-PCR Ct values correlate with cultivable virus. Indeed, it has been shown that probability of culturing virus declines to 8% in samples with Ct > 35 and to 6% ten days after onset of symptoms and it is similar in asymptomatic and symptomatic individuals (but may be longer in immunocompromised patients) [30]. Usually low Ct (<23) values are related to high viral loads, and significant excretion of infectious viruses and high Ct values (>33) correspond to low viral loads and probably moderate or low viral excretion [30].

Finally, performance of RT-PCR tests can be influenced by mutations in the primer and probe target regions in the SARS-CoV-2 genome [34]. Indeed, as in other RNA viruses, mutations and other genetic changes are likely to occur, and RNA viruses lack efficient proofreading machinery to ensure fidelity of RNA replication. Additionally, studies and regular emerging variants indicate that the SARS-CoV-2 genome is undergoing an evolutionary process through mutations and active genetic recombination. Consequently, mutations in primer and probe-targeted sequences may lead to RT-PCR false-negative results. This can be reduced by targeting two or three sequences within the viral genome, but it is also of major importance to periodically monitor the mutant sites of the viral genome by whole genome sequencing.

Other genetic material-based detections have been developed, including methods based on loop-mediated **isothermal amplification (LAMP)** [35, 36] (Table 8.1). LAMP allows to eliminate the need for sophisticated equipment of RT-PCR assays, improve rapid genetic material amplification and detection, and provide minimal specimen handling, avoiding operator's exposure to the virus and complex training. When compared with RT-PCR, these methods are less sensitive (usually >1000 copies/mL) but remain sensitive enough in case of high viral load (Ct < 33) and far more sensitive than antigenic tests. Moreover, the LAMP assay is considered a point-of-care (PoC) diagnostic test. The challenges of LAMP method are in designing sequence-specific primers as their multiplicity might lead to nonspecific amplification and the fact that it might also be affected by mutations occurring in the sequence region of the target gene causing inaccurate results [37].

Alternatively, to molecular assays, some commercially immunoassays for detecting SARS-CoV-2 viral antigens (spike (S) and nucleocapsid (N) proteins) were developed as diagnostic tools [7, 38]. **Rapid antigen detection kits** are generally characterized by suboptimal sensitivity and specificity (56–100% compared to RT-PCR) but are widely used because of their low cost and practicality especially as PoC tests (Table 8.1) [9, 39, 40].

Even if its analytical performance is being questioned, as well as its financial and logistic limitations, RT-PCR testing is still recommended as first choice of suspected cases by society guidelines in most countries. To date, there is no literature suggesting that RT-PCR, LAMP, or antigenic tests' accuracy could be different in pregnant women compared to immunocompetent nonpregnant individuals. However, concerning specimens collected during the fetal and

neonatal period, only RT-PCR should be used in order to optimize sensibility. More generally, for any specimen collected elsewhere than in the respiratory tract, only RT-PCR should be used.

8.3 Detecting the Presence of Antibodies Against SARS-CoV-2 Virus

When infected with a pathogen, the body's immune response produces antibodies that interact with specific antigen binding to them, thus helping to eliminate the pathogen. This mechanism has been used for the development of immunological diagnostic methods based on the presence of antibodies and their interactions. An antibody test detects the presence of immunoglobulin G (IgG) and immunoglobulin M (IgM) revealing if an individual has already been exposed to the virus and/or the vaccine or not. Typically, the samples used to perform serology are plasma, serum, are whole blood. Thus, serological samples have less variation compared to nasopharyngeal or other respiratory specimens because antibodies are homogeneously dispersed in the blood.

IgM are produced by host immune cells during the early stages of infection few days after initial infection while IgG are often the most abundant antibody in serum having an important role in the later stages of SARS-CoV-2 infection and in support of establishing long-term immune memory [41] (Fig. 8.1). IgM become detectable 3–4 days from symptom onset and are positive in 70% of symptomatic patients after 8–14 days [42]. IgM levels throughout the course of infection are not well characterized (there may be long-lasting IgM or reappearance of IgM few months/years after primary infection). IgG response occurs shortly later at least 7–10 days after infection; its reactivity is assumed to reach more than 98% after several weeks and persist for a long time, but the extent of this antibody response is yet to be determined [42]. The combined detection of IgM and IgG increases performances of serological assays when compared to individual detection, and about 90% of total antibodies test positive within 11–24 days [4, 37]. Therefore, serologic assays are often unable to distinguish a current infection from a prior infection except in neonates where the presence of IgM necessarily indicates a recent infection (as only maternal IgG cross the placenta). However, when an individual has compatible clinical syndrome for COVID-19 and evidence for disease with a clear exposure history to the pathogen and/or supportive laboratory and/or radiographic findings but has negative results by RT-PCR test for SARS-CoV-2, a positive serologic assay can help to confirm the diagnosis and support and guide clinical management decisions [43].

When using N protein-based assay, it may produce false-positive results, as it is the most conserved viral protein among human βcoronaviruses. Manufacturers have therefore focused on developing immunoassays for detecting serum antibodies against domains in the S protein [9]. As vaccines currently mainly target S protein, it is possible to distinguish previous exposure to the virus (anti-N and anti-S positive) from vaccination (anti-N negative and anti-S positive). There are three major types of serological diagnostic tests: **enzyme-linked immunosorbent assays (ELISA)**, **chemiluminescence immunoassays (CLIA)**, and **rapid diagnostic tests (RDT)** (Table 8.1).

A variety of immunoassays (**ELISA** and **CLIA**) has been developed. Implementation of automated serological testing has increased the quality assurance and throughput, while lowering false-positive and false-negative results [14]. Sensibility and specificity usually range from 80 to 100% [14, 44]. Test accuracy for IgG within seven days of symptom onset is usually around 25% (16.29–42.83, 95% CI) while IgM ranges from 22.5 to 47.2% (11.13–58.64, 95% CI) [45].

RDT based on immunochromatography or lateral flow immunoassays have expanded widely, adapting the immunoassay concept to be disposable, inexpensive, fast (around 15–30 min turnaround time), and qualitative (yes/no). They are considered as PoC tests as they can be used in a non-laboratory environment and require a low sample volume (usually a finger prick blood drop of 10–20 μL) [46]. Currently, most of the commercially available tests detect IgM/IgG antibodies. The overall sensitivity for IgG and IgM ranges from 0.37 (95% CI: 0.27–0.48) to 0.96 (95% CI: 0.92–0.98) and specificity from 0.91 (95% CI: 0.84–0.95) [46] to 1 (95% CI: 0.98–1) [45]. Test accuracy within seven days of symptom onset for IgG is usually around 20% (10.15–35.82, 95% CI) while IgM is around 22.8% (11.42–41.19, 95% CI) [45]. It is important to highlight that the clinical accuracy of rapid tests needs to be stringently evaluated before their use as analytical performance may be poor [9].

Serological tests play a fundamental role in diagnosis but have several intrinsic limitations that are mainly related to the individual's immune response to the pathogen, the SARS-CoV-2 variant responsible of infection, as well as the performance related to each type of kit according to the choices of the virus target made by the manufacturer. Most available serological assays (ELISA, CLIA, and RDT) measure antibody binding to SARS-CoV-2 S protein. Since not all S binding antibodies can block viral infection, these assays do not functionally measure the neutralization ability of these antibodies against SARS-CoV-2 infection [47]. **Virus neutralization assays (VNA)** are highly sensitive and specific methods that allow determining the ability of a patient's serum to inhibit viral replication. They are considered to be the gold standard for measuring specific neutralizing antibodies as their positivity is correlated with protective immunity [48]. The conventional method of this assay is based on virus inhibition by neutralizing antibodies in cell culture. Determination of the titer of neutralizing antibodies usually relies on the presence/absence of cytopathic effect, and the highest serum dilution that is able to inhibit infectivity establishes the titer. VNA tests are conducted in four steps: serum dilution, serum and virus incubation, cell culture inoculation, and detection. They require cell culture facilities, several days of work (3–5 days), and highly skilled operators. They must be performed in biosafety level-3 laboratory (BSL3), are time-consuming and labor-intensive, and are hardly standardized as compared to other serologic assays [46]. Therefore, very few laboratories can run such tests, which are not suitable for mass testing. Thus, a surrogate virus neutralization assay (sVNA) was developed for the quantification of neutralizing antibodies [49]. It is designed to detect total neutralizing antibodies in an isotype- and species-independent manner and can be completed in 1–2 h in a BSL2 laboratory. As expected, observations from these studies showed that ELISA/CLIA assays may fail in their ability in predicting neutralizing antibodies activity and therefore the results may not directly correlate with protection [50–52].

There are two main challenges related to serological testing: (1) most tests currently available do not measure neutralizing antibodies and, therefore, cannot conclude whether a previously infected person has sufficient neutralizing antibodies for immunity; and (2) many of the PoC antibody tests have poor clinical specificity, leading to a high rate of false-positive and false-negative results. RT-PCR test is the frontline diagnostic test in the early stages, and results from serological tests alone should not be used to diagnose SARS-CoV-2 infection in the first week of infection [14] (Fig. 8.1). In contrast, they are recommended from the second week of infection as antibodies are more likely to be detected after 12 or 14 days after onset of the first symptoms [53], with IgG levels generally higher than IgM levels from about four weeks after the onset of symptoms [42, 43]. Different studies suggest that 14 days after the onset of symptoms is a time period at which serological tests have high sensitivity that are able to replace RT-PCR for the effective diagnosis of COVID-19 [54–56].

Both asymptomatic and symptomatic pregnant women have detectable IgM and IgG response after SARS-CoV-2 infection. However, as in nonpregnant individuals, IgG levels are significantly higher in the symptomatic mothers compared to the asymptomatic [57–59]. The timeline of antibody response in pregnant women is similar to that of nonpregnant patients and does not deviate from classic patterns of IgM and IgG response [59]. In addition, it is important to highlight that high antibody titers have been shown to be associated with the severity of the disease [60, 61].

Concerning neonates, it was shown that their IgG levels positively correlate with maternal IgG levels [59]. Transfer ratios seem not different among infants born to mothers with asymptomatic or symptomatic illness. Interestingly, transfer ratios increase with increasing time between onset of maternal infection and delivery [62].

8.4 Interpretation of Virological and Serological Diagnostic Tests in Perinatal SARS-CoV-2 Infection

Interpreting a single positive SARS-CoV-2 RT-PCR test in a neonate may be difficult. Indeed, it may indicate either active viral replication or only transient superficial contamination by viral fragments acquired during delivery through the birth canal [63]. Persistence of a positive RT-PCR test on subsequent respiratory specimens collected at 24–48 h of life is therefore of major importance to confirm current neonatal infection. Alternatively, a positive test in a normally sterile specimen (neonatal blood, lower respiratory tract samples, cerebrospinal fluid) also confirms neonatal infection. SARS-CoV-2 has been reported to be detected by RT-PCR in the placenta in several case reports, but clinicians should be aware that the presence of a virus in the placenta is not always correlated with an active infection of the fetus/neonate [64, 65]. Similarly, umbilical cord blood may be contaminated by maternal blood usually by maternal blood cells entering the fetal circulation during uterine contractions [66]. Finally, while SARS-CoV-2 has been reported to be detected by RT-PCR in amniotic fluid in a small number of case reports, not all neonates had confirmed infection which is very different from other congenital infections where the presence of the virus in amniotic fluid always confirms fetal infection [67, 68]. Thus, a positive SARS-CoV-2 RT-PCR in cord blood, placenta, or amniotic fluid requires confirmation with either a fetal/neonatal peripheral blood sample or testing of another sterile or non-sterile sample [1].

IgG found in neonates are primarily the result of maternal IgG transfer through the placenta and hence cannot be used to diagnose in utero infection. Maternal IgM do not cross the placenta, and positive IgM in neonatal blood represents the fetal immune response to infection. However, sensitivity and specificity of IgM tests vary and are usually less reliable than RT-PCR for any virus involved in a congenital infection [69–71]. Thus, whatever the result of a serological test, it should always be confirmed on a second specimen, preferably using RT-PCR to directly detect the virus or otherwise a later serological test.

In general, definitive diagnosis of in utero infection requires a positive test close to delivery confirmed with a second positive specimen, and final diagnosis of intrapartum infection requires a negative test near the time of birth, with a later positive test in the first days after birth confirmed with a later second specimen [1].

References

1. Definition and categorization of the timing of mother-to-child transmission of SARS-CoV-2 [Internet]. [cited 2022 Jan 28]. https://www.who.int/publications/i/item/WHO-2019-nCoV-mother-to-child-transmission-2021.1.
2. Benda A, Zerajic L, Ankita A, Cleary E, Park Y, Pandey S. COVID-19 testing and diagnostics: a review of commercialized technologies for cost, convenience and quality of tests. Sensors. 2021;21:6581.
3. Kubina R, Dziedzic A. Molecular and serological tests for COVID-19. A comparative review of SARS-CoV-2 coronavirus laboratory and point-of-care diagnostics. Diagnostics. 2020;10:434.
4. Keaney D, Whelan S, Finn K, Lucey B. Misdiagnosis of SARS-CoV-2: a critical review of the influence of sampling and clinical detection methods. Med Sci. 2021;9:36.
5. Yu F, Yan L, Wang N, Yang S, Wang L, Tang Y, et al. Quantitative detection and viral load analysis of SARS-CoV-2 in infected patients. Clin Infect Dis. 2020;71:793.
6. Wang D, Hu B, Hu C, Zhu F, Liu X, Zhang J, et al. Detection of SARS-CoV-2 in different types of clinical specimens. JAMA. 2020;23:1843.
7. Interim Guidelines for Collecting and Handling of Clinical Specimens for COVID-19 Testing [Internet]. [cited 2022 Jan 28]. https://www.cdc.gov/coronavirus/2019-ncov/lab/guidelines-clinical-specimens.html.
8. WHO. Coronavirus Disease (COVID-19) Technical Guidance: Laboratory Testing for 2019-nCoV in Humans [Internet]. [cited 2022 Jan 28]. https://www.who.int/emergencies/diseases/novel-coronavirus-2019/technical-guidance/laboratory-guidance/.

9. Machado BAS, Hodel KVS, Barbosa-Júnior VG, Soares MBP, Badaró R. The main molecular and serological methods for diagnosing covid-19: an overview based on the literature. Viruses. 2021;13:40.
10. Fuk-Woo Chan J, Chik-Yan Yip C, Kai-Wang To K, Hing-Cheung Tang T, Cheuk-Ying Wong S, Leung K-H, et al. Improved molecular diagnosis of COVID-19 by the novel, highly sensitive and specific COVID-19-RdRp/Hel real-time reverse transcription-PCR assay validated in vitro and with clinical specimens. J Clin Microbiol. 2020;58:e00310.
11. Harahwa TA, Lai Yau TH, Lim-Cooke MS, Al-Haddi S, Zeinah M, Harky A. The optimal diagnostic methods for COVID-19. Diagnosis. 2020;7:349.
12. Corman VM, Landt O, Kaiser M, Molenkamp R, Meijer A, Chu DKW, et al. Detection of 2019 novel coronavirus (2019-nCoV) by real-time RT-PCR. Eurosurveillance. 2020;25(3):2000045.
13. Böger B, Fachi MM, Vilhena RO, Cobre AF, Tonin FS, Pontarolo R. Systematic review with meta-analysis of the accuracy of diagnostic tests for COVID-19. Am J Infect Control. 2021;49:21.
14. Younes N, Al-Sadeq DW, Al-Jighefee H, Younes S, Al-Jamal O, Daas HI, et al. Challenges in laboratory diagnosis of the novel coronavirus SARS-CoV-2. Viruses. 2020;12:582.
15. Teymouri M, Mollazadeh S, Mortazavi H, Naderi Ghale-Noie Z, Keyvani V, Aghababaei F, et al. Recent advances and challenges of RT-PCR tests for the diagnosis of COVID-19. Pathol Res Pract. 2021;221:153443.
16. Fang Y, Zhang H, Xie J, Lin M, Ying L, Pang P, et al. Sensitivity of chest CT for COVID-19: comparison to RT-PCR. Radiology. 2020;296:E115.
17. Joynt GM, Wu WK. Understanding COVID-19: what does viral RNA load really mean? Lancet Infect Dis. 2020;20:635.
18. Zou L, Ruan F, Huang M, Liang L, Huang H, Hong Z, et al. SARS-CoV-2 viral load in upper respiratory specimens of infected patients. N Engl J Med. 2020;382:1177.
19. Tran K, Cimon K, Severn M, Pessoa-Silva CL, Conly J. Aerosol generating procedures and risk of transmission of acute respiratory infections to healthcare workers: a systematic review. PLoS One. 2012;7:e35797.
20. Azzi L, Carcano G, Gianfagna F, Grossi P, Gasperina DD, Genoni A, et al. Saliva is a reliable tool to detect SARS-CoV-2. J Infect. 2020;81:e45.
21. Tang YW, Schmitz JE, Persing DH, Stratton CW. Laboratory diagnosis of COVID-19: current issues and challenges. J Clin Microbiol. 2020;58:e00512.
22. Kelvin Kai-Wang T, Owen Tak-Yin T, Cyril Chik-Yan Y, Kwok-Hung C, Tak-Chiu W, Jacky Man-Chun C, et al. Consistent detection of 2019 novel coronavirus in saliva. Clin Infect Dis. 2020;71:841.
23. Yeo C, Kaushal S, Yeo D. Enteric involvement of coronaviruses: is faecal–oral transmission of SARS-CoV-2 possible? Lancet Gastroenterol Hepatol. 2020;5:335.
24. Kucirka LM, Lauer SA, Laeyendecker O, Boon D, Lessler J. Variation in false-negative rate of reverse transcriptase polymerase chain reaction–based SARS-CoV-2 tests by time since exposure. Ann Intern Med. 2020;173:262.
25. Abbasi-Oshaghi E, Mirzaei F, Farahani F, Khodadadi I, Tayebinia H. Diagnosis and treatment of coronavirus disease 2019 (COVID-19): laboratory, PCR, and chest CT imaging findings. Int J Surg. 2020;79:143.
26. Marais G, Hsiao NY, Iranzadeh A, Doolabh D, Joseph R, Enoch A, Chu CY, Williamson C, Brink A, Hardie D. Improved oral detection is a characteristic of Omicron infection and has implications for clinical sampling and tissue tropism. J Clin Virol. 2022;152:105170. https://doi.org/10.1016/j.jcv.2022.105170.
27. Wölfel R, Corman VM, Guggemos W, Seilmaier M, Zange S, Müller MA, et al. Virological assessment of hospitalized patients with COVID-2019. Nature. 2020;581(7809):465–9.
28. Jang S, Rhee JY, Wi YM, Jung BK. Viral kinetics of SARS-CoV-2 over the preclinical, clinical, and postclinical period. Int J Infect Dis. 2021;102:561.
29. Louie JK, Stoltey JE, Scott HM, Trammell S, Ememu E, Samuel MC, et al. Comparison of symptomatic and asymptomatic infections due to severe acute respiratory coronavirus virus

2 (SARS-CoV-2) in San Francisco long-term care facilities. Infect Control Hosp Epidemiol. 2022;43:123.
30. Singanayagam A, Patel M, Charlett A, Bernal JL, Saliba V, Ellis J et al. Duration of infectiousness and correlation with RT-PCR cycle threshold values in cases of COVID-19, England, January to May 2020. Eurosurveillance. 2020;25:2001483.
31. Gorzalski AJ, Hartley P, Laverdure C, Kerwin H, Tillett R, Verma S, et al. Characteristics of viral specimens collected from asymptomatic and fatal cases of COVID-19. J Biomed Res. 2020;34:431.
32. Zheng S, Fan J, Yu F, Feng B, Lou B, Zou Q, et al. Viral load dynamics and disease severity in patients infected with SARS-CoV-2 in Zhejiang province, China, January-March 2020: retrospective cohort study. BMJ. 2020;369:m1443.
33. Sethuraman N, Jeremiah SS, Ryo A. Interpreting diagnostic tests for SARS-CoV-2. JAMA. 2020;323:2249.
34. Tahamtan A, Ardebili A. Real-time RT-PCR in COVID-19 detection: issues affecting the results. Expert Rev Mol Diagn. 2020;20:453.
35. Yan C, Cui J, Huang L, Du B, Chen L, Xue G, et al. Rapid and visual detection of 2019 novel coronavirus (SARS-CoV-2) by a reverse transcription loop-mediated isothermal amplification assay. Clin Microbiol Infect. 2020;26:773.
36. Nagura-Ikeda M, Imai K, Tabata S, Miyoshi K, Murahara N, Mizuno T, et al. Clinical evaluation of self-collected saliva by quantitative reverse transcription-PCR (RT-qPCR), direct RT-qPCR, reverse transcription-loop-mediated isothermal amplification, and a rapid antigen test to diagnose COVID-19. J Clin Microbiol. 2020;58:e01438.
37. Obande GA, Singh KKB. Current and future perspectives on isothermal nucleic acid amplification technologies for diagnosing infections. Infect Drug Resist. 2020;13:455.
38. Augustine R, Das S, Hasan A, Abhilash S, Salam SA, Augustine P, et al. Rapid antibody-based covid-19 mass surveillance: relevance, challenges, and prospects in a pandemic and post-pandemic world J Clin Med. 2020;9:3372.
39. Porte L, Legarraga P, Vollrath V, Aguilera X, Munita JM, Araos R, et al. Evaluation of a novel antigen-based rapid detection test for the diagnosis of SARS-CoV-2 in respiratory samples. Int J Infect Dis. 2020;99 328.
40. Diao B, Wen K, Zhang J, Chen J, Han C, Chen Y, Wang S, Deng G, Zhou H, Wu Y. Accuracy of a nucleocapsid protein antigen rapid test in the diagnosis of SARS-CoV-2 infection. Clin Microbiol Infect. 2021;27(2):289.e1–289.e4. https://doi.org/10.1016/j.cmi.2020.09.057.
41. Azkur AK, Akdis M, Azkur D, Sokolowska M, van de Veen W, Brüggen MC, et al. Immune response to SARS-CoV-2 and mechanisms of immunopathological changes in COVID-19. Allergy. 2020;75:1564.
42. Beeching NJ, Fletcher TE, Beadsworth MBJ. Covid-19: testing times. BMJ. 2020; 369:m1403.
43. Rogers R, O'Brien T, Aridi J, Beckwith CG. The COVID-19 diagnostic dilemma: a clinician's perspective. J Clin Microbiol. 2020;58:e01287.
44. Vauloup-Fellous C, Maylin S, Périllaud-Dubois C, Brichler S, Alloui C, Gordien E, et al. Performance of 30 commercial SARS-CoV-2 serology assays in testing symptomatic COVID-19 patients. Eur J Clin Microbiol Infect Dis. 2021;40:2235.
45. Makoah NA, Tipih T, Litabe MM, Brink M, Sempa JB, Goedhals D, Burt FJ. A systematic review and meta-analysis of the sensitivity of antibody tests for the laboratory confirmation of COVID-19. Future Virol. 2021. https://doi.org/10.2217/fvl-2021-0211.
46. Carter LJ, Garner LV, Smoot JW, Li Y, Zhou Q, Saveson CJ, et al. Assay techniques and test development for COVID-19 diagnosis. ACS Cent Sci. 2020;6:591.
47. Muruato AE, Fontes-Garfias CR, Ren P, Garcia-Blanco MA, Menachery VD, Xie X, et al. A high-throughput neutralizing antibody assay for COVID-19 diagnosis and vaccine evaluation. Nat Commun. 2020;11:4059.
48. Plotkin SA. Updates on immunologic correlates of vaccine-induced protection. Vaccine. 2020;38:2250.

49. Tan CW, Chia WN, Qin X, Liu P, Chen MIC, Tiu C, et al. A SARS-CoV-2 surrogate virus neutralization test based on antibody-mediated blockage of ACE2–spike protein–protein interaction. Nat Biotechnol. 2020;38:1073.
50. Luchsinger LL, Ransegnola B, Jin D, Muecksch F, Weisblum Y, Bao W, et al. Serological assays estimate highly variable SARS-CoV-2 neutralizing antibody activity in recovered COVID19 patients. J Clin Microbiol. 2020;58:e02005.
51. Therrien C, Serhir B, Bélanger-Collard M, Skrzypczak J, Shank DK, Renaud C, et al. Multicenter evaluation of the clinical performance and the neutralizing antibody activity prediction properties of 10 high-throughput serological assays used in clinical laboratories. J Clin Microbiol. 2021;59:e02511.
52. Patel EU, Bloch EM, Clarke W, Hsieh YH, Boon D, Eby Y, et al. Comparative performance of five commercially available serologic assays to detect antibodies to SARS-CoV-2 and identify individuals with high neutralizing titers. J Clin Microbiol. 2021;59:e02257.
53. Lou B, Li TD, Zheng SF, Su YY, Li ZY, Liu W, et al. Serology characteristics of SARS-CoV-2 infection since exposure and post symptom onset. Eur Respir J. 2020;56:2000763.
54. Hamilton F, Muir P, Attwood M, Noel A, Vipond B, Hopes R, et al. Kinetics and performance of the Abbott Architect SARS-CoV-2 IgG antibody assay. J Infect. 2020;81:e7.
55. Suhandynata RT, Hoffman MA, Kelner MJ, McLawhon RW, Reed SL, Fitzgerald RL. Longitudinal monitoring of SARS-CoV-2 IgM and IgG seropositivity to detect COVID-19. J Appl Lab Med. 2020;6:565.
56. Wang H, Ai J, Loeffelholz MJ, Tang YW, Zhang W. Meta-analysis of diagnostic performance of serology tests for COVID-19: impact of assay design and post-symptom-onset intervals. Emerg Microbes Infect. 2020;9:2200.
57. Brochot E, Demey B, Touzé A, Belouzard S, Dubuisson J, Schmit JL, et al. Anti-spike, anti-nucleocapsid and neutralizing antibodies in SARS-CoV-2 inpatients and asymptomatic individuals. Front Microbiol. 2020;11:584251.
58. Wajnberg A, Amanat F, Firpo A, Altman DR, Bailey MJ, Mansour M, et al. Robust neutralizing antibodies to SARS-CoV-2 infection persist for months. Science. 2020;370(6521):1227–30.
59. Kubiak JM, Murphy EA, Yee J, Cagino K, Friedlander RL, Glynn SM, et al. SARS-CoV-2 serology levels in pregnant women and their neonates. Am J Obstet Gynecol. 2021;225:73.e1.
60. Ren L, Zhang L, Chang D, Wang J, Hu Y, Chen H, et al. The kinetics of humoral response and its relationship with the disease severity in COVID-19. Commun Biol. 2020;3:780.
61. Li L, Liang Y, Hu F, Yan H, Li Y, Xie Z, et al. Molecular and serological characterization of SARS-CoV-2 infection among COVID-19 patients. Virology. 2020;551:26.
62. Flannery DD, Gouma S, Dhudasia MB, Mukhopadhyay S, Pfeifer MR, Woodford EC, et al. Assessment of maternal and neonatal cord blood SARS-CoV-2 antibodies and placental transfer ratios. JAMA Pediatr. 2021;175:594.
63. Blumberg DA, Underwood MA, Hedriana HL, Lakshminrusimha S. Vertical transmission of SARS-CoV-2: what is the optimal definition? Am J Perinatol. 2020;37:769.
64. Penfield CA, Brubaker SG, Limaye MA, Lighter J, Ratner AJ, Thomas KM, et al. Detection of severe acute respiratory syndrome coronavirus 2 in placental and fetal membrane samples. Am J Obstet Gynecol. 2020;2:100133.
65. Baud D, Greub G, Favre G, Gengler C, Jaton K, Dubruc E, et al. Second-trimester miscarriage in a pregnant woman with SARS-CoV-2 infection. JAMA. 2020;323:2198.
66. Masuzaki H, Miura K, Miura S, Yoshiura KI, Mapendano CK, Nakayama D, et al. Labor increases maternal DNA contamination in cord blood. Clin Chem. 2004;50:1709.
67. Zamaniyan M, Ebadi A, Aghajanpoor S, Rahmani Z, Haghshenas M, Aziz S. Preterm delivery, maternal death, and vertical transmission in a pregnant woman with COVID-19 infection. Prenat Diagn. 2020;40:1759.
68. Schwartz DA, Mohagheghi P, Beigi B, Zafaranloo N, Moshfegh F, Yazdani A. Spectrum of neonatal COVID-19 in Iran: 19 infants with SARS-CoV-2 perinatal infections with varying test results, clinical findings and outcomes. J Matern Neonatal Med. 2022;35:2731.

69. Kimberlin DW, Stagno S. Can SARS-CoV-2 Infection be acquired in utero?: More definitive evidence is needed. JAMA. 2020;323:1788.
70. Voordouw B, Rockx B, Jaenisch T, Fraaij P, Mayaud P, Vossen A, et al. Performance of zika assays in the context of Toxoplasma gondii, parvovirus B19, rubella virus, and cytomegalovirus (TORCH) diagnostic assays. Clin Microbiol Rev. 2019;33:e00130.
71. Schwartz DA, Morotti D, Beigi B, Moshfegh F, Zafaranloo N, Patanè L. Confirming vertical fetal infection with coronavirus disease 2019: neonatal and pathology criteria for early onset and transplacental transmission of severe acute respiratory syndrome coronavirus 2 from infected pregnant mothers. Arch Pathol Lab Med. 2020;144:1451.

Chapter 9
Vertical SARS-CoV-2 Transmission

Daniele De Luca and Maurizio Sanguinetti

9.1 Introduction

The main transmission routes of SARS-CoV-2 are represented by droplets and aerosol. However, the experience accumulated during the pandemics has shown that the vertical transmission was also possible although relatively uncommon. The rarity of this transmission has complicated its understanding since it was difficult to perform studies and investigate the matter with adequate sample size and quality. The purpose of this chapter is to comprehensively review the available knowledge on the mechanisms of SARS-CoV-2 vertical transmission.

9.2 Definitions

The term "vertical transmission" is generic as it encompasses a series of transmission routes from the mother to the fetus and the neonate. This contamination may occur (1) during the pregnancy through the placenta or through the swallowed amniotic fluid and (2) at the moment of delivery, through the contact with the

---

D. De Luca (✉)
Neonatology Department, APHP-University of Paris-Saclay, Le Kremlin-Bicêtre, France

M. Sanguinetti
Catholic University of the Sacred Heart. Rome, Italy

Department of Laboratory Medicine, "A. Gemelli" University Hospital, Rome, Italy

European Society for Clinical Microbiology and Infectious Diseases (ESCMID), Basel, Switzerland
e-mail: maurizio.sanguinetti@unicatt.it

© The Author(s), under exclusive license to Springer Nature Switzerland AG 2023
D. De Luca, A. Benachi (eds.), *COVID-19 and Perinatology*,
https://doi.org/10.1007/978-3-031-29136-4_9

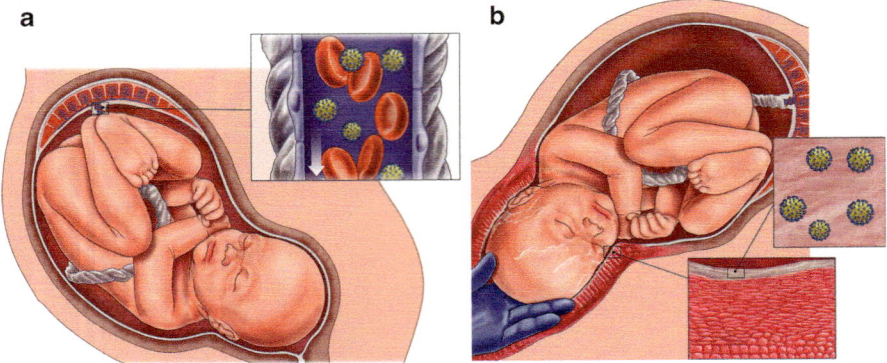

Fig. 9.1 Pathways of SARS-CoV-2 vertical transmission. (**a**, **b**) depict the in utero and intrapartum transmissions, respectively. In utero transmission (**a**) occurs through the placental circulation with SARS-CoV-2 reaching the fetus through the cord or through swallowed amniotic fluid infected through the placenta. Intrapartum transmission (**b**) occurs through the contact with the infected maternal genital mucosa or biological fluids carrying SARS-CoV-2 and covering the *perineum* at the moment of vaginal delivery. Both these transmission routes have been described, whereas, at the time of writing, SARS-CoV-2 vaginal ascending infection has not yet been described and this transmission route can only be speculated. More details in the text

maternal genital mucosal or biological fluids. These two cases correspond to the "in utero" and "intrapartum" transmission according to the World Health Organization definition [1] and are depicted in Fig. 9.1. Theoretically, the mother-to-child transmission through droplets or aerosol occurring in the first 72 h after delivery might also be considered "vertical" but has the same biological features of common environmental transmission; thus, this will not be discussed here. Finally, at the time of writing, SARS-CoV-2 vaginal ascending infection has not yet been described, and this transmission route can only be speculated but should be considered very unlikely.

Both in utero and intrapartum transmissions have been described: according to a meta-analysis published right after the first pandemic wave, they represent about 12% and 17% of neonatal infections, respectively; this accounts for approximately 40% and 60% of vertical infections, respectively (Fig. 9.2) [2]. These cases were classified with a variable level of likelihood [3] since, given the biological complexity of SARS-CoV-2 perinatal infection and the pandemic burden of care, it was not always easy to discriminate and correctly identify the moment and the exact route of transmission. In fact, this requires a significant use of resources as many different samples must be analyzed at various timepoints with techniques not always used during clinical routine in hospital laboratories [4]; thus reports have been sometimes incomplete. We have however accumulated enough knowledge to understand the pathobiological mechanisms of in utero and intrapartum transmissions, and we will describe these in detail.

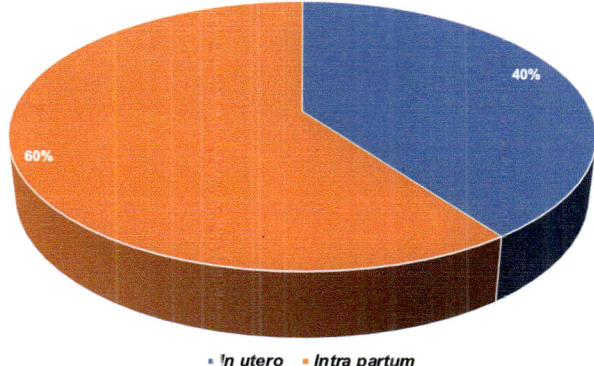

Fig. 9.2 Types and percentage of vertical infections. Distributions between in utero and intrapartum transmissions according to the meta-analysis by Raschetti et al. [2]. Taken altogether, in utero and intrapartum transmissions represent approximately 30% of neonatal SARS-CoV-2 infections (i.e., 70% of infections are acquired horizontally)

9.3 Mechanisms of In Utero SARS-CoV-2 Transmission

Early during pandemics, SARS-CoV-2 has been detected in placental tissues using electron microscopy and particularly in the syncytiotrophoblast cells at the maternofetal interface [5, 6]. This was not totally surprising if we consider that the placenta is "a lung" and represents the place where every maternofetal exchange occurs. As such, it is receiving a significant portion of cardiac output and therefore a possibly relevant viral load if viremia occurs, and this latter has been reported during SARS-CoV-2 infection, although inconstantly and in relation with the clinical severity [7–9]. Beyond a sufficient viral load, the second step needed to infect the placenta and eventually the fetus is represented by the presence of viral receptors on cellular membranes, and this has been extensively investigated in various studies.

The presence of angiotensin-converting enzyme-2 (ACE2) receptors in fetal tissues was already known before the pandemics [10]. During the first wave, a Chinese single-cell transcriptome study on the online available RNA sequencing data evaluated the cell-specific expression of ACE2 in maternal-fetal interface: ACE2 was found to be highly expressed in maternofetal interface including stromal cells and perivascular cells of decidua, cytotrophoblast, and syncytiotrophoblast [11]. ACE2 was also expressed in specific cells of the human fetal heart, liver, and lung but not in the kidney [11]. This has been finally confirmed using immunostaining by Baud and coworkers who suggested that ACE2 expression is consistently present throughout the pregnancy, irrespective of SARS-CoV-2 infection [12]. This, together with the overtime postnatal increment of ACE2 expression in some animal tissues [11], represents the basis for a possible active SARS-CoV-2 replication in placenta and in the fetus/neonate (Table 9.1).

Nonetheless, for the virus to generate an active infection, ACE2 receptor is necessary but insufficient, since the viral S-protein must be cleaved by transmembrane

Table 9.1 Factors affecting SARS-CoV-2 transplacental transmission

Favors transplacental transmission	Prevents transplacental transmission
Higher viremia	Lack of simultaneous receptor expression
Higher ACE2 expression	Deficient intracellular mechanisms of viral transport
Higher TMPRSS2 expression	Placental inflammatory reaction
Preeclampsia	Maternal vaccination
Placental abnormalities such as fetal malperfusion or associated with fetal distress	

Factors have been listed according to the available translational and clinical knowledge (on January 2021). This must only be considered qualitatively, as we cannot estimate the weight of each of these factors and evaluate the risk for each clinical case

protease serine-2 (TMPRSS2) [13]. This leads to expose a fusogenic peptide that promotes the fusion of the viral envelope with the host cell membrane, eventually allowing the endocytosis and viral replication [14]. Thus, TMPRSS2 is as necessary as ACE2 for an active SARS-CoV-2 infection, and this basic characteristic differentiates SARS-CoV-2 from SARS-CoV-1 [15]. A recent study using several techniques found that trophoblastic cells co-express ACE2 and TMPRSS2 with broad expression of furin; the same study demonstrated that the expression was colocalized in early endosomes, suggesting that SARS-CoV-2 can entry the endocytic pathways in human trophoblasts and, in fact, this was confirmed using SARS-CoV-2 pseudoviruses [16].

The situation is however more complex since the expression of ACE2 receptors is not constant and may change through the pregnancy depending on comorbidities, gestational age, and interindividual variability; of note, preeclampsia seems to increase ACE2 expression [17–20]. Moreover, TMPRSS2 expression may not follow the same pathway and, therefore, a sufficient simultaneous expression of both viral receptors may or may not occur, and this significantly influences the placental susceptibility to SARS-CoV-2 infection. Of note, all these data have been accumulating early in the pandemics, and we do not know if more recent viral strains have increased capability to infect placental tissues. The Alpha (α) and Gamma (γ) variants seem to cause more severe disease in pregnant patients [21]. At the time of writing, the omicron (o) variant is spreading and known to be less dependent by TMPRSS2, since other enzymes such as L-cathepsin may cleave its spike protein and allow to entry cells through pathways that have only been secondary so far [22, 23]. The impact of these issues on transplacental transmission has yet to be studied. The existence of viral receptors other than ACE2 has also been hypothesized. For instance, cells expressing ACE2 and TMPRSS2 also express BSG/CD147 [20] and this deserves specific studies [24].

Transplacental SARS-CoV-2 transmission exists but it is a relatively rare event. Therefore, while the aforementioned biological background for transplacental infection is ascertained, we can also speculate about the existence of some mechanisms interfering with it. First of all, a sufficient viremia should occur when there is an adequate simultaneous co-expression of both the viral receptor and the protease, and this may not often happen. Interestingly, a sex difference in the placental TMPRSS2 expression has been noticed, and this can influence the actual availability of viral receptors [25]. Second, if these factors are present, their increment does not seem to increase the risk of transplacental transmission which should be modulated by other factors: in fact, we have recently demonstrated, in a controlled study [26], that the placental viral load or the level of placental expression of ACE2 and TMPRSS2 does not significantly influence the transplacental SARS-CoV-2 passage. The expression of ACE2 can also be variable in different fetal tissues, and this may partially protect from an active infection once SARS-CoV-2 reached the fetal circulation [27]. Another interesting and protective mechanism is probably the failure to activate postentry pathways, such as endosomal escape or the lysosomal deacidification pathways [28]. Placental tissue is responding to SARS-CoV-2 infection with a number of local reactions that, as for other infections, can prevent the viral invasion and the passage to the fetal circulation [29]. For instance, the trophoblast cells may present autophagy during viral infection [30]. Also placenta may react producing a panoply of molecules including growth factors, antioxidants, interferons, and pro-inflammatory cytokines which may have a direct or indirect antiviral effect [31]. A strong local inflammatory reaction is particularly known to prevent the passage of infectious agents to the fetus, and this has been observed in pathological studies (see Chapter 7). Nevertheless, an excessive or dysregulated host inflammatory reaction can also play the opposite role and facilitate viral spread, as it is already known for severe consequences observed in nonpregnant COVID-19 patients [32]. A strong inflammatory reaction with intervillositis and necrosis has been seen in almost all cases of transplacental transmission (see also Chapter 7) [26]. Finally, in vaccinated mothers, antibodies can significantly pass to the fetus [33]. This contributes to modulate the risk of transplacental infection and eventually reduce the neonatal clinical manifestations, although this effect has not been investigated in detail yet.

The inflammatory placental reaction due to SARS-CoV-2 infection has been described in several works and is detailed in Chapter 7. Some pathological features, such as vascular malperfusion on the fetal side, may independently facilitate the transplacental transmission as they are likely to create suitable anatomical environments for the direct passage of virions to the fetal circulation. However, a pathological signature seems associated with transplacental SARS-CoV-2 passage and is represented by diffuse chronic intervillositis with positive viral staining, necrosis, and massive fibrin perivillous deposits (>50% of the placenta). These pathological abnormalities seem also associated with fetal distress, acidosis at birth, and need for neonatal critical care. The peculiar immunological and hormonal features of pregnant women might increase the risk in this particular population and support this dual hypothesis [34]. Interestingly, placentas from women affected by SARS-CoV-1 presented similar pathological findings of intervillositis, fibrin deposition, and fetal malperfusion [35]. These may be associated with intrauterine growth retardation and fetal distress, as also reported for pregnancies complicated by SARS-CoV-1 and MERS-CoV [36, 37].

Finally, as additional mechanism, it has been hypothesized that SARS-CoV-2 transplacental infection may occur through placental macrophages (Hofbauer cells) and circulating fetal monocytes carrying the virus [38]. This would be consistent with transmission of SARS-CoV-1 by infiltrating monocytes and macrophages [39, 40]. Nonetheless, an analysis of an internationally collected placenta database showed that this is only happening in a small minority of cases, if any [41]. Table 9.1 summarizes the factors facilitating or preventing transplacental SARS-CoV-2 transmission; however, this information should be considered only qualitatively. In fact, we lack large epidemiological dataset to estimate the weight of each of these factors, and we cannot evaluate the risk for each case. Also, none of these factors is suitable as screening or diagnostic tool to be applied during pregnancy or at birth. At the time of writing, we are still unaware of any link between the COVID-19 clinical severity and the odds of transplacental transmission. Similarly, it is possible that the exposure time to the virus (duration of infection) and the delay between infection and delivery might have a role, although this has been demonstrated only for the indirect consequences (e.g., prematurity, need for neonatal critical care) of maternal COVID-19 diagnosed early in the third trimester [42].

9.4 Mechanisms of Intrapartum SARS-CoV-2 Transmission

Transmission during vaginal delivery is the other main way of vertical SARS-CoV-2 infection, and there is a certain biological background supporting this transmission route. First, ACE2 receptors are upregulated in vaginal epithelium during pregnancy, making it possible for the virus to entry the genital mucosal cells [43], although we do not have any information regarding TMPRSS2 and other enzymes possibly involved in SARS-CoV-2 cellular invasion. It is also possible for SARS-CoV-2 to reach the vaginal mucosa through the exudation from the bloodstream [44]. Detection of SARS-CoV-2 in the vagina could also be due to seminal or fecal contamination [45]. This latter is facilitated by the viral shedding occurring through the stools being greater and longer compared to that occurring in other districts [46]. In this regard, SARS-CoV-2 seems similar to other coronaviruses causing severe human diseases, such as SARS-CoV-1 and MERV-CoV [46]. Conversely, while we are writing, a case of SARS-CoV-2 vaginal ascending infection has not yet been described.

Systematic review showed that approximately 10–22% of COVID-19 pregnant patients delivered vaginally [47, 48]. An Italian report from the first pandemic wave concluded that vaginal delivery may be associated with a low risk of intrapartum SARS-CoV-2 transmission to the neonate [49]. This hypothesis seems supported by more recent observational studies reporting anecdotical or very low prevalence of SARS-CoV-2-positive vaginal swabs in pregnant women affected by COVID-19 [44, 50, 51]. As certain conditions are preliminarily and simultaneously required to make an intrapartum transmission possible (for instance, sufficient plasmatic viral load, as well as vaginal expression of viral receptors) and these must occur in conjunction with a vaginal delivery, the intrapartum viral diffusion may be relatively uncommon, although we have personally witnessed some of these cases.

Anyhow, to date it is impossible to estimate the actual risk of intrapartum transmission, and its actual prevalence may be higher than originally thought for several reasons. There may be a relevant publication bias, since several cases of possible intrapartum transmission have been described particularly in the first phase of pandemics while they do not currently constitute a novelty anymore. Moreover, the diagnosis is complicated by the well-known difficulties in obtaining all the needed samples according to the WHO definition of mother-to-child transmission [1]. In fact, the aforementioned studies have been performed in small populations with variable sampling times and techniques. Therefore, it would be suitable to perform rectovaginal swabs to all pregnant women affected by COVID-19 or infected by SARS-CoV-2 in the proximity of delivery. Among all the different tests required on different samples (for instance, placenta, amniotic fluid, or cord blood), this would be the easiest to perform. The procedure is already done to screen for other infections and might be performed at the same time. Thus, rectovaginal swabs would help in determining the safety of vaginal delivery, as PCR results can be available in few hours, and also be useful to study possible sexual transmissions [52].

9.5 Consequences of SARS-CoV-2 Vertical Transmission

Once a SARS-CoV-2 vertical infection has occurred, this may cause neonatal COVID-19, whose clinical pictures are discussed in Chapter 12. The crude rate of vertical SARS-CoV-2 infection is estimated around 5% of positive pregnancies [53]. The transplacental transmission seems associated with fetal distress, acidosis with need for neonatal resuscitation, and admission to neonatal intensive care units [26]: this may be explained with the placental insufficiency caused by the infection and the strong local inflammatory reaction. The transplacental antibody transfer is discussed in Chapter 10, and if antibodies are generated after vaccination, they are more likely to reach the fetus and possibly contribute to modulate the neonatal clinical manifestations [33]. Neonates infected by SARS-CoV-2 are asymptomatic in approximately half of cases and those with clinical manifestations are usually not very ill: this seems related to the lower alveolar expression of viral receptors in neonates and children compared to adults, while there seems to be a preferential expression in upper airways [54–56]. Despite the clinical mildness, this can have an epidemiological impact in terms of SARS-CoV-2 shedding, and in fact, infants are important virus spreaders [57]. However, with the majority of adult population being vaccinated, cases of COVID-19 in neonatal and infant population appear more frequently, as this represents a significant portion of remaining nonimmune population: as a consequence, severe and critical cases of neonatal COVID-19 have also been reported [2, 58, 59]. The risk to need neonatal critical care for SARS-CoV-2 infections remains relatively low and difficult to be quantified, but it has been estimated at approximately 2% of cases [60]. However, this creates logistic and epidemiological consequences, since these patients must be isolated, preferentially in negative pressure rooms, and given full critical care, while, on the other hand, neonatal intensive care unit (NICU) beds should not be used to isolate SARS-CoV-2-positive neonates not needing critical care [61]. This has been done at the beginning of pandemics [62], when our knowledge was limited, but should be avoided to reduce the separation from parents and especially to prevent NICU bed shortage. This is particularly important since neonatal emergencies continue to occur, and catching COVID-19 during the pregnancy increases the odds of prematurity and need for NICU care [42, 63]. Also, in some settings, facilities are already insufficient as NICUs often also take care of bronchiolitis and other pediatric conditions of infants and toddlers requiring critical care [64]. A very recent clinical series has also described the occurrence of neonatal inflammatory multisystem syndrome after several weeks from SARS-CoV-2 infection [65]. Conversely, we cannot provide any clue about consequences of transplacental transmission occurring early in the pregnancy: SARS-CoV-2 does not seem to cause malformations but some anecdotical case of fetal demise have been described [66, 67], and this requires a deeper investigation. We cannot yet compare clinical consequences of in utero and intrapartum neonatal SARS-CoV-2 infections, and similarly we cannot provide any definite comparison between vertical and horizontal SARS-CoV-2 neonatal infections. However, comparing these two is one of the aims of the EPICENTRE (ESPNIC Covid pEdiatric Neonatal Registry) whose results will be available soon [68].

Conflict of Interest Authors have no conflict of interest to declare.

References

1. https://www.who.int/publications/i/item/WHO-2019-nCoV-mother-to-child-transmission-2021.1.
2. Raschetti R, Vivanti AJ, Vauloup-Fellous C, Loi B, Benachi A, De Luca D. Synthesis and systematic review of reported neonatal SARS-CoV-2 infections. Nat Commun. 2020;11:5164. https://doi.org/10.1038/s41467-020-18982-9.
3. Shah PS, Diambomba Y, Acharya G, Morris SK, Bitnun A. Classification system and case definition for SARS-CoV-2 infection in pregnant women, fetuses, and neonates. Acta Obstet Gynecol Scand. 2020;99(5):565–8.
4. Schwartz DA, Morotti D, Beigi B, Moshfegh F, Zafaranloo N, Patanè L. Confirming vertical fetal infection with COVID-19: neonatal and pathology criteria for early onset and transplacental transmission of SARS-CoV-2 from infected pregnant mothers. Arch Pathol Lab Med. 2020;144:1451.
5. Hosier H, Farhadian SF, Morotti RA, Deshmukh U, Lu-Culligan A, Campbell KH, Yasumoto Y, Vogels CBF, Casanovas-Massana A, Vijayakumar P, Geng B, Odio CD, Fournier J, Brito AF, Fauver JR, Liu F, Alpert T, Tal R, Szigeti-Buck K, Perincheri S, Larsen C, Gariepy AM, Aguilar G, Fardelmann KL, Harigopal M, Taylor HS, Pettker CM, Wyllie AL, Cruz CD, Ring AM, Grubaugh ND, Ko AI, Horvath TL, Iwasaki A, Reddy UM, Lipkind HS. SARS–CoV-2 infection of the placenta. J Clin Investig. 2020;130:4947–53. https://doi.org/10.1172/JCI139569.
6. Algarroba GN, Rekawek P, Vahanian SA, Khullar P, Palaia T, Peltier MR, Chavez MR, Vintzileos AM. Visualization of severe acute respiratory syndrome coronavirus 2 invading the human placenta using electron microscopy. Am J Obstet Gynecol. 2020;223(2):275–8. https://doi.org/10.1016/j.ajog.2020.05.023.

7. Zheng S, Fan J, Yu F, Feng B, Lou B, Zou Q, Xie G, Lin S, Wang R, Yang X, Chen W, Wang Q, Zhang D, Liu Y, Gong R, Ma Z, Lu S, Xiao Y, Gu Y, Zhang J, Yao H, Xu K, Lu X, Wei G, Zhou J, Fang Q, Cai H, Qiu Y, Sheng J, Chen Y, Liang T. Viral load dynamics and disease severity in patients infected with SARS-CoV-2 in Zhejiang province, China, January-March 2020: retrospective cohort study. BMJ. 2020;369:m1443.
8. Järhult JD, Hultström M, Bergqvist A, Frithiof R, Lipcsey M. The impact of viremia on organ failure, biomarkers and mortality in a Swedish cohort of critically ill COVID-19 patients. Sci Rep. 2021;11:7163. https://doi.org/10.1038/s41598-021-86500-y.
9. Li Y, Schneider AM, Mehta A, Sade-Feldman M, Kays KR, Gentili M, Charland NC, Gonye ALK, Gushterova I, Khanna HK, LaSalle TJ, Lavin-Parsons KM, Lilley BM, Lodenstein CL, Manakongtreecheep K, Margolin JD, McKaig BN, Parry BA, Rojas-Lopez M, Russo BC, Sharma N, Tantivit J, Thomas MF, Regan J, Flynn JP, Villani A-C, Hacohen N, Goldberg MB, Filbin MR, Li JZ. SARS-CoV-2 viremia is associated with distinct proteomic pathways and predicts COVID-19 outcomes. J Clin Invest. 2021;131:e148635. https://doi.org/10.1172/JCI148635.
10. Vento-Tormo R, Efremova M, Botting RA, Turco MY, Vento-Tormo M, Meyer KB, Park J-E, Stephenson E, Polański K, Goncalves A, Gardner L, Holmqvist S, Henriksson J, Zou A, Sharkey AM, Millar B, Innes B, Wood L, Wilbrey-Clark A, Payne RP, Ivarsson MA, Lisgo S, Filby A, Rowitch DH, Bulmer JN, Wright GJ, Stubbington MJT, Haniffa M, Moffett A, Teichmann SA. Single-cell reconstruction of the early maternal–fetal interface in humans. Nature. 2018;563:347–53. https://doi.org/10.1038/s41586-018-0698-6.
11. Li M, Chen L, Zhang J, Xiong C, Li X. The SARS-CoV-2 receptor ACE2 expression of maternal-fetal interface and fetal organs by single-cell transcriptome study. PLoS One. 2020;15:e0230295. https://doi.org/10.1371/journal.pone.0230295.
12. Gengler C, Dubruc E, Favre G, Greub G, Leval L, de Baud D. SARS-CoV-2 ACE-receptor detection in the placenta throughout pregnancy. Clin Microbiol Infect. 2021;37:489.
13. Hoffmann M, Kleine-Weber H, Schroeder S, Krüger N, Herrler T, Erichsen S, Schiergens TS, Herrler G, Wu N-H, Nitsche A, Müller MA, Drosten C, Pöhlmann S. SARS-CoV-2 cell entry depends on ACE2 and TMPRSS2 and is blocked by a clinically proven protease inhibitor. Cell. 2020;181:271–280.e8. https://doi.org/10.1016/j.cell.2020.02.052.
14. Lung Biological Network HCA, Sungnak W, Huang N, Bécavin C, Berg M, Queen R, Litvinukova M, Talavera-López C, Maatz H, Reichart D, Sampaziotis F, Worlock KB, Yoshida M, Barnes JL. SARS-CoV-2 entry factors are highly expressed in nasal epithelial cells together with innate immune genes. Nat Med. 2020;26:681–7. https://doi.org/10.1038/s41591-020-0868-6.
15. Bestle D, Heindl MR, Limburg H, Lam van V, T, Pilgram O, Moulton H, Stein DA, Hardes K, Eickmann M, Dolnik O, Rohde C, Klenk H-D, Garten W, Steinmetzer T, Böttcher-Friebertshäuser E. TMPRSS2 and furin are both essential for proteolytic activation of SARS-CoV-2 in human airway cells. Life Sci Alliance. 2020;3:e202000786. https://doi.org/10.26508/lsa.202000786.
16. Ouyang Y, Bagalkot T, Fitzgerald W, Sadovsky E, Chu T, Martínez-Marchal A, Brieño-Enríquez M, Su EJ, Margolis L, Sorkin A, Sadovsky Y. Term human placental trophoblasts express SARS-CoV-2 entry factors ACE2, TMPRSS2, and Furin. mSphere. 2021;6:e00250–21. https://doi.org/10.1128/mSphere.00250-21.
17. Taglauer E, Benarroch Y, Rop K, Barnett E, Sabharwal V, Yarrington C, Wachman EM. Consistent localization of SARS-CoV-2 spike glycoprotein and ACE2 over TMPRSS2 predominance in placental villi of 15 COVID-19 positive maternal-fetal dyads. Placenta. 2020;100:69–74. https://doi.org/10.1016/j.placenta.2020.08.015.
18. Komine-Aizawa S, Takada K, Hayakawa S. Placental barrier against COVID-19. Placenta. 2020;99:45–9. https://doi.org/10.1015/j.placenta.2020.07.022.
19. Cui D, Liu Y, Jiang X, Ding C, Poon LC, Wang H, Yang H. Single-cell RNA expression profiling of SARS-CoV-2-related ACE2 and TMPRSS2 in human trophectoderm and placenta. Ultrasound Obstet Gynecol. 2021;57:248–56. https://doi.org/10.1002/uog.22186.
20. Ashary N, Bhide A, Chakraborty P, Colaco S, Mishra A, Chhabria K, Jolly MK, Modi D. Single-cell RNA-seq identifies cell subsets in human placenta that highly expresses fac-

tors driving pathogenesis of SARS-CoV-2. Front Cell Dev Biol. 2020;8:783. https://doi.org/10.3389/fcell.2020.00783.
21. Mosnino E, Bernardes LS, Mattern J, Hipólito Micheletti B, de Castro A, Maldonado A, Vauloup-Fellous C, Doucet-Populaire F, De Luca D, Benachi A, Vivanti AJ. Impact of SARS-CoV-2 alpha and gamma variants among symptomatic pregnant women: a two-center retrospective cohort study between France and Brazil. JCM. 2022;11:2663. https://doi.org/10.3390/jcm11092663.
22. Thomas P. Peacock, Jonathan Brown Jie Zhou, Nazia Thakur, Ksenia Sukhova, Joseph Newman, Ruthiran Kugathasan, Ada W.C. Yan, Wilhelm Furnon, Giuditta De Lorenzo, Vanessa M. Cowton, Dorothee Reuss, Maya Moshe, Jessica L. Quantrill, Olivia K. Platt, Myrsini Kaforou, Arvind H. Patel, Massimo Palmarini, Dalan Bailey, Wendy S. Barclay The altered entry pathway and antigenic distance of the SARS-CoV-2 Omicron variant map to separate domains of spike protein bioRxiv 2021.12.31.474653; https://doi.org/10.1101/2021.12.31.474653.
23. Willett BJ, Grove J, MacLean OA. et al. SARS-CoV-2 Omicron is an immune escape variant with an altered cell entry pathway. Nat Microbiol 2022;7:1161–79. https://doi.org/10.1038/s41564-022-01143-7.
24. Argueta LB, Lacko LA, Bram Y, Tada T, Carrau L, Rendeiro AF, Zhang T, Uhl S, Lubor BC, Chandar V, Gil C, Zhang W, Dodson BJ, Bastiaans J, Prabhu M, Houghton S, Redmond D, Salvatore CM, Yang YJ, Elemento O, Baergen RN, tenOever BR, Landau NR, Chen S, Schwartz RE, Stuhlmann H. Inflammatory responses in the placenta upon SARS-CoV-2 infection late in pregnancy. iScience. 2022;25(5):104223. https://doi.org/10.1016/j.isci.2022.104223.
25. Shook LL, Bordt EA, Meinsohn M-C, Pepin D, De Guzman RM, Brigida S, Yockey LJ, James KE, Sullivan MW, Bebell LM, Roberts DJ, Kaimal AJ, Li JZ, Schust D, Gray KJ, Edlow AG. Placental expression of ACE2 and TMPRSS2 in maternal severe acute respiratory syndrome coronavirus 2 infection: are placental defenses mediated by fetal sex? J Infect Dis. 2021;224:S647–59. https://doi.org/10.1093/infdis/jiab335.
26. Vivanti AJ, Vauloup-Fellous C, Escourrou G, Rosenblatt J, Jouannic JM, Laurent-Bellue A, De Luca D. Factors associated with SARS-CoV-2 transplacental transmission. Am J Obstet Gynecol. 2022;227(3):541–543.e11. https://doi.org/10.1016/j.ajog.2022.05.015.
27. Beesley M, Davidson J, Panariello F, Shibuya S, Scaglioni D, Jones B, Maksym K, Ogunbiyi O, Sebire N, Cacchiarelli D, David A, De Coppi P, Gerli M. COVID-19 and vertical transmission: assessing the expression of ACE2/TMPRSS2 in the human fetus and placenta to assess the risk of SARS-CoV-2 infection. BJOG. 2022;129:256–66. https://doi.org/10.1111/1471-0528.16974.
28. Ghosh S, Dellibovi-Ragheb TA, Kerviel A, Pak E, Qiu Q, Fisher M, Takvorian PM, Bleck C, Hsu VW, Fehr AR, Perlman S, Achar SR, Straus MR, Whittaker GR, de Haan CAM, Kehrl J, Altan-Bonnet G, Altan-Bonnet N. β-coronaviruses use lysosomes for Egress instead of the biosynthetic secretory pathway. Cell. 2020;183:1520–1535.e14. https://doi.org/10.1016/j.cell.2020.10.039.
29. Delorme-Axford E, Sadovsky Y, Coyne CB. The placenta as a barrier to viral infections. Ann Rev Virol. 2014;1:133–46. https://doi.org/10.1146/annurev-virology-031413-085524.
30. Robbins JR, Bakardjiev AI. Pathogens and the placental fortress. Curr Opin Microbiol. 2012;15:36–43. https://doi.org/10.1016/j.mib.2011.11.006.
31. Joshi MG, Kshersagar J, Desai SR, Sharma S. Antiviral properties of placental growth factors: A novel therapeutic approach for COVID-19 treatment. Placenta. 2020;99:117–30. https://doi.org/10.1016/j.placenta.2020.07.033.
32. Merad M, Martin JC. Pathological inflammation in patients with COVID-19: a key role for monocytes and macrophages. Nat Rev Immunol. 2020;20:355–62. https://doi.org/10.1038/s41577-020-0331-4.
33. Gray KJ, Bordt EA, Atyeo C, Deriso E, Akinwunmi B, Young N, Baez AM, Shook LL, Cvrk D, James K, De Guzman R, Brigida S, Diouf K, Goldfarb I, Bebell LM, Yonker LM, Fasano A, Rabi SA, Elovitz MA, Alter G, Edlow AG. Coronavirus disease 2019 vaccine response in

pregnant and lactating women: a cohort study. Am J Obstet Gynecol. 2021;225(3):303.e1–303. e17. https://doi.org/10.1016/j.ajog.2021 03.023.
34. Kumar R, Yeni CM, Utami NA, Mas and R, Asrani RK, Patel SK, Kumar A, Mohd Y, Tiwari R, Natesan S, Vora KS, Nainu F, Bilal M, Dhawan M, Emran TB, Ahmad T, Harapan H, Dhama K. SARS-CoV-2 infection during pregnancy and pregnancy-related conditions: concerns, challenges, management and mitigation strategies–a narrative review. J Infect Public Health. 2021;14:863–75. https://doi.org/10.1016/j.jiph.2021.04.005.
35. Ng WF, Wong SF, Lam A, Mak YF, Yao H, Lee KC, Chow KM, Yu WC, Ho LC. The placentas of patients with severe acute respiratory syndrome: a pathophysiological evaluation. Pathology. 2006;38:210–8. https://doi.org/10.1080/00313020600696280.
36. Di Mascio D, Khalil A, Saccone G, Rizzo G, Buca D, Liberati M, Vecchiet J, Nappi L, Scambia G, Berghella V, D'Antonio F. Outcome of coronavirus spectrum infections (SARS, MERS, COVID-19) during pregnancy: a systematic review and meta-analysis. Am J Obstet Gynecol. 2020;2:100107. https://doi.org/10.1016/j.ajogmf.2020.100107.
37. Saleemuddin A, Tantbirojn P, Sirois K, Crum CP, Boyd TK, Tworoger S, Parast MM. Obstetric and perinatal complications in placentas with fetal thrombotic vasculopathy. Pediatr Dev Pathol. 2010;13:459–64. https://doi.org/10.2350/10-01-0774-OA.1.
38. Facchetti F, Bugatti M, Drera E, Tripodo C, Sartori E, Cancila V, Papaccio M, Castellani R, Casola S, Boniotti MB, Cavadini P, Lavazza A. SARS-CoV2 vertical transmission with adverse effects on the newborn revealed through integrated immunohistochemical, electron microscopy and molecular analyses of Placenta. EBioMedicine. 2020;59:102951. https://doi.org/10.1016/j.ebiom.2020.102951.
39. Gu J, Gong E, Zhang B, Zheng J, Gao Z, Zhong Y, Zou W, Zhan J, Wang S, Xie Z, Zhuang H, Wu B, Zhong H, Shao H, Fang W, Gao D, Pei F, Li X, He Z, Xu D, Shi X, Anderson VM, Leong AS-Y. Multiple organ infection and the pathogenesis of SARS. J Exp Med. 2005 202:415–24. https://doi.org/10.1084/jem.20050828.
40. Huang C, Wang Y, Li X, Ren L, Zhao J, Hu Y, Zhang L, Fan G, Xu J, Gu X, Cheng Z, Yu T, Xia J, Wei Y, Wu W, Xie X, Yin W, Li H, Liu M, Xiao Y, Gao H, Guo L, X e J, Wang G, Jiang R, Gao Z, Jin Q, Wang J, Cao B. Clinical features of patients infected with 2019 novel coronavirus in Wuhan, China. Lancet. 2020;395:497–506. https://doi.org/10.1016/S0140-6736(20)30183-5.
41. Schwartz DA, Baldewijns M, Benachi A, Bugatti M, Bulfamante G, Cheng K, Collins RRJ, Debelenko L, De Luca D, Facchetti F, Fitzgerald B, Levitan D, Linn RL, Marcelis L, Morotti D, Morotti R, Patanè L, Prevot S, Pulinx B, Saad AG, Schoenmakers S, Strybol D, Thomas K, Tosi D, Toto V, van der Meeren LE, Verdijk RM, Vivanti AJ, Zaigham M. Hofbauer Cells and COVID-19 in Pregnancy. Arch Pathol Lab Med. 2021;145(11):1328–40. https://doi.org/10.5858/arpa.2021-0296-SA.
42. Badr DA, Picone O, Bevilacqua E, Carlir A, Meli F, Sibiude J, Mattern J, Fils J-F Mandelbrot L, Lanzone A, De Luca D, Jani JC, Vivanti AJ. Severe acute respiratory syndrome coronavirus 2 and pregnancy outcomes according to gestational age at time of infection. Emerg Infect Dis. 2021;27:2535–43. https://doi.org/10.3201/eid2710.211394.
43. Narang K, Enninga EAL, Gunaratne MDSK, Ibirogba ER, Trad ATA, Elrefaei A, Theiler RN, Ruano R, Szymanski LM, Chakraborty R Garovic VD. SARS-CoV-2 infection and COVID-19 during pregnancy: a multidisciplinary review. Mayo Clin Proc. 2020;95:1750–65. https://doi.org/10.1016/j.mayocp.2020.05.011.
44. Milbak J, Holten VMF, Axelsson PB, Bendix JM, Aabakke AJM, Nielsen L, Friis MB, Jensen CAJ, Løkkegaard ECL, Olsen TE, Rode L, Clausen TD. A prospective cohort study of confirmed severe acute respiratory syndrome coronavirus 2 (SARS-CoV-2) infection during pregnancy evaluating SARS-CoV-2 antibodies in maternal and umbilical cord blood and SARS-CoV-2 in vaginal swabs. Acta Obstet Gynecol Scand. 2021;100:2268–77. https://doi.org/10.1111/aogs.14274.
45. Li D, Jin M, Bao P, Zhao W, Zhang S. Clinical Characteristics and Results of Semen Tests Among Men With Coronavirus Disease 2019. JAMA Netw Open. 2020;3:e208292. https://doi.org/10.1001/jamanetworkopen.2020.8292.

46. Cevik M, Tate M, Lloyd O, Maraolo AE, Schafers J, Ho A. SARS-CoV-2, SARS-CoV, and MERS-CoV viral load dynamics, duration of viral shedding, and infectiousness: a systematic review and meta-analysis. Lancet Microbe. 2021;2:e13–22. https://doi.org/10.1016/S2666-5247(20)30172-5.
47. Yang Z, Liu Y. Vertical transmission of severe acute respiratory syndrome coronavirus 2: a systematic review. Am J Perinatol. 2020;37:1055–60. https://doi.org/10.1055/s-0040-1712161.
48. Juan J, Gil MM, Rong Z, Zhang Y, Yang H, Poon LC. Effect of coronavirus disease 2019 (COVID-19) on maternal, perinatal and neonatal outcome: systematic review. Ultrasound Obstet Gynecol. 2020;56:15–27. https://doi.org/10.1002/uog.22088.
49. Ferrazzi E, Frigerio L, Savasi V, Vergani P, Prefumo F, Barresi S, Bianchi S, Ciriello E, Facchinetti F, Gervasi M, Iurlaro E, Kustermann A, Mangili G, Mosca F, Patanè L, Spazzini D, Spinillo A, Trojano G, Vignali M, Villa A, Zuccotti G, Parazzini F, Cetin I. Vaginal delivery in SARS-CoV-2-infected pregnant women in Northern Italy: a retrospective analysis. BJOG. 2020;127:1116–21. https://doi.org/10.1111/1471-0528.16278.
50. Fenizia C, Saulle I, Di Giminiani M, Vanetti C, Trabattoni D, Parisi F, Biasin M, Savasi V. Unlikely SARS-CoV-2 transmission during vaginal delivery. Reprod Sci. 2021;28:2939–41. https://doi.org/10.1007/s43032-021-00681-5.
51. Barber E, Kovo M, Leytes S, Sagiv R, Weiner E, Schwartz O, Mashavi M, Holtzman K, Bar J, Engel A, Ginath S. Evaluation of SARS-CoV-2 in the vaginal secretions of women with COVID-19: a prospective study. JCM. 2021;10:2735. https://doi.org/10.3390/jcm10122735.
52. Delfino M, Guida M, Patrì A, Spirito L, Gallo L, Fabbrocini G. SARS-CoV-2 possible contamination of genital area: implications for sexual and vertical transmission routes. J Eur Acad Dermatol Venereol. 2020;34:e364. https://doi.org/10.1111/jdv.16591.
53. Kotlyar AM, Grechukhina O, Chen A, Popkhadze S, Grimshaw A, Tal O, Taylor HS, Tal R. Vertical transmission of coronavirus disease 2019: a systematic review and meta-analysis. Am J Obstet Gynecol. 2021;224:35.
54. Zhao D, Chen X, Han D, Zhong J, Zhang S, Yang C. Pulmonary ACE2 expression in neonatal and adult rats. FEBS Open Bio. 2021;11:2266–72. https://doi.org/10.1002/2211-5463.13232.
55. Bunyavanich S, Do A, Vicencio A. Nasal gene expression of angiotensin-converting enzyme 2 in children and adults. JAMA. 2020;323:2427. https://doi.org/10.1001/jama.2020.8707.
56. Heinonen S, Helve O, Andersson S, Janér C, Süvari L, Kaskinen A. Nasal expression of SARS-CoV-2 entry receptors in newborns. Arch Dis Child Fetal Neonatal Ed. 2022;107:95–7. https://doi.org/10.1136/archdischild-2020-321334.
57. Paul LA, Daneman N, Schwartz KL, Science M, Brown KA, Whelan M, Chan E, Buchan SA. Association of age and pediatric household transmission of SARS-CoV-2 infection. JAMA Pediatr. 2021;175:1151. https://doi.org/10.1001/jamapediatrics.2021.2770.
58. Marsico C, Capretti MG, Aceti A, Vocale C, Carfagnini F, Serra C, Campoli C, Lazzarotto T, Corvaglia L. Severe neonatal COVID-19: challenges in management and therapeutic approach. J Med Virol. 2022;94:1701.
59. Frauenfelder C, Brierley J, Whittaker E, Perucca G, Bamford A. Infant with SARS-CoV-2 infection causing severe lung disease treated with remdesivir. Pediatrics. 2020;146:e20201701. https://doi.org/10.1542/peds.2020-1701.
60. Di Toro F, Gjoka M, Di Lorenzo G, De Santo D, De Seta F, Maso G, Risso FM, Romano F, Wiesenfeld U, Levi-D'Ancona R, Ronfani L, Ricci G. Impact of COVID-19 on maternal and neonatal outcomes: a systematic review and meta-analysis. Clin Microbiol Infect. 2021;27:36–46. https://doi.org/10.1016/j.cmi.2020.10.007.
61. De Luca D. Managing neonates with respiratory failure due to SARS-CoV-2. Lancet Child Adolesc Health. 2020;4:e8. https://doi.org/10.1016/S2352-4642(20)30073-0.
62. Yeo KT, Oei JL, De Luca D, Schmölzer GM, Guaran R, Palasanthiran P, Kumar K, Buonocore G, Cheong J, Owen LS, Kusuda S, James J, Lim G, Sharma A, Uthaya S, Gale C, Whittaker E, Battersby C, Modi N, Norman M, Naver L, Giannoni E, Diambomba Y, Shah PS, Gagliardi L, Harrison M, Pillay S, Alburaey A, Yuan Y, Zhang H. Review of guidelines and recommendations from 17 countries highlights the challenges that clinicians face caring for neonates born to mothers with COVID-19. Acta Paediatr. 2020;109:2192.

63. Metz TD, Clifton RG, Hughes BL, Sandoval G, Saade GR, Grobman WA, Manuck TA, Miodovnik M, Sowles A, Clark K, Gyamfi-Bannerman C, Mendez-Figueroa H, Sehdev HM, Rouse DJ, Tita ATN, Bailit J, Costantine MM, Simhan HN, Macones GA, Eunice Kennedy Shriver National Institute of Child Health and Human Development (NICHD) Maternal-Fetal Medicine Units (MFMU) Network. Disease severity and perinatal outcomes of pregnant patients with coronavirus disease 2019 (COVID-19). Obstet Gynecol. 2021;137 571.
64. Pozzi N, Cogo P, Moretti C, Biban P, Fedeli T, Orfeo L, Gitto E, Mosca F. The care of critically ill infants and toddlers in neonatal intensive care units across Italy and Europe: our proposal for healthcare organization. Eur J Pediatr. 2022;181:1385.
65. More K, Aiyer S, Goti A, Parikh M, Sheikh S, Patel G, Kallem V, Soni R, Kumar F. Multisystem inflammatory syndrome in neonates (MIS-N) associated with SARS-CoV2 infection: a case series. Eur J Pediatr. 2022;181:1883.
66. Shende P, Gaikwad P, Gandhewar M, Ukey P, Bhide A, Patel V, Bhagat S, Bhor V, Mahale S, Gajbhiye R, Modi D. Persistence of SARS-CoV-2 in the first trimester placenta leading to transplacental transmission and fetal demise from an asymptomatic mother. Hum Reprod. 2021;36:899.
67. Baud D, Greub G, Favre G, Gengler C, Jaton K, Dubruc E, Pomar L. Second-trimester miscarriage in a pregnant woman with SARS-CoV-2 infection. JAMA. 2020;323:2198. https://doi.org/10.1001/jama.2020.7233.
68. De Luca D, Rava L, Nadel S, Tissieres P, Gawronski O, Perkins E, Chidini G, Tingay DG, et al. Eur J Pediatr. 2020;179:1271.

Chapter 10
Transplacental Transfer of SARS-COV-2 Antibodies

Dominique A. Badr and Jacques C. Jani

The human placenta is the interface of exchange between fetus and mother. This exchange is bidirectional through the placental barrier, which has a very complex structure. Different mechanisms play a role in gas exchange, transfer of nutrients from the mother to the baby, and transfer of waste from the baby to the mother. Moreover, certain types of maternal immunoglobulins are able to cross the placental barrier into the fetal circulation and confer a passive immunity on the newborn during the first few months of life. This chapter will be a comprehensive review of the transplacental transfer of severe acute respiratory syndrome coronavirus 2 (SARS-CoV-2) antibodies and the possible factors that affect this transfer.

10.1 Mechanisms of Transfer of Molecules Across the Placental Barrier

Early during pregnancy, differentiation of the cytotrophoblast leads to the formation of the outermost layer of the placenta, named the syncytiotrophoblast, which is in direct contact with the maternal blood circulation. Fetal-maternal exchange occurs mainly through this layer via paracellular or transcellular transport mechanisms [1, 2].

Solvent drag is the movement of water across the barrier in response to changes in hydrostatic pressure. Similarly, passive transport of solutes following their concentration or electrical gradients is called simple diffusion. This process does not require

---

D. A. Badr (✉) · J. C. Jani
Department of Obstetrics and Gynecology, University Hospital Brugmann, Université Libre de Bruxelles, Brussels, Belgium
e-mail: Dominique.BADR@chu-brugmann.be; JACQUES.JANI@chu-brugmann.be

© The Author(s), under exclusive license to Springer Nature Switzerland AG 2023
D. De Luca, A. Benachi (eds.), *COVID-19 and Perinatology*,
https://doi.org/10.1007/978-3-031-29136-4_10

the presence of a transmembrane transporter. The physicochemical properties of the solute (such as molecular weight, lipophilicity, polarity, degree of ionization, etc.) and the concentrations of maternal or fetal binding proteins are the main contributors to this passive transport [3]. In contrast, facilitated diffusion is the passive movement of the substrate down its electrical or concentration gradient across the cellular membrane via a transmembrane transporter protein [4]. Nevertheless, some molecules, such as amino acids, need to be transported from the maternal to fetal circulation against their concentration gradient. This mechanism, called active transport, also occurs by specific membrane transport but requires an energy substrate [5, 6].

Another sophisticated mechanism of molecule transport is endocytosis, in which a molecule binds to a specific membrane receptor, and this molecule-receptor complex is invaginated, forming an intracellular vesicle which is transported to the other side of the barrier and released by a reverse mechanism, called exocytosis [7]. This is the mechanism of transfer of maternal antibodies from the maternal to the fetal circulation [8]. The presence of the neonatal Fc receptor (FcRn), which binds the maternal immunoglobulins, is crucial for maternal-fetal antibody transfer [7].

10.2 Immunoglobulin Structure and Types

Immunoglobulins are large proteins that comprise two heavy chains (H-chain) and two light chains (L-chain) of amino acids arranged in a Y shape (Fig. 10.1). Each branch of the Y is called a Fab fragment and the stem of the Y is called the Fc fragment. The distal portion of the Fab fragment contains a variable domain which is antigen-specific [9]. The main function of this site is to bind to the antigen and to neutralize it. On the other hand, the main functions of the Fc fragment are to activate the complement system and to bind to some specific receptors (FcR) on the surface of the phagocytic cells in order to remove the neutralized antigen via the mechanism of opsonization-phagocytosis [10, 11].

There are five categories of immunoglobulins produced by the human immune system (IgG, IgM, IgA, IgD, IgE). The sequence of amino acids in the constant domain and the structure of the protein are the main factors that vary between these categories. Immunoglobulin G is the predominant antibody in humans and it has a monomeric structure. There are four subclasses of IgG, which are IgG1, IgG2, IgG3, and IgG4, from the most to the least frequent, respectively. The structural difference between these subtypes resides in the constant domains of the heavy chains. These four subtypes vary in antigen-antibody affinity, Fc-FcR affinity, and antibody flexibility [9]. In addition, IgG2 is the main subtype produced against polysaccharide-encapsulated pathogens, whereas the remaining subtypes act mainly against protein antigens [12, 13]. Immunoglobulin M is the first antibody produced by the immune system against foreign antigens. It has a pentamer structure (five units of the Y-shaped Ig linked together by disulfide bonds at the level of the Fc fragments) which allows a rapid and potent agglutination of the antigen [14]. Immunoglobulin A is mainly responsible for mucous membrane defense, as in the intestinal and

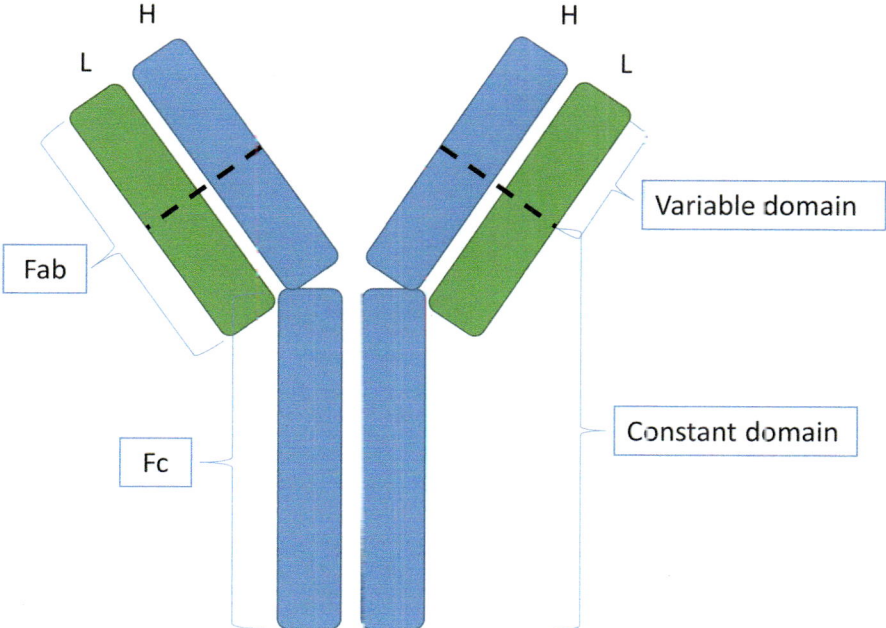

Fig. 10.1 Simplified representation of an immunoglobulin. It comprises two light chains (L) and two heavy chains (H). The arms of the Y are called Fab fragments, whereas the stem is called the Fc segment

respiratory tracts. It has two subtypes IgA1 and IgA2, and it has either a monomeric or a dimeric structure [15]. Immunoglobulin E is associated with allergic and hypersensitivity reactions and antiparasitic infections. It has the lowest serum concentration compared to the remaining classes [16]. Immunoglobulin D is also found in a low concentration in serum and its function is still unclear.

10.3 Antibody Transfer from Maternal to Fetal Circulation

The neonatal Fc receptor (FcRn), which is responsible for the transfer of immunoglobulin through the placental barrier, is IgG-specific; hence IgG is almost the only immunoglobulin that is able to cross the barrier [17, 18]. The concentration of the remaining types of maternal immunoglobulin in the fetal circulation is negligible. The half-life of IgG is 20–30 days, so the complete clearance of maternal immunoglobulins occurs at six months of life. By this time, the immune system of the newborn becomes able to produce its own immunoglobulins [19]. Many factors could play a role in increasing or decreasing IgG transfer, such as maternal IgG concentration, IgG subtypes, maternal diseases that affect placental integrity, gestational age, and birthweight [20, 21].

The fetal IgG concentration increases in parallel with the maternal IgG concentration. Nevertheless, when the maternal IgG concentration reaches 15 g/L, the FcRn becomes saturated [22, 23]. Therefore, unbound IgG molecules are degraded by intracellular lysosomes, and there is a negative correlation between maternal and fetal IgG concentrations beyond this threshold. Very high maternal IgG concentrations are detected in African women and in response to some vaccines [24–26]. Despite this decreased ratio of fetal-maternal antibody transfer, the absolute concentration of maternal IgG in the fetal circulation remains significantly higher in comparison to patients with maternal IgG concentration below the threshold [20].

Studies that compare maternal and fetal IgG subclass concentration have shown that transfer of IgG also depends on the IgG subclasses [20, 27–29]. The concentration of IgG subclasses was studied in 107 fetuses and their corresponding mothers (91 fetuses between 17 and 36 weeks of gestation, by cordocentesis, and 16 fetuses between 37 and 41 weeks of gestation, at delivery) [27]. The fetal-maternal transfer ratio of IgG1, IgG3, and IgG4 increased exponentially throughout pregnancy, whereas the ratio of IgG2 increased linearly. At the end of pregnancy, fetal IgG1 concentration exceeded maternal concentration; fetal IgG3 and IgG4 concentrations matched maternal concentrations, whereas fetal IgG2 concentration was below maternal concentration. Hence, IgG1 is the IgG most transferred from the maternal to the fetal circulation, followed by IgG4 and then IgG3 and finally IgG2. Nevertheless, a recent study suggests that the transfer of IgG2 may not be as low as previously described, and the order of IgG subclasses is rather as follows: IgG1 > IgG3 > IgG4 = IgG2 [30].

Moreover, some maternal diseases or conditions, such as maternal infections, malnutrition, diabetes mellitus, and hypertension, can cause an alteration of the maternal-fetal IgG transfer. The most studied maternal infectious diseases are human immunodeficiency virus (HIV) and malaria infection. These two infections can cause a decrease of IgG transfer either by inducing hypergammaglobulinemia (IgG > 15 g/L) or by causing direct injuries to the placental barrier [31–33].

Gestational age may also affect the transfer of IgG, which begins as early as 13 weeks of gestation and then increases linearly during the second and early third trimesters [34]. A sharp increase of IgG transfer occurs after 36 weeks of gestation, and the concentration of IgG in the fetal circulation is 20–30% higher than that of the maternal circulation at term [27, 28, 34]. This may be due to the high expression of the FcRn in the placental barrier at term [35]. Hence, many studies have shown that premature babies have a lower specific IgG in comparison to babies born at term [26, 36, 37].

Moreover, birthweight, per se, could play a role in IgG transfer even if the baby is born at term. Some studies have demonstrated that small newborns have a lower IgG concentration in comparison to their normal weighted newborn peers [38–40]. Furthermore, reduced IgG transfer seems to affect notable IgG1 and IgG2 subclasses [26, 35, 41, 42], thereby increasing the susceptibility of newborns with intrauterine growth restriction to infections caused mainly by polysaccharide-encapsulated pathogens [20]. It is still not clear whether alterations of the antibody-receptor interaction or maternal diseases that led to intrauterine growth restriction, such as preeclampsia and diabetes, are responsible for this observation.

10.4 Transfer of SARS-CoV-2 Antibodies After Maternal Infection

In response to infection by SARS-CoV-2 virus, human B lymphocytes produce a wide range of antibodies. The most studied antibodies are those targeted against the spike (S) protein, receptor-binding domain (RBD) of the spike protein, and nucleocapsid (N) core. Spike protein of the virus is composed of two distinct parts: subunit S1, which contains the RBD, and subunit S2. The interaction between the spike protein and the angiotensin-converting enzyme 2 (ACE2) receptor facilitates host cell infection. Antibodies against subunits S1 and S2 have also been studied [43, 44].

B lymphocytes start to produce IgM antibodies 7–14 days after the onset of COVID-19 symptoms, with a later production of IgG antibodies. Nevertheless, IgG may be found in 44–56% of patients at day 7 after the onset of symptoms and in 95% at day 20 [45].

The transplacental antibody transfer of IgG following maternal infection has been highlighted by several research teams around the world [46–60]. A summary of relevant studies is presented in Table 10.1. Anti-SARS-CoV-2 antibodies in maternal and umbilical cord blood were measured in almost all of these studies. Moreover, the ratio of fetal to maternal IgG, called transplacental IgG transfer ratio (TR), was calculated in the majority of them. Many factors that affect immunity transfer following COVID-19 infection were identified. They include maternal IgG concentration, time between maternal infection and delivery, gestational age at infection, severity of the COVID-19 infection, and maternal viral load.

10.4.1 Maternal IgG Concentration

As described earlier in this chapter, neonatal IgG titers correlate with maternal IgG titers. This is also valid for anti-SARS-CoV-2 IgG titers, such as anti-S and anti-N [49, 55, 59]. SARS-CoV-2 infection does not induce hypergammaglobulinemia; hence the correlation between maternal and neonatal antibody levels during COVID-19 infection is not studied when total maternal IgG exceeds 15 g/L.

10.4.2 Time Between Maternal Infection and Delivery

Maternal anti-SARS-CoV-2 antibodies start to increase many days following COVID-19 infection as explained earlier. Mothers who are infected a few days before delivery are theoretically not able to confer effective immunity on their neonates. However, it is well established that maternal and neonatal antibody titers increase in parallel with the number of days from the onset of symptoms, once the immunity transfer begins [47, 58]. Nevertheless, these titers may decrease after a certain period [54], subsequent to the waning of maternal immunity with time.

Table 10.1 Summary of studies that examined the incidence of transplacental anti-SARS-CoV-2 immunity transfer following SARS-CoV-2 infection during pregnancy and the factors that affect this transfer

Author, year Period	Type	Participants	Immunity measurement	Main results
Zeng, 2020 [46] February–March 2020	Retrospective cohort, monocenter	6 women with positive RT-PCR and their neonates	IgM and IgG anti-SARS-CoV-2	• IgG concentrations were elevated in 5/6 neonates. • One newborn and his mother had negative IgG. • IgM was detected in two infants.
Edlow, 2020 [47] April–June 2020	Prospective cohort, multicenter	37 women with positive RT-PCR, 40 women with negative RT-PCR, and their neonates	IgM and IgG anti-SARS-CoV-2 S RBD and anti-SARS-CoV-2 N	• IgG anti-SARS-CoV-2 S RBD was detected in 24/37 women and 23/37 neonates. • IgG anti-SARS-CoV-2 N was detected in 26/37 women and 22/37 neonates. • TR was 0.72 for anti-SARS-CoV-2 S RBD and 0.74 for anti-SARS-CoV-2 N. • TR was significantly negatively correlated with maternal viral load, but it did not differ significantly by maternal disease severity or maternal medical comorbidities. • Maternal and cord blood anti-SARS-CoV-2 antibody titers were significantly correlated with number of days from symptom onset.
Flannery, 2021 [48] April–August 2020	Prospective cohort, monocenter	83 seropositive women and their neonates among 1471 tested women	IgM and IgG anti-SARS-CoV-2 S RBD	• IgG was detected in 72/83 neonates. • In 11/83 seronegative neonate: five mothers had only IgM+, and six mothers had low IgG. • TR more than 1.0 was observed regardless of disease severity. • TR increased with increasing time between onset of maternal infection and delivery.
Kubiak, 2021 [49] March–May 2020	Retrospective cohort, monocenter	88 seropositive women (10 IgM+, 24 IgM and IgG+, and 54 IgG+) and 50 of their neonates	Semiquantitative detection of anti-SARS-CoV-2 IgG and IgM	• 39/50 neonates had IgG (14 to IgM+ IgG+ mothers, 24 to IgG+ mothers, and 1 to IgM+ mother). • Maternal IgG levels and maternal use of oxygen support were predictive of the neonatal IgG levels.

Table 10.1 (continued)

Author, year Period	Type	Participants	Immunity measurement	Main results
Egerup, 2021 [50] April–July 2020	Prospective cohort, monocenter	28 seropositive among 1313 tested women, 17 seropositive among 1206 tested neonates	Anti-SARS-CoV-2 IgG and IgM	• 17/21 neonates with seropositive mothers and 3/1131 with seronegative mothers had positive IgG. • None had IgM antibodies.
Rathberger, 2021 [51] April–December 2020	Prospective longitudinal cohort, monocenter	15 women with positive RT-PCR and their neonates	IgM, IgG, and IgA anti-SARS-CoV-2 S RBD	• 73% of the women and 1/3 of the neonates developed IgG+. • A long interval between infection and birth is favorable for IgG transfer. • At 6–12 weeks after birth, all infants showed declining or vanishing antibody titers.
Joseph, 2021 [52] April–December 2020	Prospective cohort, monocenter	32 women with positive RT-PCR and their neonates	IgM, IgA, and IgG anti-SARS-CoV-2 S RBD	• 32/32 women and 29/32 neonates had IgG+. • 30/32 women and 8/32 neonates had functional neutralizing antibody. • TR was 0.81. • Symptomatic infection was associated with a higher maternal IgG. • Maternal IgG were not significantly higher in patients who delivered more than 14 days after a positive PCR test result compared with those who delivered within 14 days.
Atyeo, 2021 [53] NA	Cohort, multicenter	22 women with positive RT-PCR, 33 women with negative RT-PCR, and their neonates	IgG anti-SARS-CoV-2 RBD, anti-SARS-CoV-2 S, and anti-SARS-CoV-2 N	• Anti-SARS-CoV-2 IgG have a decreased transplacental transfer. • The glycosylation of anti-SARS-CoV-2 S IgG is altered in pregnant women. • SARS-CoV-2 infection during the third trimester is associated with elevated maternal IgG levels. • Anti-SARS-CoV-2 IgG transfer is efficient after second-trimester infection.

(continued)

Table 10.1 (continued)

Author, year Period	Type	Participants	Immunity measurement	Main results
Poon, 2021 [54] March 2020–January 2021	Prospective cohort, monocenter	20 women with positive RT-PCR (14 recovered and 6 active infection) and their neonates	IgG and IgM SARS-CoV-2 S1 and N	• 13/14 recovered women and 2/6 women with active infection had IgG+. • Maternal IgG concentrations at delivery increased with increasing viral load during infection and decreased with increasing infection-to-delivery interval. • 12/13 neonates had IgG+. • The median TR of IgG was 1.3 and it decreases with increasing viral load during infection.
Song, 2021 [55] April 2020–March 2021	Prospective longitudinal cohort, monocenter	145 women with positive RT-PCR and 147 neonates	IgG and IgM SARS-CoV-2 S RBD and N	• 84/129 mothers and 83/144 neonates were seropositive. • IgG levels significantly correlated between the maternal and cord blood. • IgG TR was significantly higher when the first maternal positive PCR was 60–180 days before delivery compared with <60 days. • Infant IgG seroreversion rates increased over follow-up periods at 1–4, 5–12, and 13–28 weeks. • The IgG seropositivity in the infants was positively related to IgG levels in the cord blood and persisted up to six months of age.
Conti, 2021 [56] November 2020–May 2021	Prospective cohort, monocenter	28 women with positive RT-PCR and their neonates	IgM, IgA, and IgG anti-SARS-CoV-2 S RBD	• 16/28 women had IgG+, 17 IgA+, and 14 IgM+. • Transplacental transfer of IgG antibodies occurred in only one neonate.
Zambrano, 2021 [57] NA	Retrospective cohort, monocenter	32 seropositive women (21 IgG+ and 11 IgM+) among 100 tested women and their neonates	IgG and IgM SARS-CoV-2 S and N	• 21/21 of neonates with IgG+ mothers had IgG. • 5/21 samples showed relatively inefficient transfer of IgG. 2/21 neonates had higher concentration than their mother. 14/21 had similar concentrations. • 0/11 of neonates with IgM+ mothers and 0/68 of seronegative mothers had IgG positive.
Larcade, 2022 [58] July–October 2020	Prospective cohort, multicenter	87 women with positive RT-PCR and 57 mother-neonate dyads	IgG anti-SARS-CoV-2 S RBD	• A longer time between symptom onset and birth predicted higher maternal IgG concentration, higher IgG transfer, and higher IgG concentration in cord blood.

Table 10.1 (continued)

Author, year Period	Type	Participants	Immunity measurement	Main results
Boelig, 2022 [59]	Prospective cohort, monocenter	51 women with positive RT-PCR, 61 women with negative RT-PCR, and their neonates	IgM and IgG anti-SARS-CoV-2 S RBD, anti-SARS-CoV-2 S (N-terminal domain), anti-SARS-CoV-2 S (full length), and anti-SARS-CoV-2 N	• IgG anti-SARS-CoV-2 S RBD, anti-SARS-CoV-2 S (full length), and anti-SARS-CoV-2 N levels were high, whereas IgG anti-SARS-CoV-2 S (N-terminal domain) levels were modest in patients with a history of COVID-19.
April 2020–February 2021				• Maternal and cord blood IgG were highly correlated for both anti-SARS-CoV-2 S and anti-SARS-CoV-2 N IgG.
González-Mesa, 2022 [60]	Prospective cohort, monocenter	79 women with positive RT-PCR and their neonates	IgG and IgM anti-SARS-CoV-2 S1, IL1b, IL6, and IFN-γ	• IgG anti-SARS-CoV-2 antibodies, IL1b, IL6, and IFN-γ: positive in 100% of neonates
November 2020–May 2021				• Significant correlations between fetal CD3+ mononuclear cells and fetal IgG concentrations
				• Significant correlations between fetal IgG concentrations and fetal CD3+/CD4+, as well as CD3+/CD8+ T cell subsets

IFN-γ, interferon gamma; Ig, immunoglobulin; IL, interleukin; N, nucleocapsid protein; NA, not available; RBD, receptor-binding domain; RT-PCR, reverse transcription polymerase chain reaction; S, spike protein; SARS-CoV-2, severe acute respiratory syndrome coronavirus 2; and TR*, IgG transfer ratio
*Transfer ratio (TR) = fetal IgG level/maternal IgG level

Furthermore, IgG TR increases in line with the time between the onset of maternal infection and delivery [48, 51, 58]. When the infection occurs at less than 60 days from delivery, TR is estimated at 0.6 (95% confidence interval [95% CI] = 0.39–1.04). It increases to 1.2 (95% CI = 0.98–1.29) when the infection occurs 60–180 days before delivery, and then it decreases a little to 0.9 (95% CI 0.33–2.17) when the infection occurs at more than 180 days before delivery [55].

10.4.3 Gestational Age at Infection

High maternal IgG levels are found in infections occurring during the third trimester of pregnancy; however, transfer of specific anti-SARS-CoV-2 antibodies (anti-RBD, anti-S, anti-N, anti-S1, and anti-S2) is compromised by third-trimester infections [53]. Differences in the process of glycosylation of SARS-CoV-2-specific antibodies following third-trimester infection may impact their transfer across the placenta [61]. This alteration seems to be confined to third-trimester infection only, as IgG transfer is efficient after second-trimester infection.

10.4.4 Disease Severity

Symptomatic COVID-19 infection is associated with higher titers of maternal IgG in comparison to asymptomatic infection [52]. Moreover, neonatal IgG titers are higher in mothers who need oxygen therapy during the treatment of the acute infection [49]. In contrast, IgG TR remains around 1 regardless of the severity of maternal disease [47, 48].

10.4.5 Maternal Viral Load

Patients with high viral load on reverse transcription polymerase chain reaction (RT-PCR) testing have increased IgG titers [54]. Nevertheless, IgG TR decreases with elevated maternal viral load. A study showed that among 37 infected women, the median IgG TR was 1.3 and it decreased with increasing maternal viral load during infection [47]. The exact mechanism for this finding is still unclear.

10.5 Transfer of SARS-CoV-2 Antibodies After Maternal Vaccination

Antibodies against the S proteins are the main antibodies produced following SARS-CoV-2 vaccination. In contrast to infection, anti-SARS-CoV-2 antibodies against N protein are not produced after vaccination. Studies that examined maternal to neonatal passive immunity transfer following maternal vaccination are summarized in Table 10.2 [62–73]. The most studied vaccines during pregnancy are BNT162b2 vaccine (Pfizer-BioNTech), mRNA-1273 vaccine (Moderna), and JNJ-78436735 vaccine (Johnson & Johnson's Janssen). Similar to immunity transfer following COVID-19 infection, transfer following vaccination is affected by many factors, such as maternal IgG titers, gestational age at vaccination, time between maternal vaccination and delivery, and number of vaccine doses received.

10.5.1 Maternal IgG Titers

Neonatal IgG titers increase in parallel to the increase of maternal IgG titers [62, 65, 68]. This is similar to what is found following COVID-19 infection. In contrast, IgG TR following vaccination may reach higher levels in comparison to TR following infection. In a study comprising 129 women who received the Pfizer-BioNTech vaccine, all neonates had detectable anti-SARS-CoV-2 antibodies, and the neonatal IgG titers were 2.6 times higher than maternal titers [68]. In another study comprising 27 women, IgG TR after vaccination was greater than TR following infection [63].

Table 10.2 Summary of studies that examined the incidence of transplacental anti-SARS-CoV-2 immunity transfer following SARS-CoV-2 vaccination during pregnancy and the factors that affect this transfer

Author, year Period	Type of study	Participants	Vaccine, dose Immunity measurements	Main results
Prabhu, 2021 [62]	Prospective cohort, monocenter	122 women and their neonates	• Pfizer-BioNTech (85 women) and Moderna (37 women), at least 1 dose	• Maternal Ab production started as early as 5 days and transplacental transfer of Ab started as early as 16 days after the first vaccination dose.
January–March 2021			• Anti-SARS-CoV-2 S RBD (semiquantitative)	• Maternal IgG and TR increased over time.
				• Maternal IgG levels were linearly associated with cord blood IgG levels.
				• TR correlated with the number of weeks elapsed since maternal vaccine dose 2.
Mithal, 2021 [63]	Prospective cohort, monocenter	27 women and their 28 neonates	• Pfizer-BioNTech (18 women), Moderna (6 women), unknown (4 women), at least 1 dose	• 26/27 women and 25/28 neonates had positive IgG.
January–March 2021			• Anti-SARS-CoV-2 S RBD	• Mean TR was 1.0 ± 0.6.
				• Latency between vaccination and delivery was positively correlated with TR and neonate IgG levels.
				• TR was greater than that of SARS-CoV-2 infection.

(continued)

Table 10.2 (continued)

Author, year Period	Type of study	Participants	Vaccine, dose Immunity measurements	Main results
Gray, 2021 [64]	Prospective cohort, multicenter	131 women, of whom 84 pregnant women	• Pfizer-BioNTech (41 women), Moderna (43 women), at least 1 dose	• IgG was detected in 10/10 neonates.
December 2020–March 2021		and 10 of their neonates + 37 recovered women from Edlow et al. [47]	• Anti-SARS-CoV-2 RBD, anti-SARS-CoV-2 S, anti-SARS-CoV-2 S1, anti-SARS-CoV-2 S2	• Time from vaccination to delivery positively correlated with TR.
				• The second vaccine dose increased IgG in maternal blood.
				• Higher levels of IgG were observed in all vaccinated women compared with pregnant women with natural infection.
				• There was a significant improvement of transfer of S-, but not RBD-, specific IgG1 into the cord blood with time from second dose.
Rottenstreich, 2021 [65]	Prospective cohort, monocenter	20 women and their neonates	• Pfizer-BioNTech, 2 doses	• 20/20 of women and neonates had IgG.
February 2021			• IgG and IgM anti-SARS-CoV-2 RBD, anti-SARS-CoV-2 S	• 6/20 women and 0/20 neonates had IgM.
				• IgG concentration in cord blood correlated positively with IgG concentration in maternal blood and with time elapsed between vaccination and delivery.
Zdanowski, 2021 [66]	Retrospective cohort, monocenter	16 women and their neonates	• Pfizer-BioNTech, 2 doses	• 16/16 women and 16/16 neonates had positive IgG anti-SARS-CoV-2 S RBD.
NA			• IgG and IgM anti-SARS-CoV-2 S RBD, anti-SARS-CoV-2 N	• No woman had positive IgG anti-SARS-CoV-2 N.
				• The mean TR was 1.28.
				• IgG titers in cord blood and TR had positive correlations with the number of weeks between first-dose administration and delivery and second-dose administration and delivery.

Table 10.2 (continued)

Author, year Period	Type of study	Participants	Vaccine, dose Immunity measurements	Main results
Trostle, 2021 [67]	Prospective cohort, monocenter	36 women and their neonates	• Pfizer-BioNTech (26 women), Moderna (10 women), 2 doses	• 36/36 neonates had positive anti-SARS-CoV-2 S IgG.
NA			• IgM, IgG, and IgA anti-SARS-CoV-2 S, anti-SARS-CoV-2 N	• 0/31 neonates had positive anti-SARS-CoV-2 N. • Cord blood Ab level may correlate with the time interval between vaccine administration and delivery.
Kugelman, 2021 [68]	Prospective cohort, monocenter	129 women and 114 neonates	• Pfizer-BioNTech, 2 doses	• Mean GA for second dose administration was 24.9 weeks.
May–July 2021			• IgG anti-SARS-CoV-2 S1 RBD	• 129/129 women and 114/114 neonates had positive IgG. • Neonatal IgG titers were 2.6 times higher than maternal titers. • Maternal IgG levels were correlated with neonatal IgG levels. • For each week that passed since the second vaccine dose during the second trimester, maternal and neonatal Ab levels changed by −12.1% and −11.3%, respectively.
Rottenstreich, 2021 [69]	Prospective cohort, monocenter	171 women and their neonates	• Pfizer-BioNTech, 2 doses	• 83/171 women were immunized in early third trimester (first dose at 27–31 weeks) and 88/171 were immunized in late third trimester (first dose at 32–36 weeks).
February–April 2021			• IgG anti-SARS-CoV-2 S, anti-SARS-CoV-2 RBD	• All women and neonates had positive IgG (S and RBD). • Neonatal IgG titers and TR were higher in early- versus late third-trimester vaccination.

(continued)

Table 10.2 (continued)

Author, year Period	Type of study	Participants	Vaccine, dose Immunity measurements	Main results
Shen, 2022 [70]	Prospective cohort, monocenter	29 women and their neonates	• Moderna, at least 1 dose	• Neutralizing Ab against wild-type SARS-CoV-2 in maternal sera was lower after one dose of vaccine compared to that after two doses of vaccine.
NA			• Neutralizing Ab against both wild-type and Delta (B.1.617.2), anti-SARS-CoV-2 S1 RBD	• Neutralizing inhibition and their TR remained stable after two doses of vaccine. • The inhibition of the Delta variant was lower than that of wild-type in both maternal and neonatal sera. • After two doses, all women and neonates had positive anti-SARS-CoV-2 S1 RBD.
Gloeckner, 2022 [71]	Prospective cohort, monocenter	3 women and their neonates	• AstraZeneca and then Pfizer-BioNTech or Moderna	• High titers of IgG anti-SARS-CoV-2 S were detected in both maternal and neonatal sera (100%).
NA			• IgG anti-SARS-CoV-2 S, anti-SARS-CoV-2 N	• No IgG anti-SARS-CoV-2 N were detected.
Rottenstreich, 2022 [72]	Prospective cohort, monocenter	402 women and their neonates	• Pfizer-BioNTech, 2 doses	• 90/402 women received first dose during first trimester, 124/402 during second trimester, and 188/402 during third trimester.
February–November 2021			• IgG anti-SARS-CoV-2 S, anti-SARS-CoV-2 RBD	• IgG in maternal and neonatal sera at delivery were low in the first-trimester group, intermediate in the second-trimester group, and high in the third-trimester group. • 30/90 women received a booster dose: maternal and neonatal IgG levels were high in this subgroup.

Author, year Period	Type of study	Participants	Vaccine, dose Immunity measurements	Main results
Yang, 2022 [73]	Retrospective cohort, monocenter	1359 women and 1362 neonates	• Pfizer-BioNTech (1025 women), Moderna (301 women), or Johnson & Johnson/Janssen (33 women), at least 1 dose	• Maternal IgG were detectable at delivery regardless of timing of vaccination.
March–October 2021			• IgG anti-SARS-CoV-2 S	• Early third-trimester vaccination was associated with the highest IgG levels in maternal and cord blood.
				• Median TR dropped below 1 with vaccination initiation after 32 weeks of gestation.
				• Maternal and cord blood IgG levels in patients with early pregnancy vaccination and history of infection were comparable to those with third-trimester vaccination without a history of infection.
				• A booster dose in the third trimester was associated with maternal IgG levels greater than third-trimester vaccination in women with or without a history of infection.

Ab, antibody; GA, gestational age; Ig, immunoglobulin; N, nucleocapsid protein; NA, not available; RBD, receptor-binding domain; S, spike protein; SARS-CoV-2, severe acute respiratory syndrome coronavirus 2; and TR*, IgG transfer ratio
*Transfer ratio (TR) = fetal IgG level/maternal IgG level

10.5.2 Gestational Age at Vaccination

Antibody transfer depends also on the gestational age at which the vaccine is given. In a study comprising 171 women vaccinated with 2 doses of Pfizer-BioNTech vaccine, IgG anti-S and anti-RBD were found in all neonates; however, neonatal IgG titers and IgG TR were higher in women who received the first dose of vaccine between 27 and 31 weeks of gestation (early third trimester) in comparison to those who received the first dose between 32 and 36 weeks of gestation (late third trimester) [69]. An another study comprising 402 women who also received 2 doses of

Pfizer-BioNTech vaccine, IgG in maternal and neonatal sera at delivery were low when the vaccine was given in the first trimester, intermediate when it was given in the second trimester, and high when it was given in the third trimester [72]. Moreover, when the vaccination is initiated after 32 weeks of gestation, IgG TR drops below 1 [73]. Nevertheless, in patients who are vaccinated early in pregnancy and have a history of COVID-19 infection, maternal and neonatal IgG titers are comparable to those in patients vaccinated in the third trimester and who have no history of infection [73].

10.5.3 Time Between Maternal Vaccination and Delivery

Maternal antibody production may start as early as 5 days following SARS-CoV-2 vaccination, and transplacental antibody transfer starts 16 days after the first dose of the vaccine [62]. Maternal IgG titers, neonatal IgG titers, and IgG TR positively correlate with the time elapsed between maternal vaccination and delivery [62–67]. Moreover, there is an improvement of anti-S-specific IgG1 transfer with time [64]. This is valid in women who are mainly vaccinated during the third trimester; however, immunity waning should be taken into consideration because the decrease in maternal IgG with time will affect neonatal IgG titers. In a study comprising 129 women who received the second dose of Pfizer-BioNTech vaccine at around 24–25 weeks of gestation, maternal and neonatal IgG were decreased by 12.1% and 11.3%, respectively, for each week that passed since vaccination [68].

10.5.4 Number of Vaccine Doses

Maternal and neonatal IgG titers increase with the number of doses of vaccine received. Neonatal IgG are detected in 43.6% when the mother receives one dose and in 98.5% when she receives two doses [62, 74]. Moreover, when maternal and neonatal IgG fade following first-trimester vaccination, the administration of an additional booster vaccine dose may induce IgG titers similar to or even greater than that of third-trimester vaccination [72, 73].

10.6 Comparison of Antibody Transfer Following Infection to Antibody Transfer Following Vaccination

Some studies (summarized in Table 10.3) have compared antibody transfer after COVID-19 infection to transfer after vaccination [75–79]. The results of these studies should be interpreted with caution because of the small study samples. First, there are notable differences in specific antibody response between COVID-19 infection and vaccination. Maternal IgG for S1 and RBD are significantly higher in

Table 10.3 Summary of studies that compared transplacental anti-SARS-CoV-2 immunity transfer following SARS-CoV-2 infection to that following vaccination during pregnancy

Author, year Period	Type	Participants	Vaccine Measures	Main results
Beharier, 2021 [75]	Prospective cohort, multicenter	92 vaccinated versus 74 recovered women and their neonates	• Pfizer-BioNTech, 2 doses	• Mean duration between first dose of vaccine and delivery was 34.5 weeks and from infection to delivery 28.1 weeks.
April 2020–March 2021			• IgG anti-SARS-CoV-2 S1, S2, RBD, and N	• IgG levels in neonatal blood and TR were significantly higher when the infection occurred prior to 30 weeks of gestation in comparison to greater than 30 weeks.
				• At delivery: maternal IgG for S1 and RBD were significantly higher in vaccinated women, whereas IgG for S2 and N were significantly higher in recovered women.
				• Fetal IgG levels for S1 and RBD did not differ between the two groups.
				• TR was comparable in the two groups.
				• Immunity transfer after vaccination is rapid (15 days).
Collier, 2021 [76]	Prospective cohort, monocenter	30 vaccinated versus 22 recovered women and their neonates	• Pfizer-BioNTech (11 women) and Moderna (19 women), at least 1 dose	• Mean duration between second dose of vaccine and delivery was 21 days and from infection to delivery 41 days.
April 2020–March 2021			• IgG anti-SARS-CoV-2 RBD, neutralizing Ab	• IgG anti-SARS-CoV-2 RBD and neutralizing Ab were higher in maternal and neonatal sera of vaccinated women in comparison to those of recovered women.
Treger, 2021 [77]	Prospective cohort, monocenter	28 vaccinated versus 12 recovered women and their neonates	• Pfizer-BioNTech, 2 doses	• Mean duration between second dose of vaccine and delivery was 11.1 weeks and from infection to delivery 20.6 weeks.
NA			• IgG anti-SARS-CoV-2 S, and anti-SARS-CoV-2 N	• IgG titers at delivery were significantly higher in vaccinated in comparison to recovered women.
				• TR was high and comparable in the two groups.
				• No association between vaccination-to-delivery or infection-to-delivery interval and Ab levels.
				• Birthweight affected TR.

(continued)

Table 10.3 (continued)

Author, year / Period	Type	Participants	Vaccine / Measures	Main results
Nir, 2022 [78] / February–March 2021	Prospective cohort, monocenter	64 vaccinated versus 11 recovered women and their neonates	• Pfizer-BioNTech, 2 doses • IgG anti-SARS-CoV-2 RBD	• Mean duration between second dose of vaccine and delivery was 21.7 days and from infection to delivery 92.5 days. • 100% of vaccinated women and 98.3% of their neonates had positive IgG. • Serum IgG titers in vaccinated mothers and neonates were higher than those of recovered mothers and their neonates. • The median TR in vaccinated women was 0.77, whereas in recovered women TR was 1.26.
Shook, 2022 [79] / July–October 2021	Prospective cohort, multicenter	77 vaccinated women (+28 infants followed up for 6 months) versus 12 recovered women (+12 infants followed up for 6 months)	• Pfizer-BioNTech (52 women) and Moderna (25 women) • IgG anti-SARS-CoV-2 S	• Median duration between first dose of vaccine and delivery was 85 days and from infection to delivery 71 days. • IgG titers at delivery were significantly higher in vaccinated women in comparison to recovered women. • At six months, 16/28 (57%) infants from vaccinated mothers and 1/12 (8%) infant from recovered mothers had positive IgG.

Ab, antibody; Ig, immunoglobulin; N, nucleocapsid protein; NA, not available; RBD, receptor-binding domain; S, spike protein; SARS-CoV-2, severe acute respiratory syndrome coronavirus 2; and TR*, IgG transfer ratio
*Transfer ratio (TR) = fetal IgG level/maternal IgG level

vaccinated women, whereas maternal IgG for S2 and N are significantly higher in recovered women. Fetal IgG levels for S1 and RBD are comparable in both groups in one study [75], but fetal and maternal IgG for S and RBD are higher in vaccinated women compared to recovered women in other studies [76–79]. Second, IgG TR is comparable between vaccinated and recovered groups in two studies [75, 77]. In another study, TR in the vaccinated group was lower than in the recovered group [78]. Birthweight affects IgG TR, but there is no association between vaccination-to-delivery interval or infection-to-delivery interval and antibody titers [77]. Third, immunity transfer after vaccination is quicker than transfer following infection [75]. Lastly, passive immunity following maternal vaccination lasts longer than immunity following recovery at six months of follow-up (57% versus 8%, respectively) [79].

In summary, the transfer of antibodies against SARS-CoV-2 from the maternal to fetal circulation may protect infants during the first few months of life. Indeed, maternal vaccination is effective against COVID-19 hospitalization in 61% of infants aged less than six months [80]. The maternal antibodies transferred to the neonates may fade rapidly after birth [51, 55, 81]; however, their titer at birth is positively correlated with that at six-month follow-up [55]. Therefore, vaccination strategies that provide neonates with the highest possible level of maternal antibodies at birth and at the same time protect the mother against COVID-19 infection throughout pregnancy may be the best strategies to implement [82, 83].

References

1. Malek A, Mattison DR. Drug development for use during pregnancy: impact of the placenta. Expert Rev Obstet Gynecol. 2010;5(4):437–54.
2. Sölder E, Rohr I, Kremser C, Hutzler P, Debbage P. Imaging of placental transport mechanisms: a review. Eur J Obstet Gynecol Reprod Biol. 2009;144(Suppl 1):S114–20.
3. Roustit M, Jlaiel M, Leclercq P, Stanke-Labesque F. Pharmacokinetics and therapeutic drug monitoring of antiretrovirals in pregnant women. Br J Clin Pharmacol. 2008;66(2):179–95.
4. Nanovskaya TN, Patrikeeva S, Hemauer S, Fokina V, Mattison D, Hankins GD, et al. Effect of albumin on transplacental transfer and distribution of rosiglitazone and glyburide. J Matern Fetal Neonatal Med. 2008;21(3):197–207.
5. Unadkat DJ, Dahlin A, Vijay S. Placental drug transporters. Curr Drug Metab. 2004;5(1):125–31.
6. Cetin I, Alvino G. Intrauterine growth restriction: implications for placental metabolism and transport. A review. Estab Hypoth Curr Conc. 2009;30:77–82.
7. Fung KYY, Fairn GD, Lee WL. Transcellular vesicular transport in epithelial and endothelial cells: challenges and opportunities. Traffic. 2018;19(1):5–18.
8. Rogers Brambell FW, Halliday R, Brierley J, Hemmings WA. Transference of passive immunity from mother to young. Lancet. 1954;263(6819):964–5.
9. Schroeder HW, Cavacini L. Structure and function of immunoglobulins. J Allergy Clin Immunol. 2010;125(2):S41–52.
10. Kane SV, Acquah LA. Placental transport of immunoglobulins: a clinical review for gastroenterologists who prescribe therapeutic monoclonal antibodies to women during conception and pregnancy. Am J Gastroenterol. 2009;104(1):228. https://journals.lww.com/ajg/Fulltext/2009/01000/Placental_Transport_of_Immunoglobulins__A_Clinical.37.aspx.
11. Schneider H, Miller RK. Receptor-mediated uptake and transport of macromolecules in the human placenta. Int J Dev Biol. 2010;54(2–3):367–75.
12. Vidarsson G, Dekkers G, Rispens T. IgG Subclasses and allotypes: from structure to effector functions. Front Immunol. 2014;5:520. https://www.frontiersin.org/article/10.3389/fimmu.2014.00520.
13. Berkowska MA, Driessen GJA, Bikos V, Grosserichter-Wagener C, Stamatopoulos K, Cerutti A, et al. Human memory B cells originate from three distinct germinal center-dependent and -independent maturation pathways. Blood. 2011;118(8):2150–8.
14. Boes M. Role of natural and immune IgM antibodies in immune responses. Mol Immunol. 2000;37(18):1141–9.
15. Woof JM, Mestecky J. Mucosal immunoglobulins. Immunol Rev. 2005;206(1):64–82.
16. Chang TW, Wu PC, Hsu CL, Hung AF. Anti-IgE antibodies for the treatment of IgE-mediated allergic diseases. Advances in immunology. London: Academic Press; 2007. p. 63–119. https://www.sciencedirect.com/science/article/pii/S0065277606930028.
17. Roopenian DC, Akilesh S. FcRn: the neonatal Fc receptor comes of age. Nat Rev Immunol. 2007;7(9):715–25.

18. Akilesh S, Christianson GJ, Roopenian DC, Shaw AS. Neonatal FcR expression in bone marrow-derived cells functions to protect serum IgG from catabolism. J Immunol. 2007;179(7):4580–8.
19. Jolliff CR, Cost KM, Stivrins PC, Grossman PP, Nolte CR, Franco SM, et al. Reference intervals for serum IgG, IgA, IgM, C3, and C4 as determined by rate nephelometry. Clin Chem. 1982;28(1):126–8.
20. Wilcox CR, Holder B, Jones CE. Factors affecting the FcRn-mediated transplacental transfer of antibodies and implications for vaccination in pregnancy. Front Immunol. 2017;8:1294.
21. Palmeira P, Quinello C, Silveira-Lessa AL, Zago CA, Carneiro-Sampaio M. IgG placental transfer in healthy and pathological pregnancies. Clin Dev Immunol. 2012;2012:1–13.
22. Michaux JL, Heremans JF, Hitzig WH. Immunoglobulin levels in cord-blood serum of negroes and Caucasians. Trop Geogr Med. 1966;18(1):10–4.
23. Englund JA. The influence of maternal immunization on infant immune responses. Proc Merial Eur Vaccinol Symp MEVS. 2007;137:S16–9.
24. Hartter HK, Oyedele OI, Dietz K, Kreis S, Hoffman JP, Muller CP. Placental transfer and decay of maternally acquired antimeasles antibodies in Nigerian children. Pediatr Infect Dis J. 2000;19(7):635. https://journals.lww.com/pidj/Fulltext/2000/07000/Placental_transfer_and_decay_of_maternally.10.aspx.
25. Stach SCL, Brizot ML, Liao AW, Palmeira P, Francisco RPV, Carneiro-Sampaio MMS, et al. Placental transfer of IgG antibodies specific to klebsiella and pseudomonas LPS and to group B streptococcus in twin pregnancies. Scand J Immunol. 2015;81(2):135–41.
26. van den Berg JP, Westerbeek EAM, Berbers GAM, van Gageldonk PGM, van der Klis FRM, van Elburg RM. Transplacental transport of IgG antibodies specific for pertussis, diphtheria, tetanus, haemophilus influenzae type B, and Neisseria meningitidis serogroup C is lower in preterm compared with term infants. Pediatr Infect Dis J. 2010;29(9):801. https://journals.lww.com/pidj/Fulltext/2010/09000/Transplacental_Transport_of_IgG_Antibodies.4.aspx.
27. Malek A, Sager R, Kuhn P, Nicolaides KH, Schneider H. Evolution of maternofetal transport of immunoglobulins during human pregnancy. Am J Reprod Immunol. 1996;36(5):248–55.
28. Malek A, Sager R, Schneider H. Transport of proteins across the human placenta. Am J Reprod Immunol. 1998;40(5):347–51.
29. Hashira S, Okitsu-Negishi S, Yoshino K. Placental transfer of IgG subclasses in a Japanese population. Pediatr Int. 2000;42(4):337–42.
30. Clements T, Rice TF, Vamvakas G, Barnett S, Barnes M, Donaldson B, et al. Update on transplacental transfer of IgG subclasses: impact of maternal and fetal factors. Front Immunol. 2020;11:1920.
31. Atwell JE, Thumar B, Robinson LJ, Tobby R, Yambo P, Ome-Kaius M, et al. Impact of placental malaria and hypergammaglobulinemia on transplacental transfer of respiratory syncytial virus antibody in Papua new guinea. J Infect Dis. 2016;213(3):423–31.
32. Scott S, Cumberland P, Shulman CE, Cousens S, Cohen BJ, Brown DWG, et al. Neonatal measles immunity in Rural Kenya: the influence of HIV and placental malaria infections on placental transfer of antibodies and levels of antibody in maternal and cord serum samples. J Infect Dis. 2005;191(11):1854–60.
33. Fu C, Lu L, Wu H, Shaman J, Cao Y, Fang F, et al. Placental antibody transfer efficiency and maternal levels: specific for measles, coxsackievirus A16, enterovirus 71, poliomyelitis I-III and HIV-1 antibodies. Sci Rep. 2016;6:38874.
34. Saji F, Samejima Y, Kamiura S, Koyama M. Dynamics of immunoglobulins at the feto-maternal interface. Rev Reprod. 1999;4:81–9.
35. Okoko B, Wesumperuma H, Fern J, Yamuah L, Hart C. The transplacental transfer of IgG subclasses: influence of prematurity and low birthweight in the Gambian population. Ann Trop Paediatr. 2002;22(4):325–32.
36. Costa Carvalho B, Tavares S, Vieira HM, Barros Caronare S, Ribeiro MA, Grisardi N, et al. Niveles de inmunoglobulinas y lisozimas en sangre de cordon umbilical en recien nacidos de diversas edades gestacionales. Rev Latinoam Perinatol. 1988:98–105.

37. Silveira Lessa AL, Krebs VLJ, Brasil TB, Pontes GN, Carneiro-Sampaio M, Palmeira P. Preterm and term neonates transplacentally acquire IgG antibodies specific to LPS from Klebsiella pneumoniae, Escherichia coli and Pseudomonas aeruginosa. FEMS Immunol Med Microbiol. 2011;62(2):236–43.
38. Yeung C, Hobbs J. Serum-γG-globulin levels in normal, premature, post-mature, and "small-for-dates" newborn babies. Lancet. 1968;291(7553):1167–70.
39. Schur P. IgG subclasses. A historical perspective. Monogr Allergy. 1988;23:1–11.
40. Okoko J, Wesumperuma H, Hart C. The influence of prematurity and low birthweight on transplacental antibody transfer in a rural West African population Tropical Med Int Health. 2001;6(7):529–34.
41. Chandra R. Levels of IgG subclasses, IgA, IgM, and tetanus antitoxin in paired maternal and foetal sera: findings in healthy pregnancy and placental insufficiency. Maternofoetal Transmission Immunoglobulins. London: Cambridge University Press; 1976. p. 77–87.
42. Catty D, Drew R, Seger R. Transmission of IgG subclasses to the human foetus. Amsterdam: Elsevier; 1979.
43. Kim DS, Rowland-Jones S, Gea-Mallorquí E. Will SARS-CoV-2 infection elicit long-lasting protective or sterilising immunity? Implications for vaccine strategies (2020). Front Immunol. 2020;11:571481. https://www.frontiersin.org/article/10.3389/fimmu.2020.571481.
44. Huang Y, Yang C, Xu X, Xu W, Liu S. Structural and functional properties of SARS-CoV-2 spike protein: potential antivirus drug development for COVID-19. Acta Pharmacol Sin. 2020;41(9):1141–9.
45. Xu X, Sun J, Nie S, Li H, Kong Y, Liang M, et al. Seroprevalence of immunoglobulin M and G antibodies against SARS-CoV-2 in China. Nat Med. 2020;26(8):1193–5.
46. Zeng H, Xu C, Fan J, Tang Y, Deng Q, Zhang W, et al. Antibodies in infants born to mothers with COVID-19 pneumonia. JAMA 2020;323:1848. https://jamanetwork.com/journals/jama/fullarticle/2763854. Accessed 4 Mar 2022.
47. Edlow AG, Li JZ, Collier AY, Atyeo C, James KE, Boatin AA, et al. Assessment of maternal and neonatal SARS-CoV-2 viral load, transplacental antibody transfer, and placental pathology in pregnancies during the COVID-19 pandemic. JAMA Netw Open 2020;3(12):e2030455.
48. Flannery DD, Gouma S, Dhudasia MB, Mukhopadhyay S, Pfeifer MR, Woodford EC, et al. Assessment of maternal and neonatal cord blood SARS-CoV-2 antibodies and placental transfer ratios. JAMA Pediatr. 2021;175(5):594.
49. Kubiak JM, Murphy EA, Yee J, Cagino KA, Friedlander RL, Glynn SM, et al. Severe acute respiratory syndrome coronavirus 2 serology levels in pregnant women and their neonates. Am J Obstet Gynecol. 2021;225(1):73.e1–7.
50. Egerup P, Fich Olsen L, Christiansen A-MH, Westergaard D, Severinsen ER, Hviid KVR, et al. Severe acute respiratory syndrome coronavirus 2 (SARS-CoV-2) antibodies at delivery in women, partners, and newborns. Obstet Gynecol. 2021;137(1):49–55.
51. Rathberger K, Häusler S, Wellmann S, Weigl M, Langhammer F, Bazzano MV, et al. SARS-CoV-2 in pregnancy and possible transfer of immunity: assessment of peripartal maternal and neonatal antibody levels and a longitudinal follow-up. J Perinat Med. 2021;49(6):702–8.
52. Joseph NT, Dude CM, Verkerke HP, Irby LS, Dunlop AL, Patel RM, et al. Maternal antibody response, neutralizing potency, and placental antibody transfer after severe acute respiratory syndrome coronavirus 2 (SARS-CoV-2) infection. Obstet Gynecol. 2021;138:189. https://journals.lww.com/10.1097/AOG.0000000000004440. Accessed 4 Mar 2022.
53. Atyeo C, Pullen KM, Bordt EA, Fischinger S, Burke J, Michell A, et al. Compromised SARS-CoV-2-specific placental antibody transfer. Cell. 2021;184(3):628–642.e10.
54. Poon LC, Leung BW, Ma T, Yu FNY, Kong CW, Lo TK, et al. Relationship between viral load, infection-to-delivery interval and mother-to-child transfer of anti-SARS-CoV-2 antibodies. Ultrasound Obstet Gynecol. 2021;57(6):974–8.
55. Song D, Prahl M, Gaw SL, Narasimhan SR, Rai DS, Huang A, et al. Passive and active immunity in infants born to mothers with SARS-CoV-2 infection during pregnancy: prospective cohort study. BMJ Open. 2021;11(7):e053036.

56. Conti MG, Terreri S, Piano Mortari E, Albano C, Natale F, Boscarino G, et al. Immune response of neonates born to mothers infected with SARS-CoV-2. JAMA Netw Open. 2021;4(11):e2132563.
57. Zambrano H, Anchundia K, Aviles D, Andaluz R, Calderon N, Torres E, et al. Seroprevalence of SARS-CoV-2 immunoglobulins in pregnant women and neonatal cord blood from a highly impacted region. Placenta. 2021;115:146–50.
58. Larcade R, DeShea L, Lang GA, Caballero MT, Ferretti A, Beasley WH, et al. Maternal-fetal immunologic response to SARS-CoV-2 infection in a symptomatic vulnerable population: a prospective cohort. J Infect Dis. 2022;225(5):800–9.
59. Boelig RC, Chaudhury S, Aghai ZH, Oliver EA, Mancuso F, Berghella V, et al. Comprehensive serologic profile and specificity of maternal and neonatal cord blood SARS-CoV-2 antibodies. AJOG Glob Rep. 2022;2(1):100046.
60. González-Mesa E, García-Fuentes E, Carvia-Pontiasec R, Lavado-Fernández AI, Cuenca-Marín C, Suárez-Arana M, et al. Transmitted fetal immune response in cases of SARS-CoV-2 infections during pregnancy. Diagnostics. 2022;12(2):245.
61. Borghi S, Bournazos S, Thulin NK, Li C, Gajewski A, Sherwood RW, et al. FcRn, but not FcγRs, drives maternal-fetal transplacental transport of human IgG antibodies. Proc Natl Acad Sci U S A. 2020;117(23):12943–51.
62. Prabhu M, Murphy EA, Sukhu AC, Yee J, Singh S, Eng D, et al. Antibody response to coronavirus disease 2019 (COVID-19) messenger RNA vaccination in pregnant women and transplacental passage into cord blood. Obstet Gynecol. 2021;138:278. https://journals.lww.com/10.1097/AOG.0000000000004438. Accessed 24 Feb 2022.
63. Mithal LB, Otero S, Shanes ED, Goldstein JA, Miller ES. Cord blood antibodies following maternal coronavirus disease 2019 vaccination during pregnancy. Am J Obstet Gynecol. 2021;225(2):192–4.
64. Gray KJ, Bordt EA, Atyeo C, Deriso E, Akinwunmi B, Young N, et al. Coronavirus disease 2019 vaccine response in pregnant and lactating women: a cohort study. Am J Obstet Gynecol. 2021;225(3):303.e1–303.e17.
65. Rottenstreich A, Zarbiv G, Oiknine-Djian E, Zigron R, Wolf DG, Porat S. Efficient maternofetal transplacental transfer of anti-severe acute respiratory syndrome coronavirus 2 (SARS-CoV-2) spike antibodies after antenatal SARS-CoV-2 BNT162b2 messenger RNA vaccination. Clin Infect Dis. 2021;73(10):1909–12.
66. Zdanowski W, Waśniewski T. Evaluation of SARS-CoV-2 spike protein antibody titers in cord blood after COVID-19 vaccination during pregnancy in polish healthcare workers: preliminary results. Vaccines. 2021;9(6):675.
67. Trostle ME, Aguero-Rosenfeld ME, Roman AS, Lighter JL. High antibody levels in cord blood from pregnant women vaccinated against COVID-19. Am J Obstet Gynecol MFM. 2021;3(6):100481.
68. Kugelman N, Nahshon C, Shaked-Mishan P, Cohen N, Sher ML, Gruber M, et al. Maternal and neonatal SARS-CoV-2 immunoglobulin G antibody levels at delivery after receipt of the BNT162b2 messenger RNA COVID-19 vaccine during the second trimester of pregnancy. JAMA Pediatr. 2021;176:290. https://jamanetwork.com/journals/jamapediatrics/fullarticle/2787270. Accessed 4 Mar 2022.
69. Rottenstreich A, Zarbiv G, Oiknine-Djian E, Vorontsov O, Zigron R, Kleinstern G, et al. Timing of SARS-CoV-2 vaccination during the third trimester of pregnancy and transplacental antibody transfer: a prospective cohort study. Clin Microbiol Infect. 2021;28:419.
70. Shen C-J, Fu Y-C, Lin Y-P, Shen C-F, Sun D-J, Chen H-Y, et al. Evaluation of transplacental antibody transfer in SARS-CoV-2-immunized pregnant women. Vaccines. 2022;10(1):101.
71. Gloeckner S, Hornung F, Heimann Y, Schleussner E, Deinhardt-Emmer S, Loeffler B, et al. Newborns' passive humoral SARS-CoV-2 immunity following heterologous vaccination of the mother during pregnancy. Am J Obstet Gynecol. 2022;226(2):261–2.

72. Rottenstreich A, Zarbiv G, Oiknine-Djian E, Vorontsov O, Zigron R, Kleinstern G, et al. The effect of gestational age at BNT162b2 mRNA vaccination on maternal and neonatal SARS-CoV-2 antibody levels. Clin Infect Dis. 2022;75:e603.
73. Yang YJ, Murphy EA, Singh S, Sukhu AC, Wolfe I, Adurty S, et al. Association of gestational age at coronavirus disease 2019 (COVID-19) vaccination, history of severe acute respiratory syndrome coronavirus 2 (SARS-CoV-2) infection, and a vaccine booster dose with maternal and umbilical cord antibody levels at delivery. Obstet Gynecol. 2022;139(3):373–80.
74. Pratama NR, Wafa IA, Budi DS, Putra M, Wardhana MP, Wungu CDK. mRNA Covid-19 vaccines in pregnancy: a systematic review. PLoS One. 2022;17(2):e0261350.
75. Beharier O, Plitman Mayo R, Raz T, Nahum Sacks K, Schreiber L, Suissa-Cohen Y, et al. Efficient maternal to neonatal transfer of antibodies against SARS-CoV-2 and BNT162b2 mRNA COVID-19 vaccine. J Clin Invest. 2021;131(13):e150319.
76. Collier AY, McMahan K, Yu J, Tostanoski LH, Aguayo R, Ansel J, et al. Immunogenicity of COVID-19 mRNA Vaccines in Pregnant and Lactating Women. JAMA. 2021;325(23):2370.
77. Treger S, Shiloh SR, Ben-Valid T, Canor Paz Y, Sharvit M, Bryk G, et al. Transplacental transfer of SARS-CoV-2 antibodies in recovered and BNT162b2-vaccinated patients Am J Obstet Gynecol. 2021;226:587.
78. Nir O, Schwartz A, Toussia-Cohen S, Leibovitch L, Strauss T, Asraf K, et al. Maternal-neonatal transfer of SARS-CoV-2 immunoglobulin G antibodies among parturient women treated with BNT162b2 messenger RNA vaccine during pregnancy. Am J Obstet Gynecol MFM. 2022;4(1):100492.
79. Shook LL, Atyeo CG, Yonker LM, Fasano A, Gray KJ, Alter G, et al. Durability of anti-spike antibodies in infants after maternal COVID-19 vaccination or natural infection. JAMA. 2022;327:1087. https://jamanetwork.com/journals/jama/fullarticle/2788986. Accessed 4 Mar 2022.
80. Halasa NB, Olson SM, Staat MA, Newhams MM, Price AM, Boom JA, et al. Effectiveness of maternal vaccination with mRNA COVID-19 vaccine during pregnancy against COVID-19–associated hospitalization in infants aged <6 months — 17 states, July 2021–January 2022. MMWR Morb Mortal Wkly Rep. 2022;71(7):264–70.
81. Gao J, Li W, Hu X, Wei Y, Wu J, Luo X, et al. Disappearance of SARS-CoV-2 antibodies in infants born to women with COVID-19, Wuhan, China. Emerg Infect Dis. 2020;26(10):2491–4.
82. Badr DA, Mattern J, Carlin A, Cordier A-G, Maillart E, El Hachem L, et al. Are clinical outcomes worse for pregnant women at ≥20 weeks' gestation infected with coronavirus disease 2019? A multicenter case-control study with propensity score matching. Am J Obstet Gynecol. 2020;223(5):764–8.
83. Badr DA, Picone O, Bevilacqua E, Carlin A, Meli F, Sibiude J, et al. Severe acute respiratory syndrome coronavirus 2 and pregnancy outcomes according to gestational age at time of infection. Emerg Infect Dis. 2021;27(10):2535–43.

Part III
Neonatology

Chapter 11
COVID-19 in Neonates: Mechanisms, Clinical Features, and Treatments

Lucilla Pezza, Shivani Shankar-Aguilera, and Daniele De Luca

11.1 Introduction

Since 2019, the severe acute respiratory syndrome coronavirus-2 (SARS-CoV-2) has caused a worldwide pandemic affecting almost 400 million patients and causing approximately 7,000,000 deaths [1]. The spectrum of clinical manifestations in adults is nowadays well known. Besides respiratory features (ranging from a simple rhinitis to pneumonia and acute respiratory distress syndrome (ARDS)) [2], cardiovascular [3], neurological [4], gastroenterological [5], and dermatological [6] manifestations have also been described. They are all consequences of two main pathophysiological mechanisms: a direct viral cytopathic effect and an exaggerated host response which may also trigger important coagulation disorders [7].

The understanding of the clinical features of pediatric and neonatal COVID-19 came later, due to their lower prevalence, which makes pediatric and neonatal COVID-19 an "individual" concern more than a public health problem. Neonatal SARS-CoV-2 infections and COVID-19 have some particular features in terms of laboratory diagnosis and clinical manifestations, and we are going to elaborate them here.

L. Pezza
Paediatric Intensive Care Unit, Department of Anaesthesiology and Critical Care, University Hospital "A. Gemelli" - IRCCS, Rome, Italy

S. Shankar-Aguilera
Division of Pediatrics and Neonatal Critical Care, Paris Saclay University Hospitals, Paris Saclay University, Paris, France

D. De Luca (✉)
Neonatology Department, AFHP-University of Paris-Saclay, Le Kremlin-Bicêtre, France

© The Author(s), under exclusive license to Springer Nature Switzerland AG 2023
D. De Luca, A. Benachi (eds.), *COVID-19 and Perinatology*,
https://doi.org/10.1007/978-3-031-29135-4_11

11.2 Transmission of SARS-CoV-2 Infection to Newborn Infants

Besides the classical environmental transmission through droplets and aerosol, which remains most common and leading to 70% of cases [8], a vertical (from mother-to-child) transmission has also been ascertained and accounts for approximately 30% of cases. SARS-CoV-2 has thus been integrated into the family of vertically transmittable viruses, whose last entry was the Zika virus. Vertical transmission can be divided in two main subtypes as follows:

- **In utero transmission:** Angiotensin-converting enzyme-2 (ACE2) receptors are expressed in human placenta, which receives a significant portion of cardiac output and, therefore, a possibly relevant viral load if viremia occurs in pregnant women. Transmembrane serine protease 2 ((TMPRSS2) responsible of the cleavage of viral S-protein needed for cellular invasion) is also expressed in placental tissues, and these represent the basis for the transplacental transmission whose mechanisms are described in detail in Chap. 9.
- **Intrapartum transmission:** A vaginal delivery may be associated with intrapartum SARS-CoV-2 transmission as ACE2 receptors are expressed on the vaginal epithelium and the virus can also reach vaginal secretions as exudate from the bloodstream or through the contact with other biological fluids. This transmission route has also been described and details are available in Chap. 9.

Conversely, an ascending (from vaginal mucosa to the uterine cavity) vertical infection has never been suspected at the time of writing, and transmission through the breast milk has never been formally demonstrated. In fact, the virus has been detected by RT-PCR in human milk but only with a very low viral load [9] and without any proof of actual capacity to replicate. Indeed, neonatal infection transmitted through breast milk has not yet been documented, and breastfeeding does not represent a significant risk factor for neonatal SARS-CoV-2 infections [8]. Moreover, antibodies against SARS-CoV-2 induced by maternal vaccination are passed on through the milk and can protect during infancy [10, 11], a period for which dedicated vaccines are not yet available. More details about these issues are available in Chap. 9. Therefore, breastfeeding with correct hygienic precautions (frequent handwashing and appropriate use of masks) is encouraged [8]. The practice of expressing breast milk is also encouraged if the mother is very sick or in case direct breastfeeding is anyway not possible.

11.3 Diagnostic Criteria for Neonatal SARS-COV-2 Infection

The diagnosis of neonatal infection can be challenging because it is relatively rare, it may present with very variable clinical signs or be asymptomatic (see below), and thus it requires a high suspicion index [8]. Furthermore, due to the multiple possible transmission routes, several tests performed on different samples may be necessary to refine the diagnosis and not always available in every clinical laboratory. To overcome these problems, the World Health Organization (WHO) issued, by expert consensus, some criteria and degree of likeliness for the diagnosis of in utero, intrapartum, and horizontally (environmentally) transmitted neonatal SARS-CoV-2 infections [12].

Table 11.1 describes the WHO criteria for the diagnosis of in utero SARS-CoV-2 transmission: this obviously requires (1) maternal infection, (2) evidence of in utero exposure to SARS-CoV-2, and (3) viral persistence or immune response in the fetus/neonate. Maternal infection should be diagnosed according to classical WHO criteria, and this criterion is fulfilled if the infection occurs *anytime* during the pregnancy. Evidence of in utero viral exposure is obtained with positivity of RT-PCR on placental tissue or samples that are usually sterile (such as amniotic fluid (if collected during caesarean section prior to rupture of membranes in a sterile manner or through amniocentesis), neonatal blood obtained within the first 24 h of life while in isolation or from cord blood). Positive results of placental immunohistochemistry for viral proteins or the presence of cord IgM or IgA against SARS-CoV-2 can also be accepted. The persistence of SARS-CoV-2 or the immune response to it in the fetus/neonate requires at least one positive RT-PCR performed within the first 48 h of life, after having cleaned the baby, on usually sterile samples (e.g., blood, bronchoalveolar lavage fluid, cerebrospinal fluid). If these latter are negative, the RT-PCR positivity of non-sterile samples (e.g. nasopharyngeal aspirate or stools) or serology can provide the proof with a lower level of certainty. As seen in Table 11.1, the combination of the different tests creates a scoring system to evaluate the certainty of the diagnosis in four grades (confirmed, possible, unlikely, indeterminate).

The diagnosis of intrapartum SARS-CoV-2 transmission conversely requires, apart from confirmed maternal infection *near to the delivery*, all the following: (1) lack of in utero exposure to SARS-CoV-2 and (2) evidence of intrapartum exposure with viral persistence or immune response in the fetus/neonate. The lack of in utero viral exposure is confirmed by the negativity of the exams described above (RT-PCR on amniotic fluid, cord, or neonatal blood, RT-PCR or immunohistochemistry of placental tissues). The evidence of intrapartum exposure with viral persistence or immune response is obtained testing the neonate within the first 48 h of life (after cleansing), by one positive RT-PCR on sterile samples or at least two positive RT-PCR on non-sterile sites (obtained 2–7 days apart from each other) or two positive serology assays (obtained 10 days apart from each other). Similar to the in utero transmission, the combination of tests determines the likelihood of the diagnosis (in three grades or categories: confirmed, possible, and unlikely). The unavailability of tests regarding in utero/intrapartum fetal exposure prevents the confirmation of this diagnosis and allows to label it as "possible" at the best. Table 11.2 resumes these concepts.

The diagnosis of horizontally (environmentally) transmitted neonatal SARS-CoV-2 infections obviously requires (1) maternal infection as above, *although the infection of another caregiver or family member can also represent a valid criterion*, (2) lack of in utero and lack of intrapartum exposure as previously defined, and (3) postnatal exposure with viral persistence or immune response in the fetus/neonate. The first two points are described above. The postnatal exposure must be obviously demonstrated by testing the baby *after* the first 48 h of life and after cleansing, by one positive RT-PCR on sterile samples or at least two positive RT-PCR on non-sterile districts (obtained 2–7 days apart from each other) or two positive serology assays (obtained 10 days apart from each other). Similar to the in utero transmission, the combination of tests determines the likelihood of the diagnosis (in three grades: confirmed, possible, and unlikely). A further indeterminate grade consists of the positivity of only one RT-PCR on a non-sterile sample or only one positive serology without further confirmation. The unavailability of tests concerning the in

Table 11.1 WHO criteria for the diagnosis of in utero SARS-CoV-2 transmission

Category	(#1) Maternal infection: Suspect, probable or confirmed case of SARS-CoV-2 infection anytime during pregnancy, as defined by WHO COVID-19 case definitions (25).	
	(#2) Evidence *in utero* fetal exposure	(#3) Viral persistence/immune response
Confirmed	One or more of following samples at *age <24 hours* **positive** for SARS-CoV-2: • RT-PCR from sterile sample[1] • Placental tissue (RT-PCR or ISH) • RT-PCR from non-sterile sample[2] • Serology (IgM or IgA)	One or more of following samples *at age 24-48 hours* **positive** for SARS-CoV-2: • RT-PCR from sterile sample[1]
Possible	One or more of following samples at *age <24 hours* **positive** for SARS-CoV-2: • RT-PCR from sterile sample[1] • Placental tissue (RT-PCR, ISH, IHC or microscopy), placental swab RT-PCR • RT-PCR from non-sterile sample[2] • Serology (IgM or IgA)	One or more of following samples *at age 24-48 hours* **positive** for SARS-CoV-2: • RT-PCR from non-sterile sample[2] OR • **Positive** serology (IgM or IgA) at *age 24 hours to <7 days*
Unlikely	One or more of following samples at *age <24 hours* **positive** for SARS-CoV-2: • RT-PCR sterile sample[1] • Placental tissue (RT-PCR, ISH, IHC or microscopy), placental swab RT-PCR • RT-PCR from non-sterile sample[2] • Serology (IgM or IgA)	All tests that were performed on samples *at age 24-48 hours* are **negative** for SARS-CoV-2: • RT-PCR from sterile sample[1] • RT-PCR from non-sterile sample[2] OR • **Negative** serology (IgM or IgA) at *age 24 hours to <7 days*
	All *in utero* fetal exposure tests (above) that were performed are **negative** for SARS-CoV-2	One or more of following samples *at age 24-48 hours* **positive** for SARS-CoV-2: • RT-PCR from sterile sample[1] • RT-PCR from non-sterile sample[2] OR • **Positive** serology (IgM or IgA) at *age 24 hours to <7 days*
Indeterminate	One or more of following samples at *age <24 hours* **positive** for SARS-CoV-2 • RT-PCR from sterile sample[1] • Placental tissue (RT-PCR, ISH, IHC or microscopy), placental swab RT-PCR • RT-PCR from non-sterile sample[2] • Serology (IgM or IgA)	**No** viral persistence/immune response tests (above) performed
	No *in utero* fetal exposure tests (above) performed	One or more of following samples *at age 24-48 hours* **positive** for SARS-CoV-2: • RT-PCR from sterile sample[1] • RT-PCR from non-sterile sample[2] OR **Positive** serology (IgM or IgA) at *age 24 hours to <7 days*

In utero SARS-CoV-2 transmission requires (#1) evidence of maternal SARS-CoV-2 infection anytime during pregnancy and (#2) in utero fetal SARS-CoV-2 exposure and (#3) SARS-CoV-2 persistence or immune response in the neonate

IHC immunohistochemistry, *ISH* in situ hybridization, *RT-PCR* reverse transcription polymerase chain reaction

Reproduced from [12]

[a]Sterile sample: amniotic fluid (sterile collection caesarean section prior to rupture of membranes or amniocentesis), neonatal blood taken within the first 24 h of life during isolation or cord blood (this latter needs confirmation with peripheral blood or other sample), lower respiratory tract samples obtained by bronchoscopic or non-bronchoscopic bronchoalveolar lavage, bronchial or tracheal aspirate, or cerebrospinal fluid

[b]Non-sterile sample: upper respiratory tract samples (e.g., naso- or oropharyngeal swab or aspirate) or other non-sterile samples (e.g., stool)

utero/intrapartum fetal exposure prevents the confirmation of this diagnosis and allows to label it as "possible" at the best. Table 11.3 resumes these concepts.

Table 11.2 WHO criteria for the diagnosis of intrapartum SARS-CoV-2 transmission

Category	(#2) Lack of *in utero* fetal exposure	(#3) Intrapartum exposure with viral persistence/immune response
	(#1) **Maternal infection:** Suspect, probable or confirmed case of SARS-CoV-2 infection near the time of birth [1] as defined by WHO COVID-19 case definitions *(25)*.	
Confirmed	At least one test obtained at *age <24 hours* was performed and **negative** for SARS-CoV-2 (all tests performed must be **negative**; otherwise classify as *in utero* exposure, above) • RT-PCR from sterile sample [2] • Placental tissue (RT-PCR, ISH, IHC or microscopy), placental swab RT-PCR • RT-PCR from non-sterile sample [3] • **Negative** serology (IgM or IgA)	One or more of following samples *at age 24-48 hours* **positive** for SARS-CoV-2: • RT-PCR from sterile sample [2] • RT-PCR from *non-sterile* sample [3] that is corroborated by a **positive** PCR on a second non-sterile sample at age >48 hours to 7 days OR • **Positive** serology (IgM or IgA) at *age 7-14 days* that is corroborated by a **positive** serology test on a second sample obtained within 10 days of the first positive test [4]
Possible	• No *in utero* fetal exposure tests (above) performed	One or more of following samples *at age 24-48 hours* **positive** for SARS-CoV-2: • RT-PCR from sterile sample [2] • RT-PCR from *non-sterile* sample [3] that is corroborated by a **positive** RT-PCR on a second non-sterile sample at age >48 hours to 7 days OR • **Positive** serology (IgM or IgA) at *age 7-14 days* that is corroborated by a **positive** serology test on a second sample obtained within 10 days of the first positive test [4]
Unlikely	• No *in utero* fetal exposure tests performed	One or more of following samples at *age 24-48 hours* **positive** for SARS-CoV-2: • RT-PCR from sterile sample [2] with a **negative** RT-PCR on second sample at age >48 hours to 7 days • RT-PCR from non-sterile sample [3] with a **negative** RT-PCR on second non-sterile sample at age >48 hours to 7 days OR • **Positive** serology (IgM or IgA) at *age 7-14 days* with **negative** serology test on a second sample obtained within 10 days of the first positive test [4]

Intrapartum SARS-CoV-2 transmission requires (#1) evidence of maternal SARS-CoV-2 infection near the time of birth[a] and (#2) evidence of lack of in utero fetal SARS-CoV-2 exposure and (#3) SARS-CoV-2 intrapartum exposure with viral persistence or immune response in the infant

IHC immunohistochemistry, *ISH* in situ hybridization, *RT-PCR* reverse transcription polymerase chain reaction

Reproduced from [12]

[a]"Near the time of birth": Available data suggest that replication of competent SARS-CoV-2 virus is not detectable after 8–10 days of illness. Thus, for transmission during the intrapartum period to the infant, SARS-CoV-2 diagnosis would need to have occurred in the woman from 14 days prior to 2 days after birth

[b]Sterile sample: amniotic fluid (sterile collection caesarean section prior to rupture of membranes or amniocentesis), neonatal blood taken within the first 24 h of life during isolation or cord blood (this latter needs confirmation with peripheral blood or other sample), lower respiratory tract samples obtained by bronchoscopic or non-bronchoscopic bronchoalveolar lavage, bronchial or tracheal aspirate, or cerebrospinal fluid

[c]Non-sterile sample: upper respiratory tract samples (e.g., naso- or oropharyngeal swab or aspirate) or other non-sterile samples (e.g., stool)

[d]Second serology sample must be IgM to corroborate initial positive IgM or IgA to corroborate initial positive IgA

Table 11.3 WHO criteria for the diagnosis of postnatal SARS-CoV-2 transmission (age >48 h and ≤28 days). Postnatal SARS-CoV-2 transmission requires: (#1) evidence of maternal SARS-CoV-2 infection near the time of birth[a] or evidence of infection in another caregiver and (#2) lack of in utero and intrapartum SARS-CoV-2 exposure and (#3) SARS-CoV-2 postnatal exposure with viral persistence or immune response in the infant

Category	Maternal infection (#1): Suspected, probable or confirmed case of SARS-CoV-2 infection near the time of birth[a] as defined by WHO COVID-19 case definitions (25).	
	(#2) Lack of *in utero*/intrapartum exposure	(#3) Early postnatal exposure with viral persistence/immune response
Confirmed	At least one test obtained at *age <48 hours* was performed and **negative** for SARS-CoV-2 (all tests performed at age <48 hours must be **negative**) • RT-PCR from sterile sample[b] • Placental tissue (RT-PCR, ISH, IHC or microscopy), placental swab RT-PCR • RT-PCR from non-sterile sample[c] • **Negative** serology (IgM or IgA) at *age <14 days*	One or more of following samples at *age ≥48 hours* **positive** for SARS-CoV-2: • RT-PCR from sterile sample[b] • RT-PCR from non-sterile sample[c] that is corroborated by a **positive** PCR on a second non-sterile sample obtained within 10 days of first positive test obtained at ≥48 hours OR • **Positive** serology (IgM or IgA) at *age >14 days* that is corroborated by a second **positive** serology test obtained within 10 days of the first positive test at age >14 days[d]
Possible	• No *in utero* fetal/intrapartum exposure tests performed	One or more of following samples at *age ≥48 hours* **positive** for SARS-CoV-2: • RT-PCR from sterile sample[b] • RT-PCR from non-sterile sample[c] that is corroborated by a **positive** PCR on a second non-sterile sample obtained within 10 days of first positive test OR • **Positive** serology (IgM or IgA) at *age >14 days* that is corroborated by a second **positive** serology test obtained within 10 days of the first positive test[d]
Unlikely	No *in utero* fetal/intrapartum exposure tests performed	One or more of following samples at *age ≥48 hours* **positive** for SARS-CoV-2: • RT-PCR from non-sterile sample[c] with **negative** RT-PCR on a second non-sterile sample obtained within 10 days of first positive test OR • **Positive** serology (IgM or IgA) at *age >14 days* with **negative** serology test on second serology test obtained within 10 days of the first positive test[d]
Indeterminate	• No *in utero* fetal/intrapartum exposure tests performed	One or more of following samples at age ≥48 hours **positive** for SARS-CoV-2: • RT-PCR from non-sterile sample[c] without a second corroboratory test OR • **Positive** serology (IgM or IgA) at *age >14 days* without a second corroboratory test[d]

IHC immunohistochemistry, *ISH* in situ hybridization, *RT-PCR* reverse transcription polymerase chain reaction
Reproduced from [12]
[a]"Near the time of birth": see above notes of Table 11.2
[b]Sterile sample: amniotic fluid (sterile collection caesarean section prior to rupture of membranes or amniocentesis), neonatal blood taken within the first 24 h of life during isolation or cord blood (this latter needs confirmation with peripheral blood or other samples), lower respiratory tract samples obtained by bronchoscopic or non-bronchoscopic bronchoalveolar lavage, bronchial or tracheal aspirate, or cerebrospinal fluid
[c]Non-sterile sample: upper respiratory tract samples (e.g., naso- or oropharyngeal swab or aspirate) or other non-sterile samples (e.g., stool)
[d]Second serology sample must be IgM to corroborate initial positive IgM or IgA to corroborate initial positive IgA

Table 11.4 Summary of sampling, timing, and types of tests to classify neonatal SARS-CoV-2 infections as in utero, intrapartum, or postnatal

		Early *in utero* exposure testing						Later exposure testing							
Time of sample collection		Birth to age <24 hours						24-48 hr	≥48 hr	24-48 hr	≥48 hr	Repeated within 10 d	24 hr - 7 d	7-14 d	Repeated within 10 d	>14 d	Repeated within 10 d
Type of sample and test		Sterile sample			Non-sterile sample		Serology (IgM/IgA)	Sterile[d] sample		Non-sterile[e] sample			Serology (IgM/IgA)			
		Neonatal blood	Amniotic fluid	Lower respiratory tract/CSF	Placenta RT-PCR/ISH	Placenta IHC/microscopy	Upper respiratory tract/other[c]									
In Utero (live birth) (maternal infection anytime during pregnancy)																
Confirmed	+	+	+	+		+										
Possible	+	+	+	+	+	+		+		+		+				
Unlikely	NEG	NEG	NEG	NEG	NEG	NEG	NEG	NEG		NEG						
Indeterminate	+	+	+	+	+	+	ND	ND		ND						
	ND	ND	ND	ND	ND	ND										
Intrapartum (maternal infection near the time of birth)																
Confirmed	NEG	NEG	NEG	NEG	NEG	NEG	+		+		+ to 7 d		+	+		
Possible	ND	ND	ND	ND	ND	ND	+		+		+ to 7 d		+	+		
Unlikely	ND	ND	ND	ND	ND	ND	+	NEG	+	NEG		+	NEG			
Early Postnatal (maternal infection near the time of birth)																
Confirmed	NEG	NEG	NEG	NEG	NEG	NEG	NEG	+	NEG	+		NEG	NEG		+	+
Possible	ND	ND	ND	ND	ND	ND	ND	+	ND	+		ND	ND		+	+
Unlikely	ND	ND	ND	ND	ND	ND	ND	+	ND	NEG		ND	ND		+	NEG
Indeterminate	ND	ND	ND	ND	ND	ND	ND	+	ND	ND		ND	ND		+	ND

CSF cerebrospinal fluid, *ISH* in situ hybridization, *IHC* immunohistochemistry, *ND* not done, *RT-PCR* reverse transcription polymerase chain reaction
d, age in days; hr, age in hours
Reproduced from [12]
[a]Lower respiratory tract: bronchoscopic or non-bronchoscopic bronchoalveolar lavage and broncho- or tracheal aspirate
[b]Upper respiratory tract: nasopharyngeal or oropharyngeal swab or aspirate
[c]Other non-sterile sites (e.g., stool)
[d]Sterile sample: neonatal blood, cerebrospinal fluid, and lower respiratory tract
[e]Non-sterile sample: upper respiratory tract or other non-sterile site. + = positive test (meets category if one or more tests are positive for early exposure plus one or more tests positive for later exposure). NEG, negative test (meets category if all tests that were performed are negative, early or later exposure). Color code: in utero, blue; dark blue, positive test; light blue, negative test. Intrapartum, orange; dark orange, positive test; light orange, negative test. Postnatal: red, dark red positive test; light red, negative test. Gray: not done

The combination of tests and their timing for the three diagnoses (in utero, intrapartum, and postnatal infection in light blue, orange, and red, respectively) are resumed in Table 11.4.

11.4 Virological Tests

As in adults, the diagnosis of SARS-CoV-2 infection in neonates is based on RT-PCR while serology has a minor role and is mainly used for research and epidemiological purposes [13]. RT-PCR in neonates is preferentially performed on nasopharyngeal aspirates rather than on classical swabs. This is the sample of choice because of the difficulty in getting a correct deep swab due to the small nostril diameter in neonates and in order to reduce the risk of false-negative results. The nasopharyngeal lavage with normal saline and sterile devices has been largely used although it has not been standardized and may be performed with different volumes and pressures [14]. Nonetheless, this technique has been demonstrated to be more accurate than swabs to diagnose other common viral respiratory infections in infants and is, therefore, well grounded [15]. Co-infections with other respiratory viruses are possible particularly during the winter season [16, 17], although the effect on the global clinical severity is unclear [18, 19]. Multiple RT-PCR including at least respiratory syncytial virus and orthomyxoviruses are advisable.

In neonates with respiratory failure needing invasive ventilation, the virological diagnosis requires a RT-PCR performed on bronchoalveolar lavage (BAL) fluid which can be obtained with a bronchoscopic or non-bronchoscopic technique and is more sensitive than the RT-PCR performed on nasopharyngeal aspirate or on simple tracheal aspirate [20–22]. The non-bronchoscopic bronchoalveolar lavage is a well-known technique and can be easily performed, but it requires a clear protocol and must be standardized (in terms of injected volume of saline, aspiration pressure, timing, and procedure). Basic procedure advices from the European Respiratory Society are available to this end [23]. Examples of standardized non-bronchoscopic BAL protocols are also available in the literature [24]. In neonates admitted to neonatal intensive care units because of their clinical severity, it is advisable to perform RT-PCR on multiple sites, notably in plasma (to detect viremia, if any) and in stools (as the viral shedding is longer in these samples [25]). Cycle thresholds for RT-PCR in neonatal samples are the same used to analyze specimens from older patients, and a threshold of 35 is recommended by the European Centre for Disease Prevention and Control [26].

11.5 Clinical Manifestations of Neonatal COVID-19

In addition to positive RT-PCR, the presence of clinical signs is needed to diagnose neonatal COVID-19. Infected neonates can be preterm or at term and infection can occur anytime during the first month of life [8]. Roughly half of neonatal infections are completely asymptomatic [8]. In the other half, the clinical features of neonatal COVID-19 are represented by several signs and are much more varied compared to the adult population (Fig. 11.1).

As demonstrated by Raschetti et al. [8], neonatal COVID-19 has a predominance of respiratory signs mainly represented by respiratory distress that is not different from adult patients; nonetheless, neonates can experience respiratory distress for many common reasons early after birth (such as hyaline membrane disease due to primary surfactant deficiency, transient tachypnea of the neonate due to delayed alveolar liquid reabsorption, early-onset sepsis, meconium aspiration, or other types of neonatal ARDS), and these may co-exist with the SARS-CoV-2 infection. Therefore, differentiating the main pathology responsible for the respiratory distress may be difficult, and clinicians should have a high index of suspicion and be

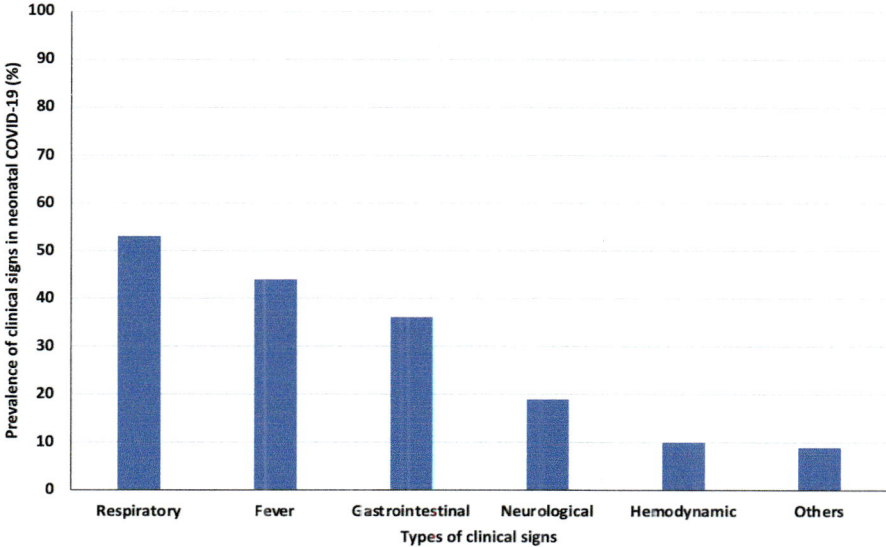

Fig. 11.1 Distribution of neonatal COVID-19 clinical features. Multiple clinical signs may be observed in one patient. The "others" category includes skin rash, hypothermia, conjunctivitis, and coagulation disorders. More details in the text. (Adapted from [8])

aware that there may be multiple causes for respiratory failure for each individual patient. Conceptually, this is not different from the identification of the ARDS caused during other outbreaks, and it has been a challenge during the H1N1 pandemic, as well [27]. Lung ultrasound is a relatively new tool that seems more accurate than chest X-rays to distinguish between viral and bacterial respiratory infections [27–29], but this cannot be the unique diagnostic test and remains a helpful imaging technique, rather than a microbiological tool (see below). Virological confirmation in neonates with respiratory distress exposed to SARS-CoV-2 requires performing an RT-PCR on a BAL (bronchoalveolar lavage) fluid or nasopharyngeal specimen as described above. Furthermore, when the clinical picture is severe enough to be classified as neonatal ARDS, the Montreux definition [30] can provide guidance to distinguish ARDS from respiratory distress syndrome due to primary surfactant deficiency.

Interestingly, we note a high prevalence of fever among neonates infected by SARS-CoV-2, whereas this is not a common sign in other neonatal infections. Nonetheless, this obviously cannot be considered a stand-alone pathognomonic sign. There are also other clinical features and both gastrointestinal and neurological signs are quite common. Gastroenteric signs mirror the viral shedding in stools that seems longer than from other sites [25], while neurological features are important as they may be very severe, such as apneas needing ventilatory support or meningeal irritation and cerebral vasculitis [31].

11.6 Severe and Critical Forms of Neonatal COVID-19

COVID-19 is known to be milder in children than in adults, although the reason behind this is not yet completely understood. The various mechanisms that have been proposed are (1) lower ACE2 receptor expression in newborn airways and lung, (2) different interaction between host immunological response and viral pathogenic mechanisms, (3) competition with other respiratory viruses commonly present in airway mucosa of infants, (4) cross-reactivity toward other coronaviruses to whom children are commonly exposed, (5) lack of chronic mild inflammation (inflammaging) in children compared to adults, and (6) relative absence of vitamin D deficiency in children. It is easily understandable that the susceptibility to develop severe COVID-19 is multifactorial as these factors may variably co-exist and they occur more or less frequently in children of different ages. It seems clear now that while adolescent may be more similar to adults in terms of developing severe COVID-19, children aged more than one year might be in a "sweet spot" compared to infants and neonates, whose immune system is not yet fully competent to adequately respond to SARS-CoV-2 invasion. As such, within the pediatric age, the first month of life (and in general during infancy) seems to be the period at a higher risk for severe and critical COVID-19 and its negative outcomes. There are no dedicated criteria to classify the severity of neonatal COVID-19, albeit, by modifying the WHO criteria for the adult population, we may consider neonatal COVID-19 as follows [32]:

- *Mild*: only minor clinical signs (e.g., conjunctivitis, runny nose, rash)
- *Moderate*: fever, mild feeding difficulties, and mild diarrhea
- *Severe*: signs requiring hospitalization (e.g., need for oxygen therapy, dehydration needing intravenous line, neurological signs needing monitoring)
- *Critical*: respiratory or hemodynamic or kidney or liver failure needing vital support, seizure, or coma

No clear epidemiological studies are yet available, but the EPICENTRE (ESPNIC Covid pEdiatric Neonatal Registry) data will be soon released and should enlighten on this [33]. Furthermore, many case series and observational studies have reported severe COVID-19 in neonates and infants presenting with ARDS [34], neurological [31] or hemodynamic compromise, and multiorgan failure syndrome [35] and death [36]. Obviously, these cases remain infrequent in terms of absolute numbers compared to adult populations, and the case of fatality rate seems approximately <0.1% [37]. Nonetheless, the existence of neonatal COVID-19 in its more severe form must be known and recognized by neonatologists. Moreover, some of the aforementioned protective mechanisms may be absent in preterm infants, and therefore it is conceivable that these patients might have be at a relatively higher risk of severe neonatal COVID-19, and we have personally observed some of these cases in our practice. It is important to note that, as maternal vaccination advances, it may become even rarer to observe clinically evident neonatal COVID-19 as antibodies induced by mRNA vaccines can reach the fetus and the neonate through the placenta and breast milk.

It is still unclear if the vertically or environmentally acquired infections are more likely to generate severe-to-critical forms of neonatal COVID-19: this question will probably be answered shortly by results from the EPICENTRE dataset [33].

11.7 Laboratory Findings in Neonatal COVID-19

Laboratory features of neonatal COVID-19 are similar to those reported in older patients. Lymphopenia is quite common (33% of cases), although relative lymphocytosis has also been described in milder cases. Raised lactate dehydrogenase (50% of cases), impaired hepatic enzymes (aspartate aminotransferase and alanine aminotransferase in 47% and 23% of cases, respectively), and anecdotally elevated phosphocreatine kinase have also been reported [38]. Coagulation disorders have been described and seem associated with the development of severe-to-critical cases in postnatal, environmentally transmitted infections [39]. C-reactive protein may be normal or transiently elevated, while conflicting data are available on procalcitonin; therefore these classical inflammatory markers do not seem very useful to discriminate COVID-19 from other neonatal infections [40, 41]. The eventual choice to measure other circulating inflammatory markers (such as ferritin and D-dimers) should be considered on a case-by-case scenario [42]. Interleukin-6 has anecdotally been found elevated in some neonates similar to adults. IL-6 has been used to guide therapy with anti-interleukin agents (tocilizumab) in adults [43], but its therapeutic role is still unclear and neonatal data on IL-6 levels are conflicting [44].

11.8 Imaging in Neonatal COVID-19

The majority of neonates with COVID-19 have radiological lung abnormalities that are nonspecific and similar to those of other common neonatal respiratory disorders [8]. Some radiological features appear comparable to those of interstitial pneumonia commonly found in adult COVID-19 patients [45]. Consistently, CT scans have revealed ground glass opacities (71%), peribronchial thickening (60%), linear or band-shaped opacities (33%), and consolidations (29%) as main abnormalities [46]. Some of these features, such as peribronchial thickening are also similar to those observed in other neonatal respiratory infections.

Lung ultrasound has been extensively used in neonates infected with SARS-CoV-2, also using wireless tablets, in order to reduce the risk of cross-contaminations [47]. First experiences with lung ultrasound showed interstitial patterns with more or less confluent B-lines as observed in other neonatal respiratory disorders [48]. More severe cases are characterized by a greater loss of lung aeration with confluent B-lines and consolidations [49]. As done in patients affected by other conditions [50], simultaneous studies have shown that ultrasound findings correlate well with CT abnormalities [51]. The evolution of ultrasound pattern in a patient is easy to study with the classical neonatal lung ultrasound score [52] and is variable overtime being influenced by the co-existence of other disorders [48]. While several studies have demonstrated the diagnostic and predictive power of lung ultrasound in adult COVID-19 patients, scanty data are available for neonates: however, lung ultrasound seems to be able to detect more lung abnormalities than conventional radiology, particularly in neonates without respiratory clinical manifestations of COVID-19 [49].

11.9 Delayed M anifestations of Neonatal SARS-COV-2 Infection: MIS-N

Since the decreasing phase of the first pandemic wave, an increased prevalence of Kawasaki-like disease was observed in children after some weeks from SARS-CoV-2 infection. This phenomenon quickly appeared multiform since it might present as myocarditis, vasculitis, macrophage activation syndrome, and serositis or a variable overlap of these [53], and it has been named as multisystem inflammatory syndrome in children (MIS-C) or pediatric inflammatory multisystem syndrome (PIMS). The trademark of MIS-C is a significant inflammation leading to multiorgan injury and possibly failure, but its exact physiopathology is far from being completely understood. In fact, MIS-C development seems significantly linked to the presence of circulating anti-SARS-CoV-2 antibodies and autoantibodies against several antigens induced by the viral infection, while an active SARS-CoV-2 infection is lacking [54]. In some genetically susceptible children, autoantibodies triggered by SARS CoV-2 bind to several receptors causing hyperinflammatory status, macrophage activation, and variably extended organ injury [55].

Thus, MIS-C always occurs in children previously infected by SARS-CoV-2. However, a similar syndrome has also been described in neonates (and called MIS-N), and interestingly, these patients might have been previously infected or not by SARS-CoV-2 [56]. In fact, MIS-N can occur in neonates after a vertically or horizontally transmitted SARS-CoV-2 infection but can also develop in neonates having received maternal antibodies and autoantibodies through the placental circulation without any actual transmission of the virus [56].

As such, MIS-N expands the possible clinical manifestations related to SARS-CoV-2 infection and makes the spectrum quite complex. The various possibilities are resumed in Fig. 11.2.

Diagnosing MIS-N is not easy as it presents with a large variety of clinical signs that can partially overlap with those of an active SARS-CoV-2 infection that must be excluded. The diffusion of the vaccination program may reduce its incidence as antibodies induced by mRNA vaccines are extremely selective toward an epitope of the spike protein and do not cross-react inducing the production of autoantibodies [57].

The US Centers for Disease Control defines MIS-C as the presence of fever plus one of the following symptoms: stomach pain, bloodshot eyes, diarrhea, dizziness

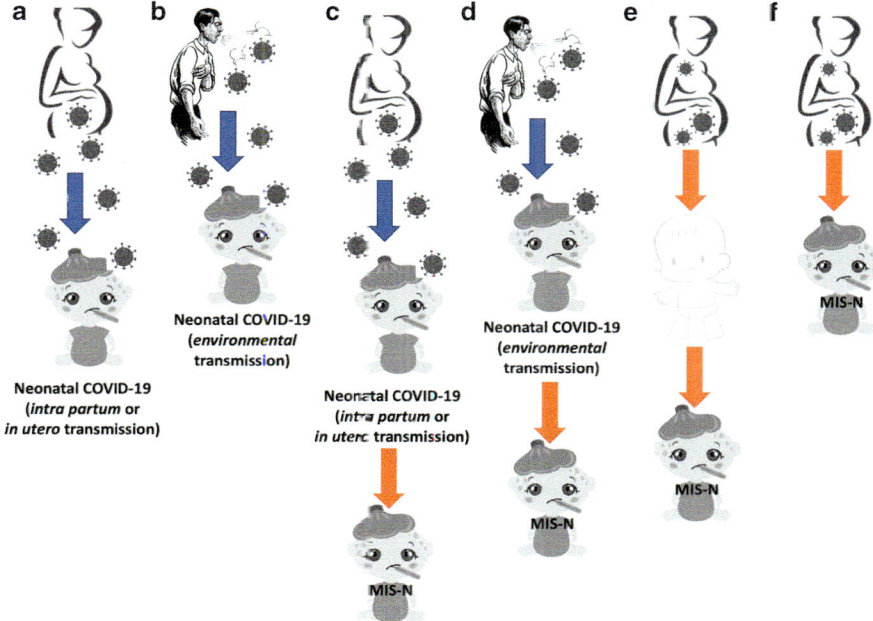

Fig. 11.2 Spectrum of neonatal clinical disorders directly or indirectly related to SARS-CoV-2. Panel (**a**) represents a woman with COVID-19 during the pregnancy and vertical (either in utero or intrapartum) transmission of SARS-CoV-2 infection to the neonate. Panel (**b**) depicts a case of horizontal (environmental) transmission of SARS-CoV-2 infection to a newborn infant from a caregiver (for instance, the mother, the father, or a family member). Panels (**c**) and (**d**) represent the cases described in Panels (**a**) and (**b**), respectively, followed by the development of MIS-N 2–6 weeks after the resolution of SARS-CoV-2 infection and caused by the development of dysregulated inflammation and autoimmunity in the neonate. Panels (**e**) and (**f**) represent a pregnant woman with SARS-CoV-2 infection during the pregnancy but without vertical transmission of the virus; conversely, antibodies anti-SARS-CoV-2 and autoantibodies induced by the infection are transmitted through the placenta and trigger an early (within 72 h from birth, Panel **f**) or late (after 72 h from birth, Panel **e**) development of MIS-N in the offspring. In the case illustrated in Panel (**e**), the neonate is originally healthy early from birth. Blue and orange arrows depict the transmission of SARS-CoV-2 and antibodies, respectively. The time needed to develop MIS-N is variable and the arrow size is purely indicative. More details in the text

or lightheadedness (signs of low blood pressure), skin rash, and vomiting [58]. By adapting this definition to newborn patients, several authors have proposed criteria to define MIS-N, albeit there is no consensus yet on a MIS-N clinical definition. However, we can globally consider MIS-N in a neonate if all the following criteria are fulfilled [56, 57]:

- Laboratory or clinical evidence of SARS-CoV-2 infection in the mother or in a caregiver or, alternatively, evidence of previous SARS-CoV-2 infection in the neonate irrespective of the transmission route.
- Severe illness requiring hospitalization with fever and/or involvement of at least two organs (e.g., cardiac, renal, respiratory, hematologic, gastrointestinal, der-

matologic, neurological injury). The cardiac involvement such as myocarditis, arrhythmias, or coronary aneurism may be sufficient to fulfil this criterion even in absence of other organ involvements.
- Laboratory evidence of systemic inflammation (e.g., increased C-reactive protein, fibrinogen, procalcitonin, D-dimer, ferritin, interleukine-6, or other inflammatory markers, elevated neutrophils or reduced lymphocytes, low albumin) *in absence of active SARS-CoV-2 infection* (negative RT-PCR and negative IgM anti-SARS-CoV-2, while IgG may be positive).
- Exclusion of alternative diagnosis (e.g., birth asphyxia, viral or bacterial sepsis-confirmed blood culture, neonatal lupus syndrome or maternal autoimmune diseases resulting in neonatal atrioventricular conduction abnormalities).

It is evident that the clinical manifestations of MIS-N are very variable as MIS-N can appear as conjunctivitis and skin rash, myocarditis with shock, vasculitis, arrhythmias, pericarditis, coronary aneurisms, encephalopathy with seizures, coagulation disorders, respiratory failure, persistent pulmonary hypertension, feeding intolerance, and/or acute kidney failure [56, 57, 59–63]. The interval between SARS-CoV-2 infection or exposure to maternal antibodies and the development of MIS-N is quite variable too, since some cases may develop after just a few days and others after weeks. MIS-N cases have also been temporally classified between those with an early (within 72 h from birth) and those with a late (after 72 h from birth) onset [56, 57]. Therefore, MIS-N remains a diagnostic challenge, and neonatologists should keep a high index of suspicion, in order to discriminate it from SARS-CoV-2 infection and other more common neonatal disorders and to eventually treat it correctly. The treatment has been provided with immunomodulant agents such as steroids and immunoglobulins (IgG) in addition to vital support when needed.

11.10 Treatment

11.10.1 General Principles

Supportive care, including temperature control with paracetamol, upper airway cleansing and humidification, attentive hydration, and nutrition have represented the main therapeutic intervention for neonatal COVID-19 so far and particularly for mild-to-moderate cases. Antibiotics should be avoided unless a co-infection is reasonably suspected. Moderate cases may require hospitalization for clinical observation, while severe-to-critical case requires vital function monitoring in a neonatal intensive care unit (NICU). All hospitalizations, particularly those occurring on units taking care of very sick or preterm infants, should be done in adequate negative pressure isolation rooms with strict hygiene protocols. Conversely, asymptomatic neonates and mild cases should not be hospitalized in order to keep the mother-neonate bonding and prevent shortage of neonatal intensive care beds [64, 65]. A clear protocol for isolation/deisolation and resource optimization should be available in each center [66].

11.10.2 Vital Support

Respiratory support should be provided according to usual protocols and titrated according to clinical severity as suggested by the European Society for Pediatric and Neonatal Intensive Care (ESPNIC) PEMVECC (Paediatric Mechanical Ventilation Consensus Conference) guidelines [67]. According to these latter and the patient severity, all modes of respiratory support can be used. It is important to place a high-capacity HEPA (high-efficiency particulate air) filter (Fig. 11.3) on the expiratory limb of all ventilatory circuits to reduce diffusion of viral particles in the environment and contamination of the ventilators.

Heated humidified high-flow nasal cannula were considered a risky aerosol technique in the beginning of pandemics but have finally proven to be as safe as other noninvasive respiratory support techniques, if adequate personal protective equipments are used [68]. Conversely, their drawbacks (inconstant and unpredictable pressure delivery) should be balanced against their comfort and availability of more complex respiratory techniques. The use of neonatal helmets to deliver continuous positive airway pressure should always be considered as gold standard to deliver a constant pressure level [69] and might be useful to reduce the viral load in the

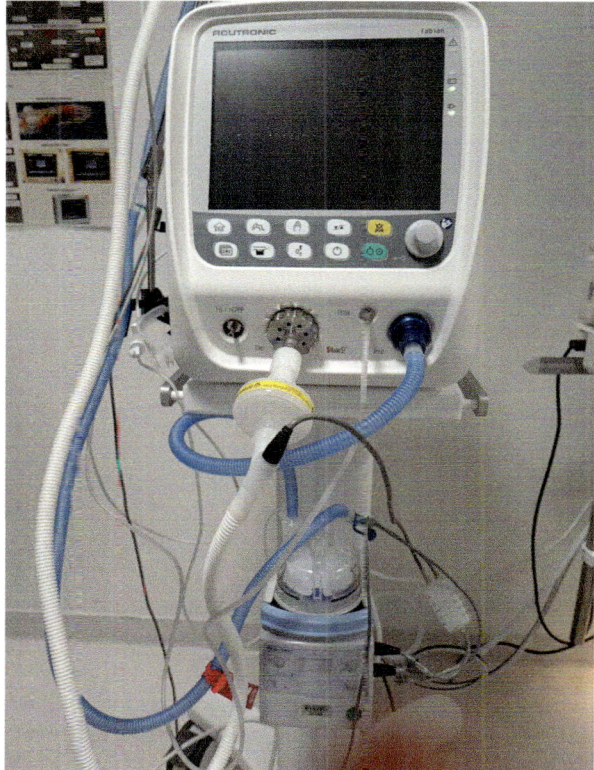

Fig. 11.3 Illustrative picture of the ventilator circuit with inbuilt HEPA filter on the expiratory limb

vicinity of the patient. Second-line vital support measures (surfactant bolus, inhaled nitric oxide, extracorporeal membrane oxygenation) have been used in some cases of severe neonatal ARDS. These therapeutics have been managed according to standard principles.

Hemodynamic support, extracorporeal renal replacement therapy, and maintenance of balanced coagulation (including the use of heparin and fresh frozen plasma or coagulation factors) should be provided and managed as usual, in the absence of specific data to refine these therapies for patients with neonatal COVID-19. A close hemodynamic monitoring with point-of-care ultrasound is also advisable as this technique may allow to reduce the risk of cross-contamination and ESPNIC guidelines are available to this end [70]. It is strongly recommended to consult with an expert neonatal/pediatric intensivist and/or a pediatric infectious disease specialist to treat these cases as this may require both expertise in advanced neonatal critical care and on COVID-19 which may not be easily available in each center.

11.10.3 Specific Antiviral Therapies

There are not yet any neonatal data available on molnupiravir and nirmatrelvir/ritonavir, the two antivirals recently introduced to treat COVID-19 in adults. Conversely, there are some case reports of neonates treated with other drugs, particularly in the beginning of the pandemic. Some of these therapeutics (e.g., hydroxychloroquine, azithromycin, and convalescent plasma) have subsequently proven to be ineffective; therefore we will not treat them here.

Remdesivir has been used in cases of severe and critical neonatal COVID-19, particularly with respiratory failure, both in term and preterm infants, following two different dose regimens [34, 71–73]. It has a US Federal Drug Administration authorization for use in patients weighting at least 3.5 kg [74], and the UK National Institute of Health and Care Excellence guidelines suggest to use it in hospitalized children of any age with need for supplemental oxygen [75]. Kidney and liver function monitoring is mandatory during the treatment and consultation with expert neonatal critical care physicians and/or the manufacturer is advisable.

Anti-SARS-CoV-2 monoclonal antibodies are available since several months, but the experience regarding their use in neonates is lacking. Bamlanivimab/etesevimab is the only drug of this class to have a US Federal Drug Administration authorization for the treatment of mild-to-moderate neonatal COVID-19 in patients at high risk of disease progression (because of prematurity, comorbidities, or immunosuppression) within the first days of infection or the onset of clinical signs [76]. Its efficacy is however dependent on the viral strain and is significantly reduced or absent against δ and o variants, and no neonatal case report has formally described its use. Casirivimab/imdevimab and sotrovimab have no neonatal authorization and no formally described neonatal experience, but their use seems very safe in pregnancy [77].

11.10.4 Anti-inflammatory Drugs

These drugs have been used to modify the dysregulated host inflammatory response that contribute to the physiopathology of more severe cases. Their use should logically be reserved to advanced cases where the contribution of the excessive host response is evident, and this may be infrequent in neonates. However, critical cases needing vital support represent the typical patients to treat with these drugs. The commonest drug of this type is dexamethasone: it has been relatively often used in neonatal COVID-19 due to large experience accumulated with this drug in neonatal critical care. The American Academy of Pediatrics recommends a dose <0.2 mg/kg/day in preterm infants in order to reduce the risk of negative neurological outcomes [78]. Lower doses have been used to treat neonates with severe COVID-19 [42]. Hydrocortisone has also been used in some cases [59] and has the advantage to be well known in neonatal care and less harmful for preterm infants from a neurological point of view [78]. There are no data about the use of betamethasone to treat neonatal COVID-19: this molecule is widely used for boost fetal lung maturation antenatally also in pregnant women affected by COVID-19, but dexamethasone or hydrocortisone should be preferred to treat severe neonatal COVID-19.

Baricitinib, a monoclonal antibody acting as JAK-1 inhibitor without direct antiviral activity, has no neonatal authorization, and its use has never been described. Tocilizumab is a recombinant and humanized IgG monoclonal antibody against interleukin-6 and has been widely used in adult COVID-19 patients. There are no formally described neonatal cases although tocilizumab can reach the fetus through the placental circulation and seems to have a good safety profile when used in pregnant patients [79, 80]. Two interleukin-1 inhibitors, anakinra and canakinumab, have been used to treat adults with COVID-19-related respiratory failure at risk of disease progression, but there are no neonatal data, even though anakinra has a European marketing authorization for use in infants older than eight months affected by periodic auto-inflammatory febrile syndromes.

Intravenous immunoglobulins-G (IVIG) represent an old drug that has been efficaciously used in neonates with autoimmune or alloimmune perinatal disorders and, with conflicting results, for severe sepsis. IVIG have multiple and complex immunomodulatory and anti-inflammatory effects [81] which might theoretically be useful in severe-to-critical neonatal COVID-19 and in cases of COVID-19-related MIS-N. In these latter cases, their use could be particularly interesting if they present with Kawasaki-like clinical features, since IVIG provide significant clinical benefit in the actual Kawasaki disease [82]. Some cases of neonatal COVID-19 even not presenting as MIS-N have been treated with IVIG, but the efficacy, dose, and timing of treatment are unclear [83].

Finally, interferons have also been used to treat some neonates [8], due to the physiopathological role of these molecules in COVID-19 pathogenesis [84]. However, the usefulness of interferons and other immunomodulating therapies not mentioned here is not ascertained even in adults [85], and it should not be used in neonates out of a research setting.

Table 11.5 reports the dosing regimens and main data for the drug used to treat neonatal COVID-19 and having the strongest background [86].

Table 11.5 Practical summary of drugs to treat neonatal COVID-19

Drug	Auth	Dose	Timing	Notes	Ref.
Remdesivir (neonates ≥3.5 kg)	Yes	Load 5 mg/kg on day 1 followed by 2.5 mg/kg/day	For 5–15 days, starting ASAP	For neonates hospitalized for COVID-19 or not hospitalized but at a high risk of disease progression	[34, 60–63]
Remdesivir (neonates <3.5 kg)	No	Load 2.5–5 mg/kg on day 1 followed by 1.25 mg/kg/day	For 4–15 days, starting ASAP	For neonates hospitalized for COVID-19 or not hospitalized but at a high risk of disease progression	[34, 60–63]
Bamlanivimab/ etesevimab	Yes	12 mg/kg and 24 mg/kg, respectively (always together)	Once. Start within ten days from the infection or onset of clinical signs	Should not be used if respiratory failure already evident. Needs viral sequencing (inactive on δ and o variants) and monitoring after infusion for an hour	[64]
Dexamethasone	–	0.15–0.2 mg/kg/day	Start if supplemental oxygen or any vital support is needed		[34, 65, 66]
Hydrocortisone	–	0.5 mg/kg/bid for seven days and then 0.5 mg/kg/day for three days	Start if supplemental oxygen or any vital support is needed		[67]
IgG immunoglobulins	–	400 mg/kg/day*	When MIS-N is evident		[72]

Only drugs with regulatory approval or formally described neonatal use published in case reports are listed. –: no specific authorization but drugs already in use in neonatal care. *: other dosing schedules are possible and have been used for other neonatal indications. More details are available in the text. Information in the table should not be taken as binding: readers should check the doses with the literature, current regulatory authorities' statements, and/or manufacturers. ASAP, as soon as possible; Auth, US Federal Drug Administration authorization for neonatal use (no other regulatory agencies have given any authorization at the time of writing); bid, *bis in die*

Conflict of Interest Authors have no conflict of interest to declare.

References

1. Our World in Data. n.d.. https://ourworldindata.org/explorers/coronavirus-data-explorer. Accessed 8 Feb 2022.
2. Boban M. Novel coronavirus disease (COVID-19) update on epidemiology, pathogenicity, clinical course and treatments. Int J Clin Pract. 2021;75(4):e13868. https://doi.org/10.1111/ijcp.13868. Epub 2020 Dec 6. PMID: 33244856; PMCID: PMC7744921.
3. Dhakal BP, Sweitzer NK, Indik JH, Acharya D, William P. SARS-CoV-2 infection and cardiovascular disease: COVID-19 heart. Heart Lung Circ. 2020;29(7):973–87. https://doi.org/10.1016/j.hlc.2020.05.101. Epub 2020 Jun 5. PMID: 32601020 PMCID: PMC7274628.
4. Aghagoli G, Gallo Marin B, Katchur NJ, Chaves-Sell F, Asaad WF, Murphy SA. Neurological involvement in COVID-19 and potential mechanisms: a review. Neurocrit Care. 2021;34(3):1062–71. https://doi.org/10.1007/s12028-020-01049-4. PMID: 32661794; PMCID: PMC7358290.
5. Yeo C, Kaushal S, Yeo D. Enteric involvement of coronaviruses: is faecal-oral transmission of SARS-CoV-2 possible? Lancet. Gastroenterol Hepatol. 2020;5(4):335–7. https://doi.org/10.1016/S2468-1253(20)30048-0. Epub 2020 Feb 20. PMID: 32087098; PMCID: PMC7130008.
6. Genovese G, Moltrasio C, Berti E, Marzano AV. Skin manifestations associated with COVID-19: current knowledge and future perspectives. Dermatology. 2021;237(1):1–12. https://doi.org/10.1159/000512932. Epub 2020 Nov 24. PMID: 33232965; PMCID: PMC7801998.
7. Lotfi M, Rezaei N. SARS-CoV-2: a comprehensive review from pathogenicity of the virus to clinical consequences. J Med Virol. 2020;92(10):1864–74. https://doi.org/10.1002/jmv.26123. Epub 2020 Jun 19. PMID: 32492197; PMCID: PMC7300719.
8. Raschetti R, Vivanti AJ, Vauloup-Fellous C, Loi B, Benachi A, De Luca D. Synthesis and systematic review of reported neonatal SARS-CoV-2 infections. Nat Commun. 2020;11(1):5164. https://doi.org/10.1038/s41467-020-18982-9.
9. Groß R, Conzelmann C, Müller JA, Stenger S, Steinhart K, Kirchhoff F, Münch J. Detection of SARS-CoV-2 in human breastmilk. Lancet. 2020;395(10239):1757–8. https://doi.org/10.1016/S0140-6736(20)31181-8. Epub 2020 May 21. Erratum in: Lancet. 2020;396(10253):758.
10. Gray KJ, Bordt EA, Atyeo C, Deriso E, Akinwunmi B, Young N, Baez AM, Shook LL, Cvrk D, James K, De Guzman R, Brigida S, Diouf K, Goldfarb I, Bebell LM, Yonker LM, Fasano A, Rabi SA, Elovitz MA, Alter G, Edlow AG. Coronavirus disease 2019 vaccine response in pregnant and lactating women: a cohort study. Am J Obstet Gynecol. 2021;225(3):303.e1–303.e17. https://doi.org/10.1016/j.ajog.2021.03.023.
11. Shook LL, Atyeo CG, Yonker LM, Fasano A, Gray KJ, Alter G, Edlow AG. Durability of anti-spike antibodies in infants after maternal COVID-19 vaccination or natural infection. JAMA. 2022;327:1087. https://doi.org/10.1001/jama.2022.1206.
12. World Health Organization. Definition and categorization of the timing of mother-to-child transmission of SARS-CoV-2: scientific brief, 8 February 2021 (No. WHO/2019-nCoV/mother-to-child_transmission/2021.1). Geneva: World Health Organization; 2021.
13. Mattern J, Vauloup-Fellous C, Zakaria H, Benachi A, Carrara J, Letourneau A, Bourgeois-Nicolaos N, De Luca D, Doucet-Populaire F, Vivanti AJ. Post lockdown COVID-19 seroprevalence and circulation at the time of delivery, France. PLoS One. 2020;15(10):e0240782. https://doi.org/10.1371/journal.pone.0240782.
14. Schwartz DA, De Luca D. The public health and clinical importance of accurate neonatal testing for COVID-19. Pediatrics. 2021;147(2):e2020036871. https://doi.org/10.1542/peds.2020-036871. PMID: 33479163.
15. Macfarlane P. RSV testing in bronchiolitis: which nasal sampling method is best? Arch Dis Child. 2005;90:634–5.
16. Akhtar Z, Islam MA, Aleem MA, Mah-E-Muneer S, Ahmmed MK, Ghosh PK, Rahman M, Rahman MZ, Sumiya MK, Rahman MM, Shirin T, Alamgir ASM, Banu S, Rahman M, Chowdhury F. SARS-CoV-2 and influenza virus coinfection among patients with severe

acute respiratory infection during the first wave of COVID-19 pandemic in Bangladesh: a hospital-based descriptive study. BMJ Open. 2021;11(11):e053768. https://doi.org/10.1136/bmjopen-2021-053768.
17. Rotulo GA, Casalini E, Brisca G, Piccotti E, Castagnola E. Unexpected peak of bronchiolitis requiring oxygen therapy in February 2020: could an undetected SARS-CoV2-RSV co-infection be the cause? Pediatr Pulmonol. 2021;56(6):1803–5. https://doi.org/10.1002/ppul.25331.
18. Huang Y, Skarlupka AL, Jang H, Blas-Machado U, Holladay N, Hogan RJ, Ross TM. SARS-CoV-2 and influenza A virus co-infections in Ferrets. J Virol. 2021;96:e0179121. https://doi.org/10.1128/JVI.01791-21.
19. Hashemi SA, Safamanesh S, Ghasemzadeh-Moghaddam H, Ghafouri M, Azimian A. High prevalence of SARS-CoV-2 and influenza A virus (H1N1) coinfection in dead patients in Northeastern Iran. J Med Virol. 2021;93(2):1008–12. https://doi.org/10.1002/jmv.26364.
20. Dargaville PA, South M, McDougall PN. Comparison of two methods of diagnostic lung lavage in ventilated infants with lung disease. Am J Respir Crit Care Med. 1999;160(3):771–7. https://doi.org/10.1164/ajrccm.160.3.9811048.
21. Winichakoon P, Chaiwarith R, Liwsrisakun C, Salee P, Goonna A, Limsukon A, Kaewpoowat Q. Negative nasopharyngeal and oropharyngeal swabs do not rule out COVID-19. J Clin Microbiol. 2020;58(5):e00297–20. https://doi.org/10.1128/JCM.00297-20.
22. Wang W, Xu Y, Gao R, Lu R, Han K, Wu G, Tan W. Detection of SARS-CoV-2 in different types of clinical specimens. JAMA. 2020;323(18):1843–4. https://doi.org/10.1001/jama.2020.3786.
23. de Blic J, Midulla F, Barbato A, Clement A, Dab I, Eber E, Green C, Grigg J, Kotecha S, Kurland G, Pohunek P, Ratjen F, Rossi G. Bronchoalveolar lavage in children. ERS Task Force on bronchoalveolar lavage in children. European Respiratory Society. Eur Respir J. 2000;15(1):217–31. https://doi.org/10.1183/09031936.00.15121700.
24. De Luca D, Minucci A, Tripodi D, Piastra M, Pietrini D, Zuppi C, Conti G, Carnielli VP, Capoluongo E. Role of distinct phospholipases A2 and their modulators in meconium aspiration syndrome in human neonates. Intensive Care Med. 2011;37(7):1158–65. https://doi.org/10.1007/s00134-011-2243-z.
25. Oliva S, Cucchiara S, Locatelli F. Children and fecal SARS-CoV-2 shedding: just the tip of the Iceberg of Italian COVID-19 outbreak? Dig Liver Dis. 2020;52(11):1219–21. https://doi.org/10.1016/j.dld.2020.06.039.
26. ECDC. n.d.. https://www.ecdc.europa.eu/en/all-topics-z/coronavirus/threats-and-outbreaks/covid-19/laboratory-support/questions. Accessed 8 Feb 2022.
27. Tsung JW, Kessler DO, Shah VP. Prospective application of clinician-performed lung ultrasonography during the 2009 H1N1 influenza A pandemic: distinguishing viral from bacterial pneumonia. Crit Ultrasound J. 2012;4(1):16. https://doi.org/10.1186/2036-7902-4-16.
28. Yousef N, De Luca D. The role of lung ultrasound in viral lower respiratory tract infections. Am J Perinatol. 2018;35(6):527–9. https://doi.org/10.1055/s-0038-1637758.
29. Caiulo VA, Gargani L, Caiulo S, Fisicaro A, Moramarco F, Latini G, Picano E. Lung ultrasound in bronchiolitis: comparison with chest X-ray. Eur J Pediatr. 2011;170(11):1427–33. https://doi.org/10.1007/s00431-011-1461-2.
30. De Luca D, van Kaam AH, Tingay DG, Courtney SE, Danhaive O, Carnielli VP, Zimmermann LJ, Kneyber MCJ, Tissieres P, Brierley J, Conti G, Pillow JJ, Rimensberger PC. The Montreux definition of neonatal ARDS: biological and clinical background behind the description of a new entity. Lancet Respir Med. 2017;5(8):657–66. https://doi.org/10.1016/S2213-2600(17)30214-X.
31. Vivanti AJ, Vauloup-Fellous C, Prevot S, Zupan V, Suffee C, Do Cao J, Benachi A, De Luca D. Transplacental transmission of SARS-CoV-2 infection. Nat Commun. 2020;11(1):3572. https://doi.org/10.1038/s41467-020-17436-6.
32. WHO Working Group on the Clinical Characterisation and Management of COVID-19 infection. A minimal common outcome measure set for COVID-19 clinical research. Lancet Infect Dis. 2020;20(8):e192–7. https://doi.org/10.1016/S1473-3099(20)30483-7.

33. De Luca D, Rava L, Nadel S, Tissieres P, Gawronski O, Perkins E, Chidini G, Tingay DG. The EPICENTRE (ESPNIC Covid pEdiatric Neonatal Registry) initiative: background and protocol for the international SARS-CoV-2 infections registry. Eur J Pediatr. 2020;179(8):1271–8. https://doi.org/10.1007/s00431-020-03690-9.
34. Frauenfelder C, Brierley J, Whittaker E, Perucca G, Bamford A. Infant with SARS-CoV-2 infection causing severe lung disease treated with remdesivir. Pediatrics 2020;146(3):e20201701. https://doi.org/10.1542/peds.2020-1701.
35. Cui Y, Tian M, Huang D, Wang X, Huang Y, Fan L, Wang L, Chen Y, Liu W, Zhang K, Wu Y, Yang Z, Tao J, Feng J, Liu K, Ye X, Wang R, Zhang X, Zha Y. A 55-day-old female infant infected with 2019 novel coronavirus disease: presenting with pneumonia, liver injury, and heart damage. J Infect Dis. 2020;222(11):1775–81. https://doi.org/10.1093/infdis/jiaa113.
36. Rashidian T, Sharifi N, Fathnezhad-Kazemi A, Mirzamrajani F, Nourollahi S, Ghaysouri A. Death of a neonate with suspected coronavirus disease 2019 born to a mother with coronavirus disease 2019 in Iran: a case report. J Med Case Rep. 2020;14(1):186. https://doi.org/10.1186/s13256-020-02519-1.
37. Di Nardo M, van Leeuwen G, Loreti A, Barbieri MA, Guner Y, Locatelli F, Ranieri VM. A literature review of 2019 novel coronavirus (SARS-CoV2) infection in neonates and children. Pediatr Res. 2021;89(5):1101–8. https://doi.org/10.1038/s41390-020-1065-5.
38. Cui X, Zhao Z, Zhang T, Guo W, Guo W, Zheng J, Zhang J, Dong C, Na R, Zheng L, Li W, Liu Z, Ma J, Wang J, He S, Xu Y, Si P, Shen Y, Cai C. A systematic review and meta-analysis of children with coronavirus disease 2019 (COVID-19). J Med Virol. 2021;93(2):1057–69. https://doi.org/10.1002/jmv.26398.
39. Akin IM, Kanburoglu MK, Tayman C, Oncel MY, Imdadoglu T, Dilek M, Yaman A, Narter F, Er I, Kahveci H, Erdeve O, Koc E, Neo-Covid Study Group. Epidemiologic and clinical characteristics of neonates with late-onset COVID-19: 1-year data of Turkish Neonatal Society. Eur J Pediatr. 2022;181:1933–42. https://doi.org/10.1007/s00431-021-04358-8.
40. Henry BM, Lippi G, Plebani M. Laboratory abnormalities in children with novel coronavirus disease 2019. Clin Chem Lab Med. 2020;58(7):1135–8. https://doi.org/10.1515/cclm-2020-0272.
41. Vakili S, Savardashtaki A, Jamalnia S, Tabrizi R, Nematollahi MH, Jafarinia M, Akbari H. Laboratory findings of COVID-19 infection are conflicting in different age groups and pregnant women: a literature review. Arch Med Res. 2020;51(7):603–7. https://doi.org/10.1016/j.arcmed.2020.06.007.
42. Briana D, Syridou G, Papaevangelou V. Perinatal COVID-19. Pediatr Infect Dis J. 2021;40(12):e504–6. https://doi.org/10.1097/INF.0000000000003356.
43. Galván-Román JM, Rodríguez-García SC, Roy-Vallejo E, Marcos-Jiménez A, Sánchez-Alonso S, Fernández-Díaz C, Alcaraz-Serna A, Mateu-Albero T, Rodríguez-Cortes P, Sánchez-Cerrillo I, Esparcia L, Martínez-Fleta P, López-Sanz C, Gabrie L, Del Campo Guerola L, Suárez-Fernández C, Ancochea J, Canabal A, Albert F, Rodríguez-Serrano DA, Aguilar JM, Del Arco C, de Los Santos I, García-Fraile L, de la Cámara R, Serra JM, Ramírez E, Alonso T, Landete P, Soriano JB, Martín-Gayo E, Fraile Torres A, Zurita Cruz ND, García-Vicuña R, Cardeñoso L, Sánchez-Madrid F, Alfranca A, Muñoz-Calleja C, González-Álvaro I, REINMUN-COVID Group. IL-6 serum levels predict severity and response to tocilizumab in COVID-19: an observational study. J Allergy Clin Immunol. 2021;147(1):72–80.e8. https://doi.org/10.1016/j.jaci.2020.09.018.
44. Soraya GV, Ulhaq ZS. Interleukin-6 levels in children developing SARS-CoV-2 infection. Pediatr Neonatol. 2020;61(3):253–4. https://doi.org/10.1016/j.pedneo.2020.04.007.
45. White A, Mukherjee P, Stremming J, Sherlock LG, Reynolds RM, Smith D, Asturias EJ, Grover TR, Dietz RM. Neonates hospitalized with community-acquired SARS-CoV-2 in a Colorado Neonatal Intensive Care Unit. Neonatology. 2020;117(5):641–5. https://doi.org/10.1159/000508962.
46. Ghodsi A, Bijari M, Ali Alamdaran S, Sateri A, Mahmoudabadi E, Reza Balali M, Ghahreman S. Chest computed tomography findings of COVID-19 in children younger than 1 year: a systematic review. World J Pediatr. 2021;17:234–41. https://doi.org/10.1007/s12519-021-00424-1.

47. Buonsenso D, Pata D, Chiaretti A. COVID-19 outbreak: less stethoscope, more ultrasound. Lancet Respir Med. 2020;8(5):e27. https://doi.org/10.1016/S2213-2600(20)30120-X.
48. Gregorio-Hernández R, Escobar-Izquierdo AB, Cobas-Pazos J, Martínez-Gimeno A. Point-of-care lung ultrasound in three neonates with COVID-19. Eur J Pediatr. 2020;179(8):1279–85. https://doi.org/10.1007/s00431-020-03706-4.
49. Guitart C, Suárez R, Girona M, Bobillo-Perez S, Hernández L, Balaguer M, Cambra FJ, Jordan I, KIDS-Corona Study Group, Kids Corona Platform. Lung ultrasound findings in pediatric patients with COVID-19. Eur J Pediatr. 2021;180(4):1117–23. https://doi.org/10.1007/s00431-020-03839-6.
50. De Luca D. Semiquantitative lung ultrasound scores are accurate and useful in critical care, irrespective of patients' ages: the power of data over opinions. J Ultrasound Med. 2020;39(6):1235–9. https://doi.org/10.1002/jum.15195.
51. Giorno EPC, De Paulis M, Sameshima YT, Weerdenburg K, Savoia P, Nanbu DY, Couto TB, Sa FVM, Farhat SCL, Carvalho WB, Preto-Zamperlini M, Schvartsman C. Point-of-care lung ultrasound imaging in pediatric COVID-19. Ultrasound J. 2020;12(1):50. https://doi.org/10.1186/s13089-020-00198-z.
52. Brat R, Yousef N, Klifa R, Reynaud S, Shankar Aguilera S, De Luca D. Lung ultrasonography score to evaluate oxygenation and surfactant need in neonates treated with continuous positive airway pressure. JAMA Pediatr. 2015;169(8):e151797. https://doi.org/10.1001/jamapediatrics.2015.1797.
53. Belot A, Antona D, Renolleau S, Javouhey E, Hentgen V, Angoulvant F, Delacourt C, Iriart X, Ovaert C, Bader-Meunier B, Kone-Paut I, Levy-Bruhl D. SARS-CoV-2-related paediatric inflammatory multisystem syndrome, an epidemiological study, France, 1 March to 17 May 2020. Euro Surveill. 2020;25(22):2001010. https://doi.org/10.2807/1560-7917.ES.2020.25.22.2001010.
54. Consiglio CR, Cotugno N, Sardh F, Pou C, Amodio D, Rodriguez L, Tan Z, Zicari S, Ruggiero A, Pascucci GR, Santilli V, Campbell T, Bryceson Y, Eriksson D, Wang J, Marchesi A, Lakshmikanth T, Campana A, Villani A, Rossi P, CACTUS Study Team, Landegren N, Palma P, Brodin P. The immunology of multisystem inflammatory syndrome in children with COVID-19. Cell. 2020;183(4):968–981.e7. https://doi.org/10.1016/j.cell.2020.09.016.
55. Nakra NA, Blumberg DA, Herrera-Guerra A, Lakshminrusimha S. Multi-system inflammatory syndrome in children (MIS-C) following SARS-CoV-2 infection: review of clinical presentation, hypothetical pathogenesis, and proposed management. Children. 2020;7(7):69. https://doi.org/10.3390/children7070069.
56. Pawar R, Gavade V, Patil N, Mali V, Girwalkar A, Tarkasband V, Loya S, Chavan A, Nanivadekar N, Shinde R, Patil U, Lakshminrusimha S. Neonatal multisystem inflammatory syndrome (MIS-N) associated with prenatal maternal SARS-CoV-2: a case series. Children. 2021;8(7):572. https://doi.org/10.3390/children8070572.
57. More K, Aiyer S, Goti A, Parikh M, Sheikh S, Patel G, Kallem V, Soni R, Kumar P. Multisystem inflammatory syndrome in neonates (MIS-N) associated with SARS-CoV2 infection: a case series. Eur J Pediatr. 2022;181:1883–98. https://doi.org/10.1007/s00431-022-04377-z.
58. CDC. n.d.. https://www.cdc.gov/mis/about.html. Accessed 8 Feb 2022.
59. Shaiba LA, Hadid A, Altirkawi KA, Bakheet HM, Alherz AM, Hussain SA, Sobaih BH, Alnemri AM, Almaghrabi R, Ahmed M, Arafah MA, Jarallah A, Bukhari EE, Alzamil FA. Case report: neonatal multi-system inflammatory syndrome associated with SARS-CoV-2 exposure in two cases from Saudi Arabia. Front Pediatr. 2021;9:652857. https://doi.org/10.3389/fped.2021.652857.
60. Khaund Borkotoky R, Banerjee Barua P, Paul SP, Heaton PA. COVID-19-related potential multisystem inflammatory syndrome in childhood in a neonate presenting as persistent pulmonary hypertension of the newborn. Pediatr Infect Dis J. 2021;40(4):e162–4. https://doi.org/10.1097/INF.0000000000003054.
61. Divekar AA, Patamasucon P, Benjamin JS. Presumptive neonatal multisystem inflammatory syndrome in children associated with coronavirus disease 2019. Am J Perinatol. 2021;38(6):632–6. https://doi.org/10.1055/s-0041-1726318.

62. McCarty KL, Tucker M, Lee G, Pandey V. Fetal inflammatory response syndrome associated with maternal SARS-CoV-2 infection. Pediatrics. 2021;147(4) e2020010132. https://doi.org/10.1542/peds.2020-010132.
63. Kappanayil M, Balan S, Alawani S. Mohanty S, Leeladharan SP, Gangadharan S. Jayashankar JP, Jagadeesan S, Kumar A, Gupta A, Kumar RK. Multisystem inflammatory syndrome in a neonate, temporally associated with prenatal exposure to SARS-CoV-2: a case report. Lancet Child Adolesc Health. 2021;5(4):304–8. https://doi.org/10.1016/S2352-4642(21)00055-9.
64. De Luca D. Managing neonates with respiratory failure due to SARS-CoV-2. Lancet Child Adolesc Health. 2020;4(4):e8. https //doi.org/10.1016/S2352-4642(20)30073-0.
65. de Winter JP, De Luca D, Tingay DG. COVID-19 surveillance for all newborns at the NICU; conditio sine qua non? Eur J Pediatr. 2020;179(12):1945–7. https://doi.org/10.1007/s00431-020-03773-7.
66. Chidini G, Villa C, Calderini E, Marchisio P, De Luca D. SARS-CoV-2 Infection in a pediatric department in Milan: a logistic rather than a clinical emergency. Pediatr Infect Dis J. 2020;39(6):e79–80. https://doi.org/10.1097/INF.0000000000002687.
67. Kneyber MCJ, de Luca D, Calderini E, Jarreau PH, Javouhey E, Lopez-Herce J, Hammer J, Macrae D, Markhorst DG, Medina A, Pons-Odena M, Racca F, Wolf G, Biban P, Brierley J, Rimensberger PC, Section Respiratory Failure of the European Society for Paediatric and Neonatal Intensive Care. Recommendations for mechanical ventilation of critically ill children from the Paediatric Mechanical Ventilation Consensus Conference (PEMVECC). Intensive Care Med. 2017;43(12):1764–80. https://doi.org/10.1007/s00134-017-4920-z.
68. Singh A, Khanna P, Sarkar S. High-flow nasal cannula, a boon or a bane for COVID-19 patients? An evidence-based review. Curr Anesthesiol Rep. 2021;11:101–6 https://doi.org/10.1007/s40140-021-00439-4.
69. Frassoni E, Shankar-Aguilera S, Yousef N, De Luca D. Helmet-delivered respiratory support in neonate with severe facial malformation. J Paediatr Child Health. 2017;53(8):825. https://doi.org/10.1111/jpc.13635.
70. Singh Y, Tissot C, Fraga MV, Yousef N, Cortes RG, Lopez J, Sanchez-de-Toledo J, Brierley J, Colunga JM, Raffaj D, Da Cruz E, Durand P, Kenderessy P, Lang HJ, Nishisaki A, Kneyber MC, Tissieres P, Conlon TW, De Luca D. International evidence-based guidelines on Point of Care Ultrasound (POCUS) for critically ill neonates and children issued by the POCUS Working Group of the European Society of Paediatric and Neonatal Intensive Care (ESPNIC). Crit Care. 2020;24(1):65. https://doi.org/10.1186/s13054-020-2787-9.
71. Wardell H, Campbell JI, Van der Pluym C, Dixit A. Severe acute respiratory syndrome coronavirus 2 infection in febrile neonates. J Paediatr Infect Dis Soc. 2020;9(5):630–5. https://doi.org/10.1093/jpids/piaa084.
72. Saikia B, Tang J, Robinson S, Nichani S, Lawman KB, Katre M, Bandi S. Neonates with SARS-CoV-2 infection and pulmonary disease safely treated with remdesivir. Pediatr Infect Dis J. 2021;40(5):e194–6. https://doi.org/10.1097/INF.0000000000003081.
73. Cursi L, Calo Carducci FI, Chiurchiu S, Romani L, Stoppa F, Lucignani G, Russo C, Longo D, Perno CF, Cecchetti C, Lombardi MH, D'Argenio P, Lancella L, Bernardi S, Rossi P. Severe COVID-19 complicated by cerebral venous thrombosis in a newborn successfully treated with remdesivir, glucocorticoids, and hyperimmune plasma. Int J Environ Res Public Health. 2021;18(24):13201. https://doi.org/10.3390/ijerph182413201.
74. FDA. n.d.. https://www.fda.gov/media/137564/download. Accessed 8 Feb 2022.
75. NICE. n.d.. https://www.nice.org.uk/guidance/ng191. Accessed 8 Feb 2022.
76. FDA. n.d.. https://www.fda.gov/media/145801/download. Accessed 8 Feb 2022.
77. Mayer C, Van Hise K, Caskey R, Naqvi M, Burwick RM. Monoclonal antibodies casirivimab and imdevimab in pregnancy for coronavirus disease 2019 (COVID-19). Obstet Gynecol. 2021;138(6):937–9. https://doi.org/10.1097/AOG.0000000000004603.
78. Watterberg KL, American Academy of Pediatrics, Committee on Fetus and Newborn. Policy statement--postnatal corticosteroids to prevent or treat bronchopulmonary dysplasia. Pediatrics. 2010;126(4):800–8. https //doi.org/10.1542/peds.2010-1534.

79. Jiménez-Lozano I, Caro-Teller JM, Fernández-Hidalgo N, Miarons M, Frick MA, Batllori Badia E, Serrano B, Parramon-Teixidó CJ, Camba-Longueira F, Moral-Pumarega MT, San Juan-Garrido R, Cabañas Poy MJ, Suy A, Gorgas Torner MQ. Safety of tocilizumab in COVID-19 pregnant women and their newborn: a retrospective study. J Clin Pharm Ther. 2021;46(4):1062–70. https://doi.org/10.1111/jcpt.13394.
80. Tada Y, Sakai M, Nakao Y, Maruyama A, Ono N, Koarada S. Placental transfer of tocilizumab in a patient with rheumatoid arthritis. Rheumatology (Oxford). 2019;58(9):1694–5. https://doi.org/10.1093/rheumatology/kez155.
81. Nimmerjahn F, Ravetch JV. The antiinflammatory activity of IgG: the intravenous IgG paradox. J Exp Med. 2007;204(1):11–5. https://doi.org/10.1084/jem.20061788.
82. Lee PY, Day-Lewis M, Henderson LA, Friedman KG, Lo J, Roberts JE, Lo MS, Platt CD, Chou J, Hoyt KJ, Baker AL, Banzon TM, Chang MH, Cohen E, de Ferranti SD, Dionne A, Habiballah S, Halyabar O, Hausmann JS, Hazen MM, Janssen E, Meidan E, Nelson RW, Nguyen AA, Sundel RP, Dedeoglu F, Nigrovic PA, Newburger JW, Son MBF. Distinct clinical and immunological features of SARS-CoV-2-induced multisystem inflammatory syndrome in children. J Clin Invest. 2020;130(11):5942–50. https://doi.org/10.1172/JCI141113.
83. Pakdel M, Pouralizadeh N, Faramarzi R, Boskabadi H, Mamouri G. Neonates with Covid-19 infection: is there any different treatment process? J Pediatr Surg Case Rep. 2022;77:102148. https://doi.org/10.1016/j.epsc.2021.102148.
84. Nakhlband A, Fakhari A, Azizi H. Interferon-alpha position in combating with COVID-19: a systematic review. J Med Virol. 2021;93(9):5277–84. https://doi.org/10.1002/jmv.27072.
85. van de Veerdonk FL, Giamarellos-Bourboulis E, Pickkers P, Derde L, Leavis H, van Crevel R, Engel JJ, Wiersinga WJ, Vlaar APJ, Shankar-Hari M, van der Poll T, Bonten M, Angus DC, van der Meer JWM, Netea MG. A guide to immunotherapy for COVID-19. Nat Med. 2022;28(1):39–50. https://doi.org/10.1038/s41591-021-01643-9.
86. De Luca D, Vauloup-Fellous C, Benachi A, Masturzo B, Manzoni P, Vivanti A. The essentials about neonatal SARS-CoV-2 infection and COVID-19: a narrative review. Am J Perinatol. 2022;39:S18.

Chapter 12
Impact of COVID on Prematurity

Helena Blakeway and Asma Khalil

12.1 Introduction

The COVID-19 pandemic continues to cause worldwide suffering and death, impacting healthcare across the globe [1]. One group who have particularly suffered are pregnant women with more and more evidence coming to light of poorer maternal and neonatal outcomes [2]. These include preterm birth, stillbirth and pre-eclampsia. Moreover, pregnant women are more likely to suffer severe COVID-19 disease with higher incidence of admission to hospital, intensive care unit (ICU) and death [3].

The impact of the COVID-19 pandemic on maternal and neonatal outcomes has been twofold, both direct and indirect. Indirectly, factors such as reduced healthcare services, fear of attending hospitals and isolation have led to poorer outcomes alongside the direct effect of the SARS-CoV-2 virus itself.

Preterm birth (birth before 37 weeks' gestation) is one of the leading causes of neonatal deaths worldwide [4]. Preterm birth can occur spontaneously or can be a medical decision to protect maternal and/or neonatal well-being [4]. This is important to distinguish when considering the effect of the COVID-19 pandemic on

---

H. Blakeway
Fetal Medicine Unit, Department of Obstetrics and Gynaecology, St. George's Hospitals NHS Foundation Trust, London, UK
e-mail: helena.blakeway@nhs.net

A. Khalil (✉)
Fetal Medicine Unit, Department of Obstetrics and Gynaecology, St. George's Hospitals NHS Foundation Trust, London, UK

Vascular Biology Research Centre, Molecular and Clinical Sciences Research Institute, St George's University of London, London, UK

Fetal Medicine Unit, Liverpool Women's Hospital, University of Liverpool, Liverpool, UK
e-mail: akhalil@sgul.ac.uk

© The Author(s), under exclusive license to Springer Nature Switzerland AG 2023
D. De Luca, A. Benachi (eds.), *COVID-19 and Perinatology*,
https://doi.org/10.1007/978-3-031-29136-4_12

prematurity as the association may be both due to the virus itself causing preterm labour and due to clinical decisions to deliver early. COVID-19 disease is also associated with other adverse maternal and neonatal outcomes including preeclampsia and stillbirth [2]. High risk of stillbirth or preeclampsia could be some of the indications to deliver early, thus increasing the incidence of preterm birth.

12.2 Evidence so Far

Initially, after the first wave of the pandemic in 2020, evidence emerged of a possible decrease in the incidence of preterm birth. In the Netherlands, a decrease in the incidence of preterm birth was observed after March 9, 2020, when national lockdown measures were imposed, in comparison to data from October 2010 to March 2020 [5]. Further data from the USA showed evidence of a decrease in preterm birth during the early COVID-19 pandemic when compared with the same time period in 2019 (9.9% vs. 12.6%; OR 0.76; 95% CI 0.58–0.99). There were no differences in subgroup analysis of spontaneous or iatrogenic preterm birth [6].

This finding was mirrored in England with a national cohort study that compared births between March 2020 and February 2021 with the same period one year earlier. They found evidence of a very small decrease in the preterm birth rate. This was with the exception of women from ethnic minority backgrounds where existing differences were exacerbated. This study only included singleton births [7].

It was hypothesised that this early decrease in the incidence of preterm birth was possibly due to reduced exposure to environmental pollutants and infections due to lockdown restrictions or a reduction in iatrogenic preterm birth early in the pandemic due to antenatal appointments being reduced where indications of preterm birth are noted. Another hypothesis is that studies focussing on singleton births will have missed multiple pregnancies that are over 50% more likely to result in preterm birth [7].

However, opposing evidence rapidly started emerging of an increase in preterm birth associated with COVID-19 disease. A systematic review that synthesised evidence from April to June 2020 found an increase in iatrogenic preterm birth with the most common indication being severe COVID-19-associated pneumonia or maternal decompensation [8].

In Nepal, an increase in preterm birth was noted during lockdown in 2020 when compared to pre-lockdown (20.0% vs. 16.7%, respectively, $p = 0.002$) [9]. This increase could have been due to increased psychosocial stress caused by COVID-19, delay in accessing healthcare due to cutback in services and travel restrictions or SARS-CoV-2 infection itself [9].

The Spanish Obstetric Emergency Group observed an increase in preterm birth associated with SARS-CoV-2 infection in pregnancy across a cohort of 78 centres in Spain. Pregnant women with SARS-CoV-2 infection were compared to noninfected pregnant women, and preterm birth was almost twice as common in infected pregnant women (11.1% vs. 5.8%, $p < 0.001$) [10]. This was mostly due to an increase in iatrogenic preterm deliveries due to maternal illness caused by COVID-19 disease [10].

Evidence has also emerged of more severe SARS-CoV-2 infection in turn causing more severe adverse maternal and neonatal outcomes including preterm birth. Pregnant women with severe or critical COVID-19 infection had a much higher risk of preterm birth when compared with pregnant women with asymptomatic COVID-19 disease (41.8% vs. 11.9%) [11]. This is important as it highlights the role of the COVID-19 vaccine in preventing severe disease in pregnancy.

12.3 Other Adverse Pregnancy Outcomes

Increasingly, evidence is emerging of the adverse impact SARS-COV-2 infection could have on other maternal and perinatal outcomes.

It is now widely accepted that the COVID-19 pandemic has caused an increase in stillbirth. In the UK, a large-scale analysis of 342,080 pregnant women of whom 3527 had confirmed SARS-CoV-2 infection; stillbirth (along with preterm birth) occurred more often in infected women [12]. The underlying mechanism is still unclear; however, placental histology has consistently shown features of maternal vascular malperfusion likely caused by hypoxic events [13]. Maternal vascular malperfusion is caused by poor or abnormal uterine perfusion which leads to a sequela of changes in the placenta including fibrin deposition, villous infarction and villous thrombosis. These changes may not directly cause stillbirth; however, they certainly contribute to increasing the risk of foetal death and other adverse pregnancy outcomes. Severe SARS-CoV-2 infection in pregnancy causes maternal hypoxia which could cause maternal vascular malperfusion via uterine ischaemia and thus placental hypoxia [14].

These changes are also associated with preeclampsia, and like preterm birth and stillbirth, evidence has emerged of an association between COVID-19 disease and preeclampsia. This association appears to be unrelated to the severity of COVID-19 infection [15]. Researchers have shown that preeclampsia and COVID-19 infection are associated not only independently but also in an additive fashion with preterm birth [15].

It is important to note that the increase in preterm birth could be directly linked to the increase in stillbirth and preeclampsia caused by COVID-19 disease as these are both indications for iatrogenic preterm birth.

In a meta-analysis of COVID-19 disease in pregnancy, the authors have demonstrated an increase in the risk of foetal growth restriction (FGR) and preterm premature rupture of membranes (PPROM) [16]. Researchers have found incidences of PPROM to be as high as 9.9% in COVID-19-infected individuals. Prior to the COVID-19 pandemic, the incidence of PPROM was shown to be around 3%. The incidence of FGR is estimated to be between 4% and 7%. It is often associated with preeclampsia and has been shown to increase up to 12.5% in pregnant women with COVID-19 infection [16]. These results are yet to be replicated in other studies.

12.4 Mechanism of Prematurity Associated with COVID-19 in Pregnancy

Research studies initially highlighted a reduction in the preterm birth rate caused by the COVID-19 pandemic. This was in all pregnant women as opposed to pregnant women who had COVID-19 disease. Researchers found that this was mainly evident in medically indicated preterm birth which could have been due to fewer face-to-face antenatal appointments and fewer pregnant women attending triage [17].

There appears to be higher incidence of adverse maternal and neonatal outcomes depending on the gestational age at the time of SARS-CoV-2 infection. Adverse obstetric outcomes increase when infected by COVID-19 disease after 20 weeks' gestation, and increased adverse neonatal outcomes occur when infected after 26 weeks' gestation [18].

There have been several theories hypothesised about why preterm birth has increased during the pandemic. Predominantly, the increase in preterm birth appears to be iatrogenic—a medical decision to deliver early in order to prevent further harm to the pregnant women and/or the baby [10, 19]. This includes caesarean delivery without labour and induction of labour [20]. Pregnant women are at increased risk of severe COVID-19 disease with increased likelihood of being admitted to intensive care unit, intubation, receipt of extracorporeal membrane oxygenation and death [21]. Therefore, iatrogenic preterm birth may be indicated when pregnant women are deteriorating due to COVID-19 disease and either the mother, the foetus, or both are compromised [22]. This could explain the increase in preterm birth.

Another reason preterm birth may be medically indicated is due to severe preeclampsia or preeclampsia-like manifestations. As discussed, COVID-19 infection in pregnancy is associated with preeclampsia. Preterm birth is indicated in pregnant women with severe hypertension which is difficult to control or those with low platelet count or evidence of coagulopathy [23]. As this is more common in pregnant women with SARS-CoV-2 infection, the association between COVID-19 disease and preterm birth may be confounded by the association between COVID-19 disease and preeclampsia.

Foetal complications or demise are also an indication for iatrogenic preterm birth [20]. COVID-19 disease is associated with stillbirth, and therefore the increase in iatrogenic preterm birth may be due to foetal distress caused by COVID-19 disease, meaning a decision is made to deliver early. A pregnant woman with severe COVID-19 disease and hypoxia causing foetal distress may have a preterm birth to protect the foetus. Of note, the increase in the risk of neonatal adverse outcome noted in a national cohort study in England was mainly mediated through preterm birth [12].

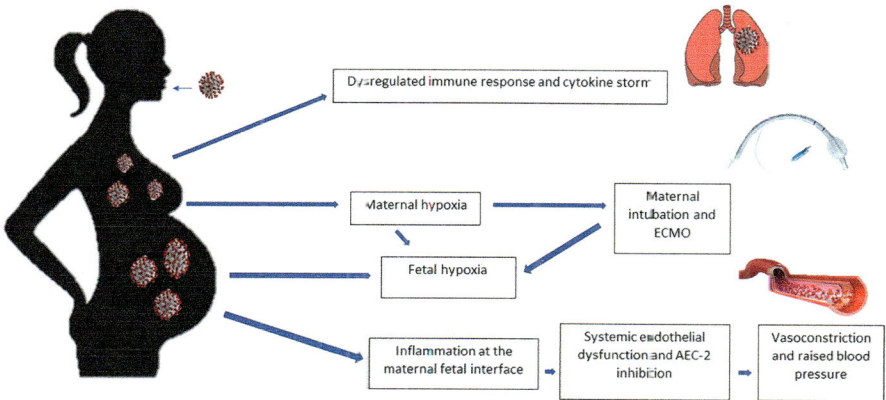

Fig. 12.1 SARS-CoV-2 infection in pregnancy: inflammatory response at the maternal-foetal interface

There is also evidence of an increase in spontaneous preterm birth. Infection is a recognised cause of preterm birth and is thought to cause up to 50% of extreme preterm birth (birth before 28 weeks) [24]. SARS-CoV-2 infection causes mass inflammation with increased proinflammatory cytokines and chemokines [25]. In preterm labour, proinflammatory cytokines in turn stimulate production of prostaglandins by amnion and decidua which triggers labour [24]. This could be a possible mechanism by which COVID-19 disease leads to preterm birth.

SARS-CoV-2 infection in pregnancy is associated with preterm premature rupture of membranes (PPROM) [16]. PPROM precedes around 50% of all preterm births and oxidative stress has been shown to play a role in the pathophysiology of PPROM [26]. In moderate and severe COVID-19, oxygen therapy is used to treat hypoxaemia. This induces oxidative stress and causes generation of reactive oxygen species [27]. This can cause an unbalanced redox state in the amniotic fluid which is associated with PPROM and could be part of the mechanism by which COVID-19 disease causes PPROM and thus preterm birth.

Interestingly, the majority of neonates born to women infected with SARS-CoV-2 test negative for the virus; however, there is evidence of inflammatory response at the maternal-foetal interface [28]. Research into the maternal-foetal immune response found higher levels of pro-inflammatory cytokines in both mothers and their neonates as well as dysregulated immune and non-immune processes in neonates. As well as this, there is evidence of enhanced maternal T-cell function and foetal stromal cell function at the maternal-foetal interface (Fig. 12.1). However, in the majority of SARS-CoV-2-infected mothers, the virus was not detected in the placenta, amniotic fluid or the neonates, and no IgM response was triggered in the foetus. It appears that only in severe disease can SARS-CoV-2 cross the placenta indicating that there are mechanisms by which the virus can do this [28].

12.5 Direct Versus Indirect Effect

To understand the impact of the COVID-19 pandemic on preterm birth, both the direct and indirect effects of the pandemic must be considered. Direct effects are those caused by SARS-CoV-2 infection itself, as shown by changes in placental pathology caused by the virus. Indirect effects are those caused by changes in health seeking behaviour and availability of healthcare services which may in turn lead to adverse pregnancy outcomes.

The indirect effect of the pandemic is shown by an increase in preterm birth in pregnant women during the pandemic who did not test positive for COVID-19 during pregnancy. This is shown by a large systematic review and meta-analysis of maternal, foetal and neonatal outcomes in the pandemic which included 40 studies of pregnant women in the pandemic [2]. This systematic review looked at maternal and neonatal outcomes for pregnant women as a whole rather than just pregnant women who had COVID-19 disease.

During the pandemic, many healthcare services were scaled back or withdrawn, including maternity services across the world [29]. This meant that women had fewer face-to-face appointments as well as fewer appointments overall. Appointments were instead conducted over the phone or by video call, meaning pregnant women were often not physically seen or examined. This meant that there were fewer opportunities for pregnant women to raise concerns or for healthcare professionals to notice abnormal signs or symptoms.

Moreover, at the peak of the pandemic, there were daily news reports and footage released showing hospitals overwhelmed by COVID-19-positive patients [30]. Governments across the world ran extensive public health campaigns, repeatedly telling people to stay at home and not attend hospital unless they urgently needed to. Furthermore, reports of high levels of staff isolating and redeployment of staff from areas such as maternity to COVID-19 wards were broadcast alongside news reports of long ambulance waiting times and burnt-out staff [31]. Pregnant women may have stayed at home even when experiencing signs or symptoms of adverse pregnancy outcomes due to an altruistic wish not to be a burden on an already struggling health service or add the pressure on hospitals and hospital staff [32].

Another reason pregnant women may have avoided going into hospital is due to fear of catching SARS-CoV-2 infection. Initially, early in the pandemic, little was known about the effect of SARS-CoV-2 infection in pregnancy, and many pregnant women made the decision to shield. Evidence quickly started to emerge that

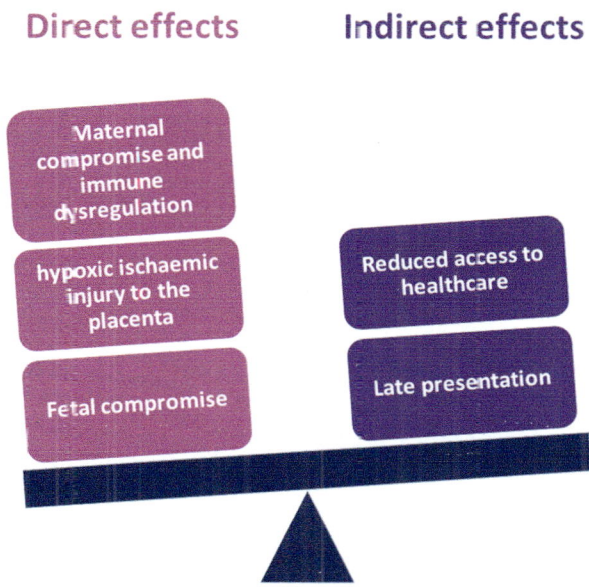

Fig. 12.2 Direct versus indirect effects of SARS-CoV-2 infection in pregnancy

COVID-19 infection in pregnancy was dangerous, and this further encouraged pregnant women to stay at home and shield [33]. Moreover, pregnant women were excluded from the initial randomised control trials into COVID-19 vaccinations [34]. This meant many pregnant women were vaccinated much later than their non-pregnant counterparts as there was limited information on the safety and efficacy of COVID-19 vaccines in pregnancy. All of these factors contributed to extreme hesitancy exercised by pregnant women to attend hospital for fear of COVID-19 [35].

Another reason that pregnant women may not have accessed healthcare during the pandemic is reduced transport facilities or a desire to avoid public transport. As mentioned above, pregnant women were hesitant to risk exposing themselves to COVID-19 disease and thus may have not travelled to hospital due to an inability to get to hospital without using public transport. Many public transport services were also significantly reduced during the pandemic due to little demand, making it harder for pregnant women to get to hospital [36].

Though undoubtedly, SARS-CoV-2 infection itself contributes directly to adverse pregnancy outcomes, there is no doubt that indirect effects of the pandemic, particularly reduced access to healthcare, have contributed to the increase in adverse pregnancy outcomes (Fig. 12.2).

Table 12.1 Preterm birth and COVID-19 in pregnancy: Bradford-Hill Criteria

Bradford-Hill Criteria in a nutshell	
Strength	Research repeatedly shows evidence of an association
Consistency	Earlier reports from the pandemic showed a possible decrease in COVID-19 and stillbirth, preterm birth and preeclampsia; however, later evidence repeatedly shows an increase.
Specificity	These conditions are all specific to pregnancy; however, there is overlap with the risk factors for COVID-19.
Temporality	SARS-CoV-2 infection in pregnancy precedes preterm birth and stillbirth. Evidence suggests that preeclampsia precedes COVID-19.
Biological gradient	Severe COVID-19 leads to more severe adverse pregnancy outcomes.
Plausibility	Placental changes and endothelial dysfunction have been found in SARS-CoV-2-infected pregnant patients.
Coherence	Experimental evidence and epidemiological evidence concur.
Experimental evidence	RCTs are not possible but further prospective cohort studies should take place.
Analogous evidence	Meta-analyses have taken place showing evidence of an association.
Reversibility	Pregnancy outcomes after COVID-19 vaccination are similar to pre-pandemic data.

12.6 Does COVID-19 Cause Preterm Birth, Preeclampsia and Stillbirth?

12.6.1 Bradford-Hill Criteria (Table 12.1)

12.6.1.1 Strength

Evidence is repeatedly showing an association between SARS-CoV-2 infection and adverse pregnancy outcomes including preterm birth, preeclampsia and stillbirth. As discussed previously in the 'evidence so far' discussion, evidence initially pointed to a decrease in preterm birth but has since pointed towards an increase in the incidence of preterm birth.

12.6.1.2 Consistency

Research varies—some show a decrease in incidence, some show no change and some show increase.

A systematic review published in 2020 of 24 studies including 324 pregnant women found no association between COVID-19 disease in pregnancy with preeclampsia and preterm birth [37]. This review was unable to draw firm conclusions, however, due to small sample sizes, inability to perform a meta-analysis and risk of bias [37].

A further systematic review of 42 studies including 438,548 people who were pregnant found that when compared with no SARS-CoV-2 in pregnancy, there was evidence of an association between COVID-19 and preeclampsia (OR 1.33, 95% CI 1.03–1.73), stillbirth (OR 2.11, 95% CI 1.14–3.90) and preterm birth (OR 1.82, 95% CI 1.38–2.39). When this association was assessed in severe versus mild

COVID-19, the association with preeclampsia (OR 4.16, 95% CI 1.55–11.15) and preterm birth (OR 4.29, 95% CI 2.41–7.63) was stronger [38].

The researchers performed sensitivity analysis which showed their results were reproducible and consistent and publication bias was assessed by using funnel plots. They used the Newcastle-Ottawa Scale to assess for bias and found that 95% of the included studies had low risk of bias and 5% had moderate risk [38].

In summary, although early evidence initially pointed to no association between COVID-19 in pregnancy, since then, much more evidence has emerged that points towards an association between COVID-19 in pregnancy and poor maternal and neonatal outcomes.

12.6.1.3 Specificity

Preterm birth, stillbirth and preeclampsia are all complications that are specific to pregnancy. Risk factors for preterm birth include previous preterm birth, maternal diabetes mellitus, antepartum bleeding, late commencement of prenatal care and Black and Hispanic ethnicity [39].

Some of these risk factors overlap with the risk factors for developing severe COVID-19 disease in pregnancy: diabetes mellitus and Black and Hispanic ethnicity [3]. This overlap between the risk factors for both conditions highlights that there is a potential for confounding of the association between COVID-19 disease in pregnancy and adverse pregnancy outcomes.

The INTERCOVID study, a prospective cohort study of the effects of COVID-19 in pregnancy and the neonatal period with 2184 pregnant women of which 725 had confirmed COVID-19 infection, adjusted their analysis of the association between COVID-19 and preeclampsia for risk factors known to be associated with preeclampsia. They found that even though there was a small reduction in the risk ratio, the results still showed evidence of a significant association between COVID-19 and preeclampsia, independent of confounding variables [15].

The systematic review by Wei et al. of 42 studies used unadjusted estimates for meta-analysis which may mean the effect sizes were overestimated. The researchers used the I^2 statistic to assess for heterogeneity in included studies and performed sensitivity analysis to exclude studies with moderate risk of bias [38].

12.6.1.4 Temporality

SARS-CoV-2 infection in pregnancy, by definition, precedes the outcomes of preterm birth and stillbirth. A systematic review of 111 studies including 42,752 pregnant women with COVID-19 performed comparative analysis between COVID-19-positive patients and confirmed negative patients and found that there was an increased risk of preterm birth and stillbirth in COVID-19-positive patients. They also found evidence of an increase in preeclampsia incidence among COVID-19-positive pregnant women; however it is unclear whether the diagnoses of COVID-19 infection preceded the diagnosis of preeclampsia. As a result, it is difficult to draw robust conclusions from this study [40].

The INTERCOVID study, a prospective longitudinal study, enrolled 2184 pregnant women of which 725 had confirmed COVID-19 infection. Pregnant women were followed from diagnosis of COVID-19 until hospital discharge [15]. The researchers found that COVID-19 is strongly associated with preeclampsia. They found that women with preeclampsia were mostly diagnosed with COVID-19 disease from 33 to 37 weeks' gestation whereas in women without preeclampsia, pregnant women were diagnosed with COVID-19 disease throughout pregnancy with a gradual, constant increase in diagnoses with increasing gestational age. Most commonly, pregnant women were diagnosed with COVID-19 in the last week of pregnancy. Although the pathophysiology of preeclampsia is not fully understood, researchers believe that it starts early in pregnancy in the first and early second trimesters [15]. Therefore, it is unlikely that COVID-19 infection this late in pregnancy would be on the etiologic pathway of preeclampsia. This points to preeclampsia leading to COVID-19 rather than the opposite.

12.6.1.5 Biological Gradient

Evidence shows more severe outcomes in pregnant women who suffered more severe SARS-CoV-2 infection. In the aforementioned systematic review by Wei et al., 28 studies compared confirmed SARS-CoV-2 infection with no infection in pregnancy. Thirteen studies compared severe versus mild COVID and the 12 remaining studies compared symptomatic versus asymptomatic SARS-CoV-2 infection. When the researchers compared mild COVID-19 with severe COVID-19, severe COVID-19 was strongly associated with preeclampsia and preterm birth (OR 4.16, 95% CI 1.55–11.15; $I^2 = 0\%$; based on five studies and OR 4.29, 95% CI 2.41–7.63; $I^2 = 61\%$; ten studies, respectively) [38].

A systematic review by Conde-Agudelo et al. of 790,954 pregnant women (15,524 with SARS-CoV-2 infection in pregnancy) also found that the association between SARS-CoV-2 infection in pregnancy was stronger in symptomatic patients versus asymptomatic patients (odds ratio, 1.59; 95% confidence interval, 1.21–2.10; and odds ratio, 2.11; 95% confidence interval, 1.59–2.81, respectively) [41].

This points to a dose-response relationship and provides more evidence to support a causal relationship between SARS-CoV-2 infection and adverse maternal outcomes.

12.7 Plausibility

As discussed, the exact mechanism by which SARS-CoV-2 caused preterm birth is unknown. This is also true for stillbirth and preeclampsia.

Like preterm birth, SARS-CoV-2 infection appears to cause placental changes in cases of stillbirth. SARS-CoV-2 appears to cause widespread placental destruction causing placental insufficiency. Researchers who studied 68 placentas from 64 stillbirths and four neonatal deaths found evidence of villous trophoblast necrosis and fibrin deposition in all of the placentas [42]. Almost all of the placentas (97%) also showed signs of histiocytic intervillositis. These together with villous trophoblast necrosis and fibrin deposition are the elements that define SARS-CoV-2 placentitis which causes severe destructive placental disease. They also found multiple intervillous thrombi in 37% of placentas. The researchers also performed 30 autopsies which highlighted that almost two-thirds (63%) showed signs of intrauterine hypoxia and asphyxia, but no other significant foetal abnormalities. It is hypothesised that the placental destruction caused by SARS-CoV-2 infection in turn leads to placental malperfusion and insufficiency. This causes hypoxic-ischaemic injury and is likely the cause of intrauterine death [42].

COVID-19 and preeclampsia appear to share similar disease pathophysiology—both appear to cause systemic endothelial dysfunction. SARS-CoV-2 gains access to cells via the ACE-2 receptor. ACE-2 is involved in the renin-angiotensin-aldosterone system in which it opposes ACE [43]. The end product of the renin-angiotensin-aldosterone system is angiotensin II. Angiotensin II leads to the increase in blood pressure via multiple mechanisms including vasoconstriction. Under normal circumstances, ACE-2 works to reduce the amount of angiotensin II by converting it to angiotensin which is a vasodilator and thus lowers the blood pressure. It has been hypothesised that this is the mechanism by which SARS-CoV-2 infection causes blood pressure dysfunction as lower amounts of ACE-2 lead to higher levels of angiotensin II circulating [43].

12.8 Coherence

As mentioned, laboratory evidence has shown systemic endothelial dysfunction and hypoxic ischaemic injury which results from SARS-CoV-2 infection [42]. This is consistent with the epidemiological data.

12.9 Experimental Evidence

It is neither feasible nor ethical to perform randomised control trials to examine this association. Evidence from cohort and case-control studies has shown an increase in COVID-19 disease and the adverse pregnancy outcomes mentioned: stillbirth, preterm birth and preeclampsia. Further prospective cohort studies could provide more evidence particularly as each new variant of COVID-19 disease emerges.

12.10 Analogous Evidence

As mentioned above, a meta-analysis of 42 studies involving 438,548 pregnant women identified higher incidence of preterm birth, stillbirth and preeclampsia in pregnant women with SARS-CoV-2 infection compared to non-infected pregnant women [38].

12.11 Reversibility

Vaccination against COVID-19 along with treatments for SARS-CoV-2 infection should reduce the risk of COVID-19 if SARS-CoV-2 infection does cause preeclampsia, stillbirth and preterm birth. Evidence from cohort studies has shown that women who received vaccination in pregnancy had similar pregnancy and neonatal outcomes to unvaccinated pregnant women without COVID-19 infection [35, 44].

12.12 Clinical Implications

It is interesting to consider the clinical implications of COVID-19 disease in pregnancy and the evidence that it may cause preterm birth. Countries have dealt with this differently, and there is variation in national and international guidelines.

In the early days of the pandemic, labour and delivery guidance were released. In this guidance, it was suggested that pregnant women who test positive were considered for induction of labour. This management has not been taken up in most countries, and induction of labour tends to only take place if there is maternal or foetal compromise [45].

There is also debate about prophylactic steroid use in pregnant women with SARS-CoV-2 infection. Corticosteroids are used in both COVID-19 treatment and in preterm birth to aid lung maturation. They are recommended in mechanically ventilated or oxygen requiring pregnant women with COVID-19. In most research, it is recommended to assess each individual case and discuss with the wider MDT (multi disciplinary team) before prescribing corticosteroids in COVID-19-positive pregnant women [46].

12.13 The Case for COVID Vaccination in Pregnancy

The WHO has called for all pregnant women to be fast-tracked to receive vaccines in the initial vaccine and subsequent booster rollout [47]. However, this is a long overdue and as is often the case, pregnant women were neglected in initial research into the COVID-19 vaccine. The initial randomised controlled trials into the COVID-19 vaccine excluded pregnant women, and for a long time, only limited information was available for pregnant women about the safety and efficacy of the COVID-19 vaccine [48].

The COVID-19 vaccines have been shown to reduce COVID-19 infection and severity, making hospital admission and admission to ICU (intensive care unit) much less likely if pregnant women are infected with SARS-COV-2 [49]. However, hesitancy and poor uptake of COVID-19 vaccine in pregnant women remain a problem. In August 2021, only 23% of women aged 35–39 who gave birth in Scotland had received both doses of COVID-19 vaccination according to data from the Public Health Scotland [50].

Given the considerable risks of SARS-CoV-2 infection in pregnancy both to the pregnant woman and to the foetus, it is paramount that pregnant women are encouraged to accept COVID-19 vaccine. Research has shown that COVID-19 vaccination in pregnancy has no effect on maternal and neonatal outcomes and is safe in pregnancy [51]. Although data from randomised controlled trials has not yet been published (they are underway [52, 53]), systematic review and meta-analysis, synthesising evidence from multiple cohort and case-control studies has been undertaken. Given COVID-19 vaccine is likely to be safe in pregnancy [51], it is really vital to educate pregnant women and prioritise them in vaccine rollout efforts as the potential adverse consequences of SARS-CoV-2 infection in pregnancy are great and may be stopped by receipt of a vaccine.

One of the reasons pregnant women have been hesitant to accept a COVID-19 vaccine is lack of information. This includes lack of information and guidance from healthcare professionals including midwives and doctors [35]. Medical professionals have a duty to educate themselves on the COVID-19 vaccine in pregnancy in order to be able to communicate with pregnant women and guide their decision-making.

Unfortunately, however, there is health inequity in vaccine availability. The percentage of population who have had one dose of a COVID-19 vaccine is much lower in low-income and middle-income (LMIC) countries when compared to high-income countries, despite lower vaccine hesitancy in LMIC. Conversely, maternal mortality due to COVID-19 is much higher in LMIC—almost a tenfold increase in Mexico (149 per 100,000) compared to the USA (15 per 100,000) [21, 54]. As a result, the number needed to treat to benefit with a COVID vaccine is much lower in LMIC. This is a huge opportunity for health equity, and the global health community must respond and ensure vaccination is readily available in LMIC.

12.14 Lessons Learned from the COVID-19 Pandemic

As the acute phase of the COVID-19 pandemic passes, it is important to reflect and consider lessons learned from the pandemic. One particular lesson is that pregnant women must not be overlooked as individuals. As pregnant women are predominantly young, fit and healthy, this can lead them to be overlooked in research and care in evolving situations. For example, as discussed, pregnant women were excluded from the initial randomised control trials into the COVID-19 vaccine in pregnancy. This led to slow uptake of the COVID-19 vaccine amongst pregnant women and thus may have led to multiple adverse outcomes including preeclampsia, preterm birth and stillbirth that could have potentially been prevented. Although this is a lesson to be learned from the pandemic, it is not a new phenomenon—pregnant women are often overlooked in research although they are a vulnerable population [54].

Another lesson to be learned is the importance of communication and messaging for pregnant women. Many pregnant women were unsure whether they needed to shield or not in the early days of the pandemic and later they were unsure whether or not to accept a COVID-19 vaccine [55]. Although healthcare professionals were also limited by the dearth of information available about SARS-CoV-2 infection when it first emerged, it is important to recognise that we are in positions of authority to guide and help pregnant women and we have a duty to educate ourselves in order to help in the decision-making and advise pregnant women where possible.

References

1. Ritchie H, Ortiz-Ospina E, Beltekian D. Coronavirus pandemic (COVID-19). 2021. https://ourworldindata.org/coronavirus. Accessed 1 Feb 2022.
2. Chmielewska B, Barratt I, Townsend R, et al. Effects of the COVID-19 pandemic on maternal and perinatal outcomes: a systematic review and meta-analysis [published correction appears in Lancet Glob Health. 2021;9(6): e758]. Lancet Glob Health. 2021;9(6):e759–72. https://doi.org/10.1016/S2214-109X(21)00079-6.
3. Mahase E. Covid-19: pregnant women with virus are more likely to need intensive care, study finds. BMJ. 2020;370:m3391. https://doi.org/10.1136/bmj.m3391.
4. Simmons LE, Rubens CE, Darmstadt GL. Preventing preterm birth and neonatal mortality: exploring the epidemiology, causes, and interventions. Semin Perinatol. 2010;34(6):408–15. https://doi.org/10.1053/j.semperi.2010.09.005, ISSN 0146-0005.
5. Klumper J, Kazemier BM, Been JV, et al. Association between COVID-19 lockdown measures and the incidence of iatrogenic versus spontaneous very preterm births in the Netherlands: a retrospective study. BMC Pregnan Childb. 2021;21:767. https://doi.org/10.1186/s12884-021-04249-8.
6. Berghella V, Boelig R, Roman A, Burd J, Anderson K. Decreased incidence of preterm birth during coronavirus disease 2019 pandemic. Am J Obstet Gynecol MFM. 2020;2(4):100258. https://doi.org/10.1016/j.ajogmf.2020.100258.
7. Gurol-Urganci I, Waite L, Webster K, et al. Obstetric interventions and pregnancy outcomes during the COVID-19 pandemic in England: a nationwide cohort study. PLoS Med. 2022;19(1):e1003884. https://doi.org/10.1371/journal.pmed.1003884.
8. Khalil A, Kalafat E, Benlioglu C, O'Brien P, Morris E, Draycott T, Thangaratinam S, Le Doare K, Heath P, Ladhani S, von Dadelszen P, Magee LA. SARS-CoV-2 infection in pregnancy: a systematic review and meta-analysis of clinical features and pregnancy outcomes. EClinicalMedicine. 2020;25:100446. https://doi.org/10.1016/j.eclinm.2020.100446. Epub 2020. PMID: 32838230; PMCID: PMC7334039.

9. Ashish KC, Gurung R, Kinney MV, et al. Effect of the COVID-19 pandemic response on intrapartum care, stillbirth, and neonatal mortality outcomes in Nepal: a prospective observational study. Lancet Glob Health. 2020;8(10):e1273–81. https://doi.org/10.1016/S2214-109X(20)30345-4, ISSN 2214-109X.
10. Cruz Melguizo S, de la Cruz Conty ML, Carmona Payán P, et al. Pregnancy outcomes and SARS-CoV-2 infection: the Spanish Obstetric Emergency Group Study. Viruses. 2021;13(5):853. https://doi.org/10.3390/v13050853.
11. Metz TD, Clifton RG, Hughes BL, et al. Disease severity and perinatal outcomes of pregnant patients with coronavirus disease 2019 (COVID-19). Obstet Gynecol. 2021;137(4):571–80. https://doi.org/10.1097/AOG.0000000000004339.
12. Gurol-Urganci I, Jardine JE, Carroll F, et al. Maternal and perinatal outcomes of pregnant women with SARS-CoV-2 infection at the time of birth in England: national cohort study. Am J Obstet Gynecol. 2021;225(5):522.e1–522.e11. https://doi.org/10.1016/j.ajog.2021.05.016.
13. Bunnell ME, Koenigs KJ, Roberts DJ, Quade BJ, Hornick JL, Goldfarb IT. Third trimester stillbirth during the first wave of the SARS-CoV-2 pandemic: similar rates with increase in placental vasculopathic pathology. Placenta. 2021;109:72–4. https://doi.org/10.1016/j.placenta.2021.04.003.
14. Wong YP, Khong TY, Tan GC. The effects of COVID-19 on placenta and pregnancy: what do we know so far? Diagnostics. 2021;11(1):94. https://doi.org/10.3390/diagnostics11010094.
15. Papageorghiou AT, Deruelle P, Gunier RB, et al. Preeclampsia and COVID-19: results from the INTERCOVID prospective longitudinal study. Am J Obstet Gynecol. 2021;225(3):289.e1–289.e17. https://doi.org/10.1016/j.ajog.2021.05.014.
16. Bahrami R, Schwartz DA, Karimi-Zarchi M, et al. Meta-analysis of the frequency of intrauterine growth restriction and preterm premature rupture of the membranes in pregnant women with COVID-19. Turk J Obstet Gynecol. 2021;18(3):236–44. https://doi.org/10.4274/tjod.galenos.2021.74829.
17. Einarsdóttir K, Swift EM, Zoega H. Changes in obstetric interventions and preterm birth during COVID-19: a nationwide study from Iceland. Acta Obstet Gynecol Scand. 2021;100:1924–30. https://doi.org/10.1111/aogs.14231.
18. Karasek D, Baer R, McLemore M, et al. The Association of COVID-19 Infection in Pregnancy with Preterm Birth: a retrospective cohort study in California. Lancet Reg Health Am. 2021;2:100027.
19. Martinez-Perez O, Prats Rodriguez P, Muner Hernandez M, et al. The association between SARS-CoV-2 infection and preterm delivery: a prospective study with a multivariable analysis. BMC Pregnan Childb. 2021;21:273. https://doi.org/10.1186/s12884-021-03742-4.
20. Chen X, Zhang X, Li W, et al. Iatrogenic vs. spontaneous preterm birth: a retrospective study of neonatal outcome among very preterm infants. Front Neurol. 2021;12:649749. https://doi.org/10.3389/fneur.2021.649749.
21. Zambrano LD, Ellington S, Strid P, et al. Update: characteristics of symptomatic women of reproductive age with laboratory-confirmed SARS-CoV-2 infection by pregnancy status - United States, January 22-October 3, 2020. MMWR Morb Mortal Wkly Rep. 2020;69(44):1641–7. https://doi.org/10.15585/mmwr.mm6944e3.
22. Rad HS, Röhl J, Stylianou N, et al. The effects of COVID-19 on the placenta during pregnancy. Front Immunol. 2021;12:743022. https://doi.org/10.3389/fimmu.2021.743022.
23. Varnier N, Brown MA, Reynolds M, et al. Indications for delivery in pre-eclampsia. Pregnan Hypertens. 2018;11:12–7. https://doi.org/10.1016/j.preghy.2017.11.004.
24. Gravett MG, Rubens CE, Nunes TM, et al. Global report on preterm birth and stillbirth (2 of 7): discovery science. BMC Pregnan Childb. 2010;10:S2. https://doi.org/10.1186/1471-2393-10-S1-S2.
25. Mishra KP, Singh AK, Singh SB. Hyperinflammation and Immune Response Generation in COVID-19. Neuroimmunomodulation. 2020;27(2):80–6. https://doi.org/10.1159/000513198.
26. Menon R, Richardson LS. Preterm prelabor rupture of the membranes: a disease of the fetal membranes. Semin Perinatol. 2017;41(7):409–19. https://doi.org/10.1053/j.semperi.2017.07.012.

27. Chernyak BV, Popova EN, Prikhodko AS, Grebenchikov OA, Zinovkina LA, Zinovkin RA. COVID-19 and oxidative stress. Biochemistry. 2020;85(12):1543–53. https://doi.org/10.1134/S0006297920120068.
28. Garcia-Flores V, Romero R, Xu Y, et al. Maternal-fetal immune responses in pregnant women infected with SARS-CoV-2. Nat Commun. 2022;13:320. https://doi.org/10.1038/s41467-021-27745-z.
29. Jardine J, Relph S, Magee LA, von Dadelszen P, Morris E, Ross-Davie M, Draycott T, Khalil A. Maternity services in the UK during the coronavirus disease 2019 pandemic: a national survey of modifications to standard care. BJOG. 2021;128:880–9.
30. Su Z, McDonnell D, Wen J, et al. Mental health consequences of COVID-19 media coverage: the need for effective crisis communication practices. Glob Health. 2021;17:4. https://doi.org/10.1186/s12992-020-00654-4.
31. Vera San Juan N, Clark SE, Camilleri M, et al. Training and redeployment of healthcare workers to intensive care units (ICUs) during the COVID-19 pandemic: a systematic review. BMJ Open. 2022;12:e050038. https://doi.org/10.1136/bmjopen-2021-050038.
32. Khalil A, Blakeway H, Samara A, O'Brien P. COVID-19 and stillbirth: direct vs indirect effect of the pandemic. Ultrasound Obstet Gynecol. 2022;59:288–95. https://doi.org/10.1002/uog.24846.
33. GOV.UK. Coronarvrius (COVID-19): advice for pregnant employees. 2022. www.gov.uk. Accessed 1 Mar 2022.
34. Clinical Trials Arena. Lack of trials in pregnant people driving Covid-19 vaccine hesitancy. n.d. clinicaltrialsarena.com.
35. Blakeway H, Prasad S, Kalafat E, et al. COVID-19 vaccination during pregnancy: coverage and safety. Am J Obstet Gynecol. 2022;226(2):236.e1–236.e14. https://doi.org/10.1016/j.ajog.2021.08.007.
36. Marra AD, Sun L, Corman F. The impact of COVID-19 pandemic on public transport usage and route choice: evidences from a long-term tracking study in urban area. Transp Policy. 2022;116:258–68. https://doi.org/10.1016/j.tranpol.2021.12.009, ISSN 0967-070X.
37. Juan J, Gil MM, Rong Z, Zhang Y, Yang H, Poon LC. Effect of coronavirus disease 2019 (COVID-19) on maternal, perinatal and neonatal outcome: systematic review. Ultrasound Obstet Gynecol. 2020;56:15–27. https://doi.org/10.1002/uog.22088.
38. Wei SQ, Bilodeau-Bertrand M, Liu S, Auger N. The impact of COVID-19 on pregnancy outcomes: a systematic review and meta-analysis. CMAJ. 2021;193(16):E540–8. https://doi.org/10.1503/cmaj.202604.
39. ACOG. Preterm labor and birth. Preterm labor and birth. Washington, DC: ACOG; 2022. Accessed 2 Feb 2022.
40. Marchand G, Patil AS, Masoud AT, et al. Systematic review and meta-analysis of COVID-19 maternal and neonatal clinical features and pregnancy outcomes up to June 3, 2021. AJOG Glob Rep. 2022;2(1):100049. https://doi.org/10.1016/j.xagr.2021.100049.
41. Conde-Agudelo A, Romero R. SARS-CoV-2 infection during pregnancy and risk of preeclampsia: a systematic review and meta-analysis. Am J Obstet Gynecol. 2022;226(1):68–89.e3. https://doi.org/10.1016/j.ajog.2021.07.009.
42. Schwartz DA, Avvad-Portari E, Babál P. Placental tissue destruction and insufficiency from COVID-19 causes stillbirth and neonatal death from hypoxic-ischemic injury: a study of 68 cases with SARS-CoV-2 placentitis from 12 countries. Arch Pathol Lab Med. 2022;146:660. https://doi.org/10.5858/arpa.2022-0029-SA.
43. Bhalla V, Blish CA, South AM. A historical perspective on ACE2 in the COVID-19 era. J Hum Hypertens. 2020;35:935–9.
44. Lipkind HS, Vazquez-Benitez G, DeSilva M, et al. Receipt of COVID-19 vaccine during pregnancy and preterm or small-for-gestational-age at birth - Eight Integrated Health Care

Organizations, United States, December 15, 2020-July 22, 2021. MMWR Morb Mortal Wkly Rep. 2022;71(1):26–30. https://doi.org/10.15585/mmwr.mm7101e1.
45. Boelig RC, Manuck T, Oliver EA. Di Mascio D, Saccone G, Bellussi F, Berghella V. Labor and delivery guidance for COVID-19. Am J Obstetr Gynecol MFM. 2020;2(2 Suppl):100110. https://doi.org/10.1016/j.ajogmf.2020.100110, ISSN 2589-9333.
46. D'Souza R, Ashraf R, Rowe H, Zipursky J, Clarfield L, Maxwell C, Arzola C, Lapinsky S, Paquette K, Murthy S, Cheng MP, Malhamé I. Pregnancy and COVID-19: pharmacologic considerations. Ultrasound Obstet Gynecol. 2021;57:195–203. https://doi.org/10.1002/uog.23116.
47. WHO. Coronavirus disease (COVID-19): vaccines. 2022. https://www.who.int/emergencies/diseases/novel-coronavirus-2019/question-and-answers-hub/q-a-detail/coronavirus-disease-(covid-19)-vaccines?adgroupsurvey={adgroupsurvey}&gclid=CjwKCAiA4KaRBhBdEiwAZi1zzjh1CxKHnBp6GgIz3XKMm5J7eHPhF5l2PEk3tAxc9ZbzU_W4ZuJ0wxoC3kEQAvD_BwEREF. Accessed 8 Feb 2022.
48. van der Zande ISE, van der Graaf R, Oudijk MA, van Delden JJM. Vulnerability of pregnant women in clinical research. J Med Ethics. 2017;43(10):657–63. https://doi.org/10.1136/medethics-2016-103955.
49. GOV.UK. New UKHSA study provides more safety data on COVID-19 vaccines in pregnancy. 2021. https://www.gov.uk/government/news/new-ukhsa-study-provides-more-safety-data-on-covid-19-vaccines-in-pregnancy. Accessed 2 Jan 2021.
50. Iacobucci G. Covid-19 and pregnancy: vaccine hesitancy and how to overcome it. BMJ. 2021;375:2862. https://doi.org/10.1136/bmj.n2862.
51. Shimabukuro TT, Kim SY, Myers TR, et al. Preliminary Findings of mRNA Covid-19 Vaccine Safety in Pregnant Persons. N Engl J Med. 2021;384(24):2273–82. https://doi.org/10.1056/NEJMoa2104983. Published correction appears in N Engl J Med. 2021;385(16):1536.
52. National Institutes of Health. NIH begins study of COVID-19 vaccination during pregnancy and postpartum. Washington, DC: US Department of Health and Human Services; 2021. https://www.nih.gov/news-events/news-releases/nih-begins-study-covid-19-vaccination-during-pregnancy-postpartum. Accessed 1 Jan 2022.
53. US National Library of Medicine. ClinicalTrials.gov. A study of Ad26.COV2.S in healthy pregnant participants (COVID-19) (HORIZON 1). Bethesda, MD: NLM; 2021. https://clinicaltrials.gov/ct2/show/NCT04765384. Accessed 3 Jan 2022.
54. Martinez-Portilla RJ, Sotiriadis A, Chatzakis C, et al. Pregnant women with SARS-CoV-2 infection are at higher risk of death and pneumonia: propensity score matched analysis of a nationwide prospective cohort (COV19Mx). Ultrasound Obstet Gynecol. 2021;57:224–31.
55. Anderson E, Brigden A, Davies A, et al. Pregnant women's experiences of social distancing behavioural guidelines during the Covid-19 pandemic 'lockdown' in the UK, a qualitative interview study. BMC Public Health. 2021;21:1202. https://doi.org/10.1186/s12889-021-11202-z.

Chapter 13
Management of Neonatal Care During COVID19 Pandemics

Manuel Sánchez Luna and Belén Fernández Colomer

13.1 Introduction

From the beginning of the pandemic declaration of the COVID-19, much has been learned about neonatal impact of the infection. Although vertical transmission from the mother to her neonate is a potential route of infection either in utero, intrapartum, or postnatal, majority of newborn cases of COVID-19 are acquired like other respiratory virus infection. Concern about the risk of neonatal infection through the infected mother was high when no epidemiological data was available, and close contact at delivery and breastfeeding were initially prevented. But after the first

---

On behalf of the SENEO Infection Workgroup*

*Concepción de Alba Romero, Ana Alarcón Allen, Ana Baña Souto, Fátima Camba Longueira, María Cernada Badía, Zenaida Galve Pradell, María González López, M. Cruz López Herrera, Carmen Ribes Bautista, Laura Sánchez García, Elena Zamora Flores

---

M. S. Luna (✉)
Pediatrics, Complutense University of Madrid, Madrid, Spain

Research Institute Gregorio Marañón, Madrid, Spain

Spanish National Society of Neonatology (SENEO), Barcelona, Spain

Neonatology Division and NICU, Hospital General Universitario "Gregorio Marañón", Madrid, Spain
e-mail: msluna@salud.madrid.org

B. F. Colomer
Pediatrics, Oviedo University, Oviedo, Spain

Neonatology Unit, HUCA, Oviedo, Spain

Infection Workgroup of the Spanish National Society of Neonatology (SENEO), Barcelona, Spain

© The Author(s), under exclusive license to Springer Nature Switzerland AG 2023
D. De Luca, A. Benachi (eds.), *COVID-19 and Perinatology*,
https://doi.org/10.1007/978-3-031-29136-4_13

reports of the safety of close care and breastfeeding, this approach was recommended [1].

WHO encouraged to initiate and continue breastfeeding in mothers with suspected or confirmed COVID-19 [2], due to the benefits of breastfeeding, while adhering to infection prevention and control measurement by the breastfeeding mother [3], and although the virus and viral fragments have been detected in breast milk, there is a low risk of transmission of the SARS Cov2 in breastfed infants [4].

These recommendations of no separation and promoting breastfeeding were adopted in Spain by the Spanish Society of Neonatology (*Sociedad Española de Neonatología*, SENEO), and to better understand the epidemiology of the disease in newborns, a nationwide registry aimed to collect real-time data of neonates born to mothers diagnosed with COVID-19 during pregnancy or in the immediate postpartum period was prospectively conducted by the SENEO. The registry was started at the beginning of the pandemic, in March 2020, and was kept working until the end of the Omicron wave. Initial results of the first wave from 503 neonates born to 497 mothers diagnosed with COVID-19 during pregnancy or at the time of delivery indicated that there is no need of separation of mothers from neonates allowing delaying cord clamping and skin-to-skin contact, with maintenance of breastfeeding in a high percentage of newborns from COVID-19 mothers [5].

At the end of the sixth wave, similar data from the registry corroborate former results but with a substantial decrease in the rate of severe maternal disease and prematurity. In a second SENEO registry of neonates with postnatal hospital-acquired or community-acquired SARS-CoV-2 infection, most of the infected newborns appear to have a mild or asymptomatic disease during the first wave of the disease [6], and after the sixth wave, similar results were found.

In this chapter, data from the Spanish nationwide registry of neonatal COVID-19 will be presented and discussed, together with the most recent evidence of the disease in neonates.

13.2 Mothers with Perinatal COVID-19 Infection and Neonatal Outcome

A potential mechanism of perinatal transmission is well described (for more details, see also Chap. 9), and although the SARS-CoV-2 has been found in the placenta [7–9], newborn vertical infection is rare [4, 5].

Pregnant women with the COVID-19 are more likely to suffer a more serious disease compared to nonpregnant women with COVID-19, more pregnancy complications (general and obstetric), and higher cesarean delivery rate and death [10–12]. Premature delivery rate has also been significantly increased in these women mostly due to the need of gestation termination because of the severity of the maternal respiratory failure. Consequently, a higher rate of adverse outcomes in neonates to mothers with COVID-19 was also detected [10].

In a multicentric observational study of Spanish hospitals, during the first wave, 30.8% of pregnant women had pneumonia, and 4.8% women were admitted to the intensive care unit needing invasive mechanical ventilation, with five times increased risk of cesarean sections than those without pneumonia in the univariable analysis (OR: 5.0 [2.0; 12.2], p-value <0.001), and lower gestational age at delivery with a preterm birth rate of 20.6%, associated to maternal pneumonia [13].

After the first wave, in a population-based cohort study in England, between May 29, 2020, and January 31, 2021, the risk of neonatal adverse outcome was significantly higher for infants with mothers with laboratory-confirmed SARS-CoV-2 infection. But for neonates born at term, they were only more likely to have prolonged admission after birth, so neonatal morbidity was mostly related to the rate of premature delivery, with no additional adverse neonatal outcomes [14].

The Spanish Society of Neonatology (SENEO) developed a nationwide prospective online case registration system aimed to collect real-time data of neonates born to mothers diagnosed with COVID-19 during pregnancy or in the immediate postpartum period. SENEO executive committee members reviewed the literature and designed the items that should be entered into the database, which was accessible from the SENEO website to all neonatology departments in Spain.

The registry adapted the WHO classification system [3] about the vertical transmission of SARS-CoV-2 to better allow comparison of data from various studies.

The first 503 neonates born to COVID-19-positive mothers ($n = 497$) from 79 hospitals throughout Spain were recently published [5]. According to official data of the National Epidemiological Surveillance Network from the Spanish Ministry of Health, data extracted on May 29, 2020, including a total of 250,273 cases of COVID-19 notified up to May 11, 2020, with 18,975 deaths and 86,488 hospital admissions, representing the first wave of the disease.

The clinical impact of the COVID-19 in pregnant women was higher at the beginning of the pandemic and most women acquired COVID-19 during the third trimester of pregnancy, usually presented with mild symptoms (fever, cough, malaise).

At the end of the first wave, almost one-half of women (49.3%) did not present symptom at the time of delivery, and COVID-19 was detected because of the new recommendations established in the country to screen SARS CoV2 in all women admitted to the hospital for labor. Because of this new strategy, the percentage of asymptomatic women increase from 21.8% in March to 56.6% in April and up to 65.5% in May.

At this time, a total of 164 women (33%) delivered by cesarean section, one-half of them on an emergency basis and 76% due to obstetric factors. Maternal COVID-19 infection was the indication of cesarean section in 39 cases (23.8%), 81.5% of which had moderate or severe COVID-19.

Currently, the registry collected data from April 2020 to March 2022, including more than 4600 women (4720 mother-newborn dyads) with COVID-19 during pregnancy (all gestational trimester).

Asymptomatic (50.0%) and mild disease occurred in 92% of cases, but severe disease (1.6% of cases) was eight times higher than the general population in the same age group.

Table 13.1 shows the comparison of severe COVID-19 cases versus the other forms of the disease.

Global cesarean delivery rate was 23.0% (lower than pre-pandemic rates), and 76.0% of all were in severe cases (Table 13.1). Prematurity rate (10.2%) was higher than pre-pandemic years (7.4%) and was associated to more severe COVID-19 disease (Table 13.1). Of interest is that the rate of prematurity decreased along the registry period (10.6% in 2020 and 8.9% in 2021) (Fig. 13.1).

Table 13.1 Comparison of clinical and perinatal characteristics of pregnant women with severe vs. nonsevere COVID-19

	Mother severe cases ($N = 73$)	Mother nonsevere cases ($N = 4579$)	p
Mother age (median)	32 years	31 years	N.S.
COVID-19 infection during gestation	81% third trimester	74% third trimester	<0.01
Previous morbidity			
• None	42 (57.5%)	3.369 (73.5%)	0.002
• Obesity	17 (23.3%)	309 (6.7%)	<0.0001
Gestational pathology			
• None	58 (79%)	3628 (79%)	N.S.
• Preeclampsia	6 (8.2%)	156 (3.4%)	<0.05
Cesarean delivery rate	56 (76%)	994 (21%)	<0.0001
Prematurity rate	50 (68%)	381 (8.3%)	<0.0001

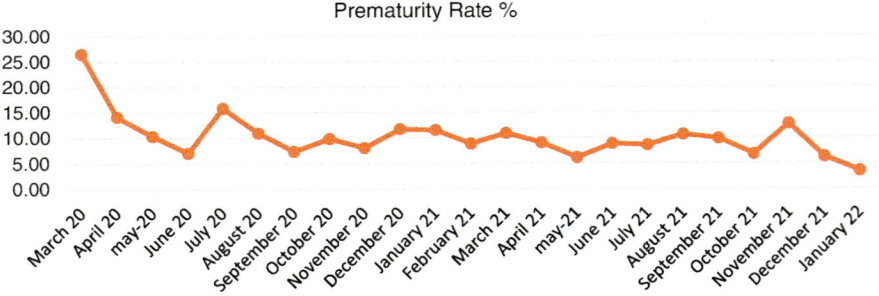

Fig. 13.1 Rate of prematurity (%) in the Spanish Registry, by month, from March 2020 to January 2022 (Data from the Spanish Registry)

13.3 Neonatal Infection

To date, SARS-CoV-2 infection rates are low in babies born to mothers with SARS-CoV-2 infection [5].

In a large systematic review and meta-analysis, SARS-CoV-2 positivity using RT-PCR was observed in 1.8% (95% confidence interval: 1.2–2.5%) of all babies ($n = 14,271$) born to mothers with a diagnosis of SARS-CoV-2 infection (140 cohort studies) [13].

In fact, the fetus and the newborn could be protected by the antibody response (including IgM, IgG, and IgA) observed in the serum and milk of mothers infected with SARS-CoV2 during pregnancy [15, 16].

It has been demonstrated that a maternal SARS-CoV-2 IgG efficiently transferred across the placenta when infection occurs more than 2 months before delivery, and it is proposed that maternally derived passive immunity may persist in infants up to 6 months of life [17].

Probably because of this, most of the neonatal cases reported are rather related to postnatal transmission by the usual mechanisms (aerosols, fomites) and by family members or caregivers in contact with the newborn.

During the first wave, the Spanish Registry showed a premature and very premature birth rates of 15.7% and 5.2%, respectively. 50% of newborns were left for skin-to-skin contact after delivery, delayed clamping of umbilical cords was performed in 42.9% of neonates, and 62% of babies born at term did not require any resuscitation.

PCR-positive mothers used facemasks and hand hygiene when having skin-to-skin contact with their newborns, the clinical course of neonates was generally favorable, and less than 40% of them required hospital admission, with the lack of hospital infrastructure for safe practice of rooming-in as the reason for admission in most of the cases, particularly during the first weeks of the pandemic COVID-19. In these cases, however, the length of hospital stay was less than 3 days [5].

During this first wave, in the first test of viral RNA (PCR of nasopharyngeal swabs) collected in the neonate at a median age of 3 h after delivery (1–12 h), there were 14 positive samples of the 469 nasopharyngeal swabs (positive rate, 3.0%).

However, repeating the test in a second PCR testing in all these 14 cases, done 24–48 h later, 12 samples gave negative results (a third PCR testing in nasopharyngeal swabs carried out in some of these cases gave also negative results). In all these cases, newborns were asymptomatic. The remaining two cases were one baby born at term by cesarean section, without skin-to-skin contact and admitted separated from his mother (mild symptoms) immediately after delivery. The baby remained asymptomatic, the first PCR test was performed at 10 h of age, and the second PCR performed at 8 days during outpatient follow-up gave negative results.

Currently, the Spanish Registry included 4,720 neonates born to women with COVID-19 during pregnancy. Eighty-five percent were healthy newborns at or near term who had no problems at birth. Rest of newborns (15%) required admission to the neonatal ward either because of their prematurity or due to other standard neonatal pathologies.

A total of 2,874 neonates were tested for SARS-CoV-2 in nasopharyngeal swabs in the first 24–48 h of life (the remained 1,846 were not tested because COVID-19 was not active in the mother at delivery).

One hundred and seven neonates resulted positive in a first PCR test (median age of 4 h after delivery), but 92 of them were considered false positives or transient colonization. Only 15 neonates were considered true positive.

Also, in a second PCR test (median age of 48 h after delivery), 27 neonates previously negative became positive.

Therefore, transmission rate was 1.4% of tested newborn (42/2,874) and 0.9% overall. Of the 42 true positive neonates, 35 remained asymptomatic (eight were admitted in the neonatal unit because of prematurity, jaundice, or congenital defect).

The remaining seven cases were all admitted in the neonatal unit, two term twins with hypoxic ischemic encephalopathy, four (three term and one preterm) with mild respiratory distress syndrome, and one preterm neonate with periventricular lesions in cranial ultrasound. Table 13.2 shows perinatal characteristics of negative versus positive neonates.

Noteworthy, the registry data showed that mothers from neonates with a positive PCR test got infected near delivery, suffered frequently more severe disease, and had lower transmission rate of antibodies (which is expected since maternal infection is very close to delivery).

There were no significant differences on the prematurity rate, although it was higher during the first wave of the pandemic (Fig. 13.1). Indeed, premature delivery was associated to the severity of COVID-19 in mothers (Fig. 13.2). Also this

Table 13.2 Comparison of perinatal characteristics of newborn with positive vs. negative SARS-CoV-2 test

	Positive PCR test in the newborn ($n = 42$)	Negative PCR test in the newborn ($n = 4678$)	p
COVID-19 infection during gestation	Third trimester—100%	Third trimester—74%	0.001
Number of days before delivery at maternal COVID-19 diagnosis (median)	5 [1–8]	60 [15–120]	0.0001
Prematurity rate (%)	9.5	10.0	N.S.
Severe maternal disease (%)	4.8%	1.5%	0.1
Cesarean delivery rate	36%	23%	0.05
Neonatal resuscitation at delivery (any)	21.4%	12.6%	0.001
Skin-to-skin care	69%	78%	0.1
Neonatal hospital admission rate	36%	18%	0.02
Positive mother IgG rate	1/12 (8%)	1205/1660 (72%)	0.0
Newborn with IgG+	5/14 (36%)	479/731 (65%)	0.003
Breastfeeding rate	69%	85%	0.005

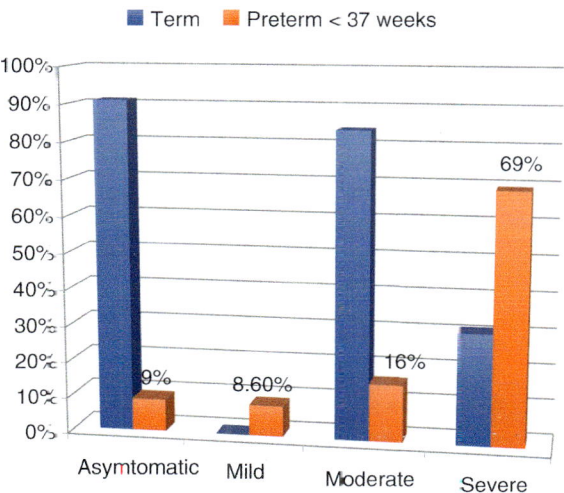

Fig. 13.2 COVID-19 severity in pregnancy and % of premature neonates <37 weeks (Data form the Spanish Registry)

relation of COVID severity in the mother and higher prematurity risk was found in other nationwide registries [18].

Compared to neonates infected with SARS-CoV-2, in the immediate perinatal period, those infected later both at home (community-acquired infection) and at the hospital (nosocomial-acquired infection) were more frequently detected.

The preliminary results of this group of later-infected neonates, from the Spanish Registry [6], during the first wave (40 cases) showed mild clinical manifestations of infection in neonates (two acquired in the community and eight nosocomial). Severe forms and requiring admission to NICU were usually associated with prematurity or concomitant pathologies [6].

Currently, there are 162 cases of neonates infected with SARS-CoV-2 (136 community-acquired and 26 nosocomial); 12 of which were detected in the follow-up from birth because they were born to COVID-19 mothers.

Of interest is that most of the community-acquired cases were during the first year of the pandemic, in 2020, and the mean age of the diagnosis was 16 days (range 10–22 days).

The focus of the infection of these children was their parents or relatives. This data is like the first analysis with an asymptomatic rate of 20% (45% in nosocomial cases) and more than 70% of mild cases (mainly in the form of upper respiratory airways infection). Only 8% (11 out of 136 community-acquired cases) required admission to NICU with the most common diagnosis as pneumonia, but none of them required invasive mechanical ventilation, with a mean stay in the ICU of 14 days (8–23 days). There was no newborn demise. Of the 26 nosocomial cases, 57% were premature newborns and 46% were asymptomatic. All cases had a good prognosis.

13.4 Neonatal Care

After the first weeks of the beginning of the pandemic, the Spanish National Society of Neonatology, following official agencies' recommendations and current evidence [2, 19–22] recommended to delay umbilical cord clamping and skin-to-skin care after delivery, avoid the separation of the mother and her newborn, and promote breast feeding [22]. This situation was later adopted by other international guidelines [1].

Figure 13.3 shows the Spanish Society of Neonatology recommendations for perinatal management of children born to COVID-19 mothers, which were based in two main principles: to avoid mother-newborn separation (if allowed by their clinical situation and regardless SARS-CoV-2 test result for the newborn) and to promote breastfeeding. In this situation, it is essential to support and to inform parents about preventive hygiene measures to get a safe practice. Neonatal testing and diagnosis should follow the WHO definition principles for neonatal SARS-CoV-2 infections (See Chap. 12).

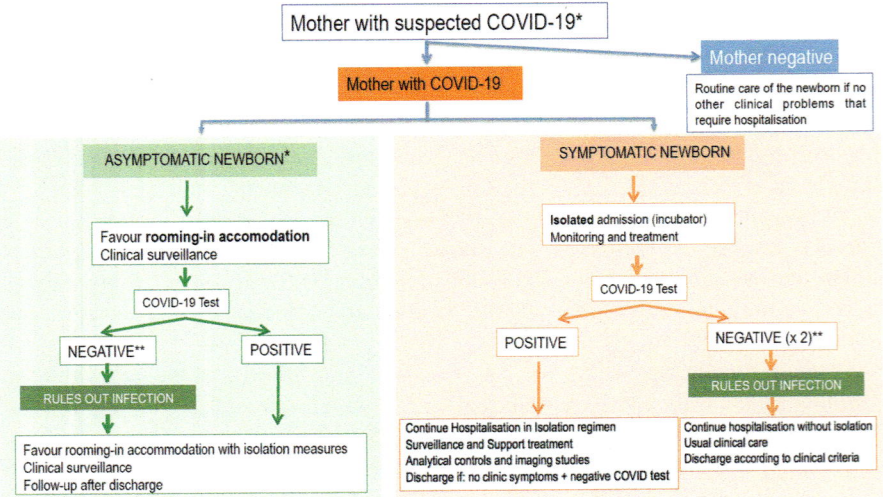

Fig. 13.3 Flow chart algorithm from the Spanish Society of Neonatology, SENEO, for neonates born to COVID-19 mothers. *In cases of mothers who are positive or under investigation, if the mother is pauci- or asymptomatic and the newborn is asymptomatic, joint accommodation with contact and droplet isolation between mother and child (hand hygiene, face mask, and cradle 2 m from the mother's bed) is recommended. If the mother is symptomatic (fever, cough, and respiratory secretions), the newborn should be admitted in isolation and separated from its mother only when the clinical conditions of the mother make this advisable. The duration of the isolation measures and mother-child separation should be analyzed individually in relation to the virological results of the child and the mother and clinical conditions of both. **In symptomatic cases under investigation of infants born to mothers with confirmed or highly suspected clinical/epidemiological infection, two negative PCR controls (at birth and after 24–48 h) are recommended to consider a case as discarded and lift isolation measures. In asymptomatic patients, one or two viral PCR controls will be performed, depending on availability. Neonatal testing and diagnosis should follow the WHO definition principles for neonatal SARS-CoV-2 infections (See Chap. 12)

Real-time analysis of cases included in this registry showed that 92% of the infected pregnant women were in good clinical condition to handle their newborn. And 85% of the neonates born to COVID-19 mother were healthy and not requiring medical care. Rooming-in recommendation was then followed by most maternity hospitals in our country.

Although some initial difficulties were faced, 97% of healthy newborns were not separated from their mother at birth (including skin-to-skin contact after childbirth), and 88% were breastfed. Infection rate was higher in newborns separated at delivery (1.8%) compared to those managed with rooming-in (0.7%), indicating at least no more risk of newborn infection when mothers and their newborns are kept together while applying necessary precautions for infection prevention control.

In a recent systematic review, 276 neonates with COVID-19 diagnosis, and 60.1% had mild or moderate disease, being fever and respiratory and gastrointestinal symptoms more frequently described. Mortality was 1.7% and mostly associated to other comorbidities [23].

Kiran More et al. described a multisystem inflammatory syndrome in 20 neonates (MIS-N) from five western hospitals in India [24]. As in the pediatric population, neonates developed respiratory distress, hypotension and shock, and encephalopathy. It is hypothesized to be caused either following transplacental transfer of SARS-CoV2 antibodies or antibodies developed in the neonate after infection with SARS-CoV-2 [24], and although it has been described by others, it is uncommon in this population of newborns, and none of our neonates develop this complication [25].

Finally, although there was an important increase in pediatric cases, including neonates, during the Omicron wave [26], we did not find this increase, being the higher number of neonatal cases registered in the first two waves.

Even more, as in other prospective registries [27], most of the maternal cases were mild, and no cases of neonatal disease were notified.

In conclusion, current data show that newborn perinatal infection is uncommon (0.9%–1.4% incidence in the National Registry). Symptomatology of these cases is mild and probably related to usual neonatal pathology and prematurity.

Care from birth should not be different from any other newborn, except for preventive strategies to protect the neonate from the infected mother. In this sense, delayed umbilical cord clamping, skin-to-skin contact care, and breastfeeding were proven to be safe for these newborns.

Clinical monitoring of these cases did not detect other effects. In neonates with COVID-19, clinical management does not differ from that of any neonate with the same symptomatology, applying the necessary support measures.

There is currently no approved specific neonatal treatment for SARS-CoV-2. It is recommended to avoid the inappropriate use of antibiotic therapy, which should be limited to cases of confirmed bacterial superinfection.

If newborn needs to be admitted to a neonatal unit, a contact and droplet isolation is recommended. If there is a risk of aerosol production, the use of rooms with negative pressure should be evaluated [28].

Conflict of Interest The authors have no conflict of interest to declare.

References

1. Puopolo K, Hudak ML, Kimberlin D, et al. Management of infants born to mothers with COVID-19. Itasca, IL: AAP; 2020.
2. World Health Organization. Breastfeeding advice during the COVID-19 outbreak. Geneva: WHO. http://www.emro.who.int/nutrition/nutrition-infocus/breastfeeding-advice-during-covid-19-outbreak.html. Accessed 15 Jun 2020.
3. World Health Organization. Definition and categorization of the timing of mother-to-child transmission of SARS-CoV-2. Scientific brief. Geneva: WHO; 2021. https://www.who.int/publications/i/item/WHO-2019-nCoV-mother-to-child-transmission-2021.1. Accessed Mar 2022.
4. Allotey J, Chatterjee S, Kew T, Gaetano A, Stallings E, Fernández-García S, Yap M, Sheikh J, Lawson H, Coomar D, Dixit A, Zhou D, Balaji R, Littmoden M, King Y, Debenham L, Llavall AC, Ansari K, Sandhu G, Banjoko A, Walker K, O'Donoghue K, van Wely M, van Leeuwen E, Kostova E, Kunst H, Khalil A, Brizuela V, Broutet N, Kara E, Kim CR, Thorson A, Oladapo OT, Zamora J, Bonet M, Mofenson L, Thangaratinam S, PregCOV-19 Living Systematic Review Consortium. SARS-CoV-2 positivity in offspring and timing of mother-to-child transmission: living systematic review and meta-analysis. BMJ. 2022;376:e067696. https://doi.org/10.1136/bmj-2021-067696.
5. Sánchez-Luna M, Fernández Colomer B, de Alba Romero C, Alarcón Allen A, Baña Souto A, Camba Longueira F, Cernada Badía M, Galve Pradell Z, González López M, López Herrera MC, Ribes Bautista C, Sánchez García L, Zamora Flores E, SENEO COVID-19 Registry Study Group. Neonates born to mothers with COVID-19: data from the Spanish Society of Neonatology Registry. Pediatrics. 2021;147(2):e2020015065. https://doi.org/10.1542/peds.2020-015065.
6. Fernández Colomer B, Sánchez-Luna M, de Alba Romero C, Alarcón A, Baña Souto A, Camba Longueira F, Cernada M, Galve Pradell Z, González López M, López Herrera MC, Ribes Bautista C, Sánchez García L, Zamora Flores E, Pellicer A, Alonso Díaz C, Herraiz Perea C, Romero Ramírez DS, de Las Cuevas Terán I, Pescador Chamorro I, Fernández Trisac JL, Arruza Gómez L, Cardo Fernández LM, García García MJ, Nicolás López M, Hortelano López M, Riaza Gómez M, Hernández González N, González Sánchez R, Zambudio Sert S, Larrosa Capacés S, Matías Del Pozo V. Neonatal infection due to SARS-CoV-2: an epidemiological study in Spain. Front Pediatr. 2020;8:580584. https://doi.org/10.3389/fped.2020.580584.
7. Penfield CA, et al. Detection of SARS-COV-2 in placental and fetal membrane samples. Am J Obstet Gynecol MFM. 2020;2:100133. https://doi.org/10.1016/j.ajogmf.2020.100133.
8. Verma S, Carter EB, Mysorekar IU. SARS-CoV2 and pregnancy: an Invisible enemy? Am J Reprod Immunol. 2020;84:e13308. https://doi.org/10.1111/aji.13308.
9. Algarroba GN, et al. Visualization of severe acute respiratory syndrome coronavirus 2 invading the human placenta using electron microscopy. Am J Obstet Gynecol. 2020;223:275–8.
10. Villar J, Ariff S, Gunier RB, et al. Maternal and neonatal morbidity and mortality among pregnant women with and without COVID-19 infection. JAMA Pediatr. 2021;175(8):817. https://doi.org/10.1001/jamapediatrics.2021.1050.
11. Zambrano LD, Ellington S, Strid P, et al. CDC COVID-19 Response Pregnancy and Infant Linked Outcomes Team. Update: characteristics of symptomatic women of reproductive age with laboratory-confirmed SARS-CoV-2 infection by pregnancy status—United States, January 22-October 3, 2020. MMWR Morb Mortal Wkly Rep. 2020;69(44):1641–7. https://doi.org/10.15585/mmwr.mm6944e3.

12. Metz T, Clifton R, Hughes R, et al. Association of SARS-CoV-2 infection with serious maternal morbidity and mortality from obstetric complications. JAMA. 2022;327(8):748–59. https://doi.org/10.1001/jama.2022.1190.
13. Carrasco I, Muñoz-Chapuli M, Vigil-Vázquez S, Aguilera-Alonso D, Hernández C, Sánchez-Sánchez C, Oliver C, Riaza M, Pareja M, Sanz O, Pérez-Seoane B, López J, Márquez E, Domínguez-Rodríguez S, Hernanz-Lobo A, De León-Luis JA, Sánchez-Luna M, Navarro ML. SARS-COV-2 infection in pregnant women and newborns in a Spanish cohort (GESNEO-COVID) during the first wave. BMC Pregnan Childb. 2021;21(1):326. https://doi.org/10.1186/s12884-021-03784-8.
14. Gurol-Urganci I, Jardine JE, Carroll F, Draycott T, Dunn G, Fremeaux A, Harris T, Hawdon J, Morris E, Muller P, Waite L, Webster K, van der Meulen J, Khalil A. Maternal and perinatal outcomes of pregnant women with SARS-CoV-2 infection at the time of birth in England: national cohort study. Am J Obstet Gynecol. 2021;225(5):522.e1–522.e11. https://doi.org/10.1016/j.ajog.2021.05.016.
15. Pace RM, Williams JE, Järvinen KM, Belfort MB, Pace CD, Lackey KA, Gogel AC, Nguyen-Contant P, Kanagaiah P, Fitzgerald T, Ferri R, Young B, Rosen-Carole C, Diaz N, Meehan C, Caffe B, Sangster MY, Topham DJ, McGuire MA, Seppo A, McGuire MK. COVID-19 and human milk: SARS-CoV-2, antibodies, and neutralizing capacity. medRxiv. 2020:2020.09.16.20196071.
16. Joseph NT, Dude CM, Verkerke HP, et al. Maternal antibody response, neutralizing potency, and placental antibody transfer after severe acute respiratory syndrome coronavirus 2 (SARS-CoV-2) infection. Obstet Gynecol. 2021 138:189–97.
17. Song D, Prahl M, Gaw SL, Narasimhan SR, Rai DS, Huang A, Flores CV, Lin CY, Jigmeddagva U, Wu A, Warrier L, Levan J, Nguyen CBT, Callaway P, Farrington L, Acevedo GR, Gonzalez VJ, Vaaben A, Nguyen P, Atmosfera E, Marleau C, Anderson C, Misra S, Stemmle M, Cortes M, McAuley J, Metz N, Patel R, Nudelman M, Abraham S, Byrne J, Jegatheesan P. Passive and active immunity in infants born to mothers with SARS-CoV-2 infection during pregnancy: prospective cohort study. BMJ Open. 2021;11(7):e053036. https://doi.org/10.1136/bmjopen-2021-053036.
18. Vousden N, Ramakrishnan R, Bunch K, Morris E, Simpson N, Gale C, O'Brien P, Quigley M, Brocklehurst P, Kurinczuk JJ, Knight M. Management and implications of severe COVID-19 in pregnancy in the UK: data from the UK Obstetric Surveillance System national cohort. Acta Obstet Gynecol Scand. 2022;101:461. https://doi.org/10.1111/aogs.14329.
19. UNICEF. n.d.. https://www.unicef.org.au/blog/news-and-insights/february-2020/novel-coronavirus-outbreak-what-parents-need-to-know.
20. Davanzo R, Moro G, Sandri F, Agosti M, Moretti C, Mosca F. Breastfeeding and coronavirus disease-2019: Ad interim indications of the Italian Society of Neonatology endorsed by the Union of European Neonatal & Perinatal Societies. Matern Child Nutr. 2020;16(3):e13010. https://doi.org/10.1111/mcn.13010. Epub 2020 Apr 26.
21. CDC. Interim guidance on breastfeeding for a mother confirmed or under investigation for COVID-19. 2020. https://www.cdc.gov/coronavirus/2019-ncov/specific-groups/pregnancy-guidance-breastfeeding.html.
22. Allattamento e infezione da SARS-CoV-2. Coronavirus disease 2019 - COVID-19. 2020.
23. García H, Allende-López A, Morales-Ruíz P, Miranda-Novales G, Villasis-Keever MÁ. COVID-19 in neonates with positive RT-PCR test. Systematic review. Arch Med Res. 2022;53:252.
24. More K, Aiyer S, Goti A, Parikh M, Shekh S, Patel G, Kallem V, Soni R, Kumar P. Multisystem inflammatory syndrome in neonates (MIS-N) associated with SARS-CoV2 infection: a case series. Eur J Pediatr. 2022;181:1883–98.
25. Ryan L, Plötz FB, van den Hoogen A, Latour JM, Degtyareva M, Keuning M, Klingenberg C, Reiss IKM, Giannoni E, Roehr C, Gale C, Molloy EJ. Neonates and COVID-19: state of the art: neonatal Sepsis series. Pediatr Res. 2022;91(2):432–9. https://doi.org/10.1038/s41390-021-01875-y.

26. Cloete J, Kruger A, Masha M, du Plessis NM, Mawela D, Tshukudu M, Manyane T, Komane L, Venter M, Jassat W, Goga A, Feucht U. Paediatric hospitalisations due to COVID-19 during the first SARS-CoV-2 omicron (B.1.1.529) variant wave in South Africa: a multicentre observational study. Lancet Child Adolesc Health. 2022;6:294. https://doi.org/10.1016/S2352-4642(22)00027-X.
27. Adhikari E, MacDonald L, SoRelle J, Morse J, Pruszynski J, Spong C. COVID-19 cases and disease severity in pregnancy and neonatal positivity associated with delta (B.1.617.2) and omicron (B.1.1.529) variant predominance. JAMA. 2022;327:1500. https://doi.org/10.1001/jama.2022.4356.
28. Sociedad Española de Neonatología (Spanish Society of Neonatology). Recommendations for management of newborns for SARS-CoV-2 infection. https://www.seneo.es/images/site/noticias/home/Recomendaciones_SENeo_COVID-19_v6_eng.pdf. Accessed Mar 2022.

Part IV
Public Health

Chapter 14
Research Networks and Accelerated Research Pathways for Perinatal Health

Mark A. Turner

14.1 Introduction

Effective care during pregnancy and afterwards has enormous impacts on individuals and on public health. Effective care is based on effective research. Research that is accurate, reproducible, inclusive, timely, and efficient is important at any time [1], but particularly during a pandemic. In the face of a public health emergency, research needs to be prioritised, accelerated, and targeted to clinical and public health needs. Each of these characteristics of research has been addressed by collaboration during the COVID-19 pandemic [2–5] although collaboration has been imperfect, particularly from an equity perspective [6]. Research networks accelerated clinical trials of therapies for COVID-19 but not completely [7]. Pandemics are not unexpected so perinatal collaborations and research can be prepared.

Research collaboration takes many forms. The collaboration journey has been described in the partnership model [8]. There are various forms of partnership. Some partnerships are focused on individual projects. These partnerships can be labelled as consortia. Some partnerships live beyond individual projects and the links between partners are reused for multiple projects. These partnerships can be labelled as networks. Some partnerships are independent of projects and researchers and use links that are permanent. These partnerships can be labelled as infrastructures.

M. A. Turner (✉)
Department of Women's and Children's Health, University of Liverpool, Liverpool, UK

Liverpool Neonatal Partnership, Liverpool, UK

Liverpool Women's NHS Foundation Trust, Liverpool, UK
e-mail: mark.turner@liverpool.ac.uk

Characteristics of successful collaboration have been described [9] and include the following: shared vision; common language, goals, and objectives; good communication between the parties and mutual respect; equal share of burdens and responsibilities; sufficient resources; consistent clinical practice; and trust—from the outset that is maintained during the work. The nature of research changed to some extent during COVID-19 [10] with more opportunities for collaboration.

Some elements of an ideal state for collaborative interventional research about COVID-19 have been described [7]. Many elements of this ideal state are also relevant to observational data. The COVID-19 pandemic was not unexpected, and many groups were prepared for this type of pandemic. Preparedness is well described for disasters in general [11] and for science [12]. Future pandemics will occur requiring sustainability, adaptability, and scalability of research.

Good research methods should be generalisable to other related topics.

This chapter considers how the perinatal research enterprise during 2020 related to the well-described characteristics of research identified in the preceding paragraphs: high-quality research, good preparation for the COVID-19 pandemic, and sustainability for future pandemics. Using selected research projects about perinatal aspects of COVID-19, this chapter reviews how perinatal research fits with these ideal characteristics by reviewing timelines and other elements of research. This chapter does not provide a complete review of all perinatal health research but focuses on exemplars to identify key themes that can inform future work. The perinatal exemplars are compared with other more general research networks. Lessons for the future are identified in the context of global initiatives relating to the COVID-19 pandemic and future outbreaks of infectious disease.

14.2 Selected Perinatal COVID-19 Research Partnerships

The illustrative examples are summarised in Table 14.1. Elements of science preparedness reported by the examples are summarised in Table 14.2. Many studies were done. For example, 90 studies of COVID-19 in pregnancy were published within 2 months of the declaration of the pandemic [15], and the most recent living review of vertical transmission includes 472 studies [16]. The studies selected here are a purposive sample of convenience representing a range of approaches to collaboration.

14.2.1 Site-Level Collaboration

The PregOuTCOV cohort study was conducted in several centres from Belgium, France, and Italy [17, 18]. The relationships between the centres had been established through personal contacts, mainly based on where hospital specialists had trained. Some of the sites had collaborated before, but this configuration of sites was

Table 14.1 Illustrative collaborations for pregnancy COVID-19 research

	1	2	3	4
	PregOuTCOV	CDC	UKOSS	WAPM
Nature of study	Site-based collaboration	Multicentre surveillance system	Population-based cohort	Multinational collaboration
Reference of first publication	16	18	13	32
Date of first publication	27/07/2020	26/06/2020	27/05/2020	14/09/2020
Dates of cohort included in first publication	01/01/2020–13/05/2020	22/01/2020–07/06/2020	01/03/2020–14/04/2020	01/02/20–30/04/20
Number of countries included in first publication	2	1	1	22
Number of centres included in first publication	4	50 states + District of Columbia + New York City	194	72
Entry criteria for first publication	Laboratory-confirmed SARS-CoV-2 infection	Laboratory-confirmed SARS-CoV-2 infection	Laboratory-confirmed SARS-CoV-2 infection or clinical definition	Singleton pregnancy. Lab confirmed of SARS-CoV-2 infection
Number of pregnancies included in first publication	83	8207	427	388
Structure	Retrospective study of hospital admissions	National Disease Surveillance System	National prospective observational cohort study using the UK Obstetric Surveillance System	Purpose-driven collaboration of sites linked through a learned society
Infrastructure	No	Yes	Yes	No
Network	No	Yes	Yes	Not clear
Project	Yes	Yes	Yes	Yes
Non-pregnant comparisons	Yes, women of reproductive age admitted with laboratory-confirmed SARS-CoV-2 infection	National Disease Surveillance System (pregnancy status and other data not recorded for some women)	None	None

(continued)

Table 14.1 (continued)

	1	2	3	4
	PregOuTCOV	CDC	UKOSS	WAPM
Non-COVID-19 comparisons	None	None	National maternity statistics	None
Neonatal outcomes	Characteristics at birth (birth weight, Apgar scores)	Nil	Linked to neonatal studies, refs. [13] and [14]	Gestational age, birth weight, death, admission to neonatal intensive care

novel. The goal of the collaboration was to pool experience from sites with similar approaches to clinical practice and was rooted in answering clinically relevant questions to inform practice at the sites. Early alignment on the scope of the study, key questions, and relevant data that resulted from similar approaches to clinical practice facilitated detailed preparation.

The perception of the investigators that this collaboration was easier in some respects than other collaborations continued during the preparation of the manuscripts. This may have resulted from the "pandemic mindset" or greater focus resulting from remote working. It was easier to work with distant colleagues with shared interests than with local colleagues. No finance was needed because the study was simple and was conducted by staff in parallel with other work. In effect, this study was funded by in-kind contributions from the health and academic institutions and the investigators. Data collection started as internal audit of experience so that the study was inherently pragmatic. Accordingly, ethics and institutional approvals were straightforward. There are no standing protocols, and no resources, such as terminologies, are available for future pandemics. However, the investigators will be able to activate a similar project during any future pandemics.

Several papers were produced [17, 18] and the results were shared through presentations given by the authors. The French government cited one of the articles when discussing when pregnant women should stop work during the pandemic.

14.2.2 National Surveillance

The US Centers for Disease Control and Prevention started surveillance for COVID-19 based on laboratory testing started on January 22, 2020 [19]. This included surveillance among women aged 15–44 years. The first report was published [20], and there were multiple updates [21].

The CDC repurposing of routine surveillance contributed to the US public health efforts during the pandemic. There was some incomplete data. Pregnancy status was recorded in 28% of the women aged 15–44 years with laboratory-confirmed cases of

Table 14.2 Preparedness for pregnancy COVID-19 research and future pandemics among the illustrative examples shown

	1 PregOuTCOV	2 CDC	3 UKOSS	4 WAPM
Identify questions that will need to be addressed for common scenarios and develop generic study protocols	Study questions developed by clinicians during the pandemic	Surveillance protocols adapted	Dormant protocol that was rapidly adapted and activated	Study questions developed by clinicians during the pandemic
Ensure that appropriate cadres of Scientists are available to respond to events	Informal links	Standing contacts in place in each healthcare setting	Standing contacts in place in each healthcare setting	Repurposing of links in place through learned society
Develop a process for activating Research response	Personal networks deployed	Standing contacts in place in each healthcare setting	Standing contacts in place in each healthcare setting	Society working group deployed
Identify and prioritise research needs	Other studies were done (so prioritisation was incomplete)	Other studies were done (so prioritisation was incomplete)	Other studies were done (so prioritisation was incomplete)	Other studies were done (so prioritisation was incomplete)
Ensure conditions for rapid data collection	Rapid set-up of a fit-for-purpose study	Standing system in place	Standing system in place	Rapid set-up of a fit-for-purpose study
Ensure rapid and appropriate ethical review	Pragmatic protocol so rapid approval	Not reported	Approvals obtained in advance National agreement to expedite approvals	Pragmatic protocol so rapid approval
Ensure mechanisms for rapid funding	No funding	Standing system in place	National agreements in place	No funding
Understand concerns of affected communities	Not reported	Not reported	Not reported	Not reported
Preparation for future pandemics	Not reported	Standing surveillance can be adapted	Standing protocol can be adapted	Not reported
Financial sustainability	No funding	Standing system in place	Limited funding between urgent research events; sustainability depends on good will of collaborators	No funding

Criteria modified from Lurie et al. [12]

SARS-CoV-2 infection. Information on race/ethnicity was not recorded in 20% of pregnant women and 30% of nonpregnant women. It was not possible to distinguish between admissions due to COVID-19 and admissions due to pregnancy-related events (e.g. delivery). This study provided large-scale indicative data that has many uses, but the extent of incomplete data means that some epidemiological precision is lost.

14.2.3 Population-Based Reporting

Population-based perinatal COVID-19 research in the UK was an amalgam of several initiatives.

Reporting relating to pregnancy was done by UKOSS, the national reporting system for rare disorders in pregnancy hosted by the National Perinatal Epidemiology Unit (NPEU) [22]. UKOSS includes one reporter in each obstetric unit who notifies the central office of cases that meet a pre-defined definition and organises gathering of data according to a pre-defined case report form. The foundations for the study were laid in 2011 following the 2009 influenza A/H1N1 pandemic [23]. Obstetric reporting was supplemented by neonatal and paediatric reporting through the British Perinatal Surveillance Unit (BPSU). Every paediatrician in the country is sent monthly prompts to report cases that meet a pre-defined definition. BPSU setup its reporting in collaboration with the national programme for surveillance of maternal deaths, stillbirths and infant deaths (MBRRACE) [24], the national paediatric intensive care registry, and the English National Institute for Health Research (NIHR) [13, 14]. NIHR includes a research funding arm and an arm that provides national research infrastructure the Clinical Research Network (CRN). The CRN maintains research staff who can access every healthcare setting.

The UKOSS COVID-19 study was open within days of the declaration of the pandemic following a 3-week preparation period during which the study was updated and information governance and ethical approvals were activated. Collaborations were already in place, and there were contacts with the public health authority at the time, Public Health England. Obstetric data fed through to the government, single national healthcare provider and professional organisations so that real time data was available from 21 March 2020 and published a couple of months later [15]. This allowed ongoing dialogue between these stakeholders about the burden of disease and the need for public health actions. UK data contributed significantly to WHO guidance in September 2020. Rapid reviews promoted optimal care [25].

In addition to the UKOSS study that was activated from dormancy, other pregnancy studies were done in the UK [26, 27]. The PAN-COVID-19 study results were pooled with a similar US study [27], although closer alignment between the studies would have increased the utility of the report: preparation between pandemics would allow optimal study design across locations. The three national observational studies addressed a range of questions but caused confusion and burden on staff at site level because of multiple methods for data capture; see Fig. 14.1. Real-world data about hospital admissions for pregnant women and neonates was also

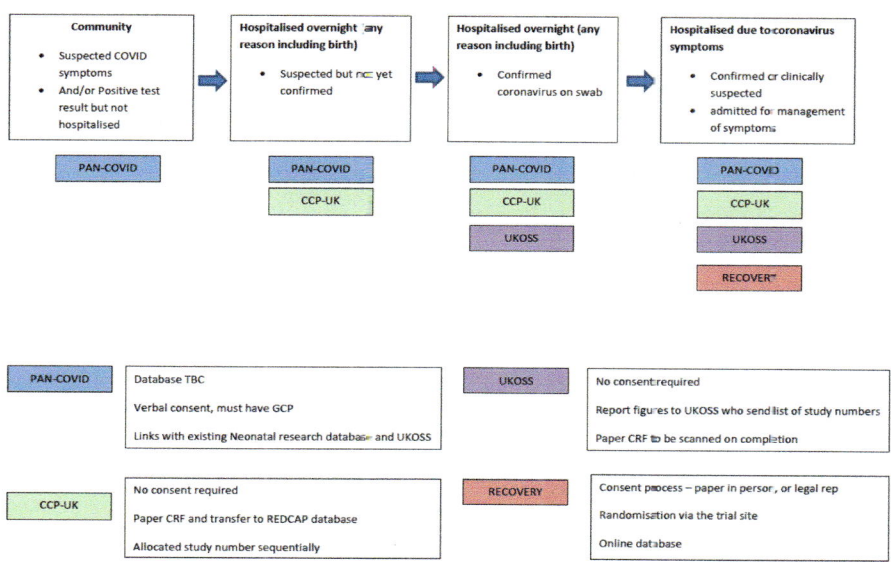

Fig. 14.1 Studies about COVID-19 recruiting pregnant women in a UK tertiary maternity unit. *PAN-COVID* Pregnancy and Neonatal Outcomes in COVID-19 study, *UKOSS* United Kingdom Obstetric Surveillance System, *CCP-UK* Clinical Characterisation Protocol (part of ISARIC), *RECOVERY* Randomised Evaluation of COVID-19 Therapy

analysed in the UK [28]. Other modes of data capture are available [29]. Pooling of relevant real-world/administrative data is underway and could be adapted to studying acute and chronic impacts of disease outbreaks and individual and societal levels [30]. In the future, it would be beneficial to learn from the range of options for data collection and rationalise data collection and analysis.

The UK demonstrated that infrastructure can be repurposed, but you need infrastructure in the first place. Each initiative that contributed to the perinatal COVID-19 research effort was precarious, despite their strengths. Dormant funding awarded following previous pandemics was available to some initiatives, but this was not sufficient and considerable personal effort and in-kind contributions were needed from individuals and institutions.

14.2.4 International Network

The World Association of Perinatal Medicine set up a COVID-19 working group that involved 22 countries with a wide range of economic circumstances. The primary paper was published in September 2020 [31]. Other papers followed [32, 33]. Guidelines were available in June 2020 [34].

Globally, WHO convened a perinatal research network with several workstreams. This programme developed a generic protocol for "A prospective cohort study investigating maternal, pregnancy and neonatal outcomes for women and neonates infected with SARS-CoV-2" [35], but it is not clear how many studies have used that protocol. WHO also developed a protocol for a living systematic review [36] that has been done [16, 37].

14.2.5 Summary of the Characteristics of the Selected Studies

The quality of the research in these and other COVID-19 studies varied. Study design ranged from a large population-based cohort to case series that were useful but had limitations due to incomplete sampling and data. All these studies showed effective collaboration in that reports were produced in a timely manner. In the absence of detailed ethnological studies, it is not clear whether the collaborations were efficient. One UK study was the product of extensive preparation for the pandemic. The other studies compensated for lack of preparation by rapidly pivoting to the pandemic using existing collaborations and resources. There was some overlap in study design and the reported variables. There is minimal evidence that these collaborations are sustainable for future pandemics. There is minimal evidence of preparation for future pandemics through shared terminologies, protocols, or infrastructure. Each of these projects was successful in its own terms. The perinatal community can clearly conduct research quickly and at scale. There are opportunities for greater benefits and impact on perinatal health particularly if preparedness and sustainability are enhanced.

14.3 Successful Planning for Pandemic Research that Is not Specific to Pregnancy

Other parts of the healthcare research effort were more prepared for the pandemic than perinatal health. Review of this experience illustrates the timelines, strengths, and challenges of an integrated approach and can inform the perinatal community.

14.3.1 The UK

In line with internationally acknowledged good practice for disaster preparedness, the UK has a 'whole systems' approach to pandemic research [11, 12]. UK COVID-19 research was underpinned by a national approach to pandemic readiness that grew out of recognition in 2007 that highly pathogenic avian flu could cause substantial disruption to society. This risk was captured on the UK Government Cabinet's risk register which was the basis for an integrated response across society.

This recognised links between infection and national security. The UK Government National Risk Registry included a hazard relating to a failure to mount an effective research response to a pandemic. In 2009, a collaboration called Flu-CIN developed a standardised case report form across 30 hospitals that enabled real-time data gathering, analysis, and presentation. The public health function (then Public Health England) gathered data in the community but lacked access to data from secondary care. In 2011, the lack of integration was noted and the International Severe Acute Respiratory and emerging Infection Consortium (ISARIC) was set up to provide a comprehensive approach to research during an outbreak of infectious disease [38]. ISARIC evolved in the light of experience in 2012 (Middle Eastern Respiratory Virus and Ebola), 2013 (H5N1 influenza), and test activations in 2018. Thus, an effective system took many years to develop with several iterative improvements.

One component of ISARIC is protocols that are prepared in advance (so-called "oven ready" protocols). These protocols are disease agnostic and ready to be deployed whenever a relevant condition is identified. The protocols were designed to minimise burden on the sites. WHO ethics committees were consulted early. A network of infectious disease, critical care, and child health professionals was established. Within that network, all agreed to not compete but pool effort for the public health interest. This agreement to pool effort was not a passive endeavour but requires constant reinforcement through robust agreements and action against people who do not follow community norms.

Pregnant women were included in data collection, but the specific features of pregnancy and the perinatal period were not included. A separate perinatal study was needed (see selected study 3 above) because the ISARIC Clinical Characterisation Protocol (CCP) does not capture: (1) babies who were not themselves infected but who might be affected by infection in a pregnant woman or (2) sufficient data about pregnancies to interpret the effects of an infection on the foetus and neonate, or vertical infection.

In the UK, initial discussions about activating ISARIC to study SARS-CoV-2 started on 17 January 2020, and work, labelled as Covid-19 clinical information network in the UK, started shortly after that [39]. By March 2020, ISARIC was fully active and providing integration within the NHS and to the governments of the UK. The NIHR CRN was deployed, and 2,600 nurses and medical students entered data. Accordingly, all healthcare settings including mental health (secure hospitals) and small community hospitals were included. This allowed identification of nosocomial infection by 21 February 2020 with immediate implications for management of the infection [39].

Biosamples were sent from all sites to two hubs: Glasgow and Liverpool. These hubs provided aliquots to well-qualified laboratories under strict material transfer agreements (MTA) and data transfer agreements (DTA). These agreements were embedded in protocol agreements which avoided endless negotiations and "special case" for individual sites. This system provided accountability for samples and recognised the contributions of sites which allows gathering the maximum number of samples. These arrangements provided the basis for international diagnostic standards, lateral flow tests, and control materials for assays used in the Oxford trial.

The following success factors to successful preparedness can be identified:

1. Decades-long political will inspired by clinical academic leadership, eminent supporters, and 'next-generation' active workers across the EU, US, and China
2. Energetic individuals who are able to focus on preparedness and activating studies when needed
3. Pooling networks—with added value to existing networks through disease agnostic protocol and trusting relationships
4. Sponsorship and sustaining funding
5. Dogged determination for fair play across the network—requires ruthlessness when people contravene agreements
6. Clear scope of activities for each stakeholder

14.3.1.1 Challenges

Work to prepare for pandemics was not helped by a lack of understanding among institutions that employed interested professionals and by funders. Institutions and funders did not understand the value of work to prepare for pandemics and did not allow time within job plans. The apparent sustainability of work in the UK is due to considerable contributions by individuals in addition to relatively modest external funding. This may be the only way to sustain perinatal health research into outbreaks.

14.3.1.2 UK Summary

Elements of the UK COVID-19 research response were prepared over 13 years and required considerable effort from publicly spirited leadership. There were large in-kind contributions from individuals and organisations. Some parts of the response were developed ad hoc which caused unnecessary duplication at site level and lack of scientific coordination.

14.3.2 The European Union (EU)

The Platform for European Preparedness Against (Re-)emerging Epidemics [40] (PREPARE) is a large-scale European network, including 27 beneficiaries that was funded by the EU FP7 Programme. PREPARE started its activities in February 2014. The work of PREPARE included an observational study on acute respiratory infection in adults, MERMAIDS [41], that was adapted to COVID-19. The presence of a pragmatic protocol was not sufficient for successful research. Problems with conducting the project included the following: regulatory complexity, lack of funding compared to other projects, lack of clinician engagement, and low numbers of recruited participants [7]. The MERMAIDS protocol did not exclude pregnant women but did not gather comprehensive perinatal data. COMBACTE (Combatting Bacterial Resistance in Europe) is part of the IMI-funded programme ND4BB (New Drugs for Bad Bugs) and focuses on improving the clinical development of antibiotics [42]. PREPARE and COMBACTE have folded into a successor organisation that will become the European Clinical Research Alliance on Infectious Diseases (ECRAID) [43]. ECRAID will generate rigorous evidence to respond to threats from infectious diseases and for diagnosis, prevention, and treatment of infection. ECRAID will build a pan-European, globally linked clinical research network. ECRAID is linked with a paediatric network but not a perinatal network.

14.3.3 Interventional Studies

Treatments for pregnant women have been investigated but not to the extent that is necessary [44]. Several well-prepared platform trials to test treatments for COVID-19 recruited pregnant women including SOLIDARITY [45], RECOVERY [46], and REMAP-CAP [47]. Experience with RECOVERY and REMAP-CAP showed that generic issues such as regulatory delays and lack of infrastructure could be overcome in some jurisdictions but not others [7]. The perinatal community needs to contribute to the success of interventional studies during protocol design and conduct. Sites that have contributed to observational studies in the COVID-19 pandemic could be useful additional contributors to interventional studies.

It is essential to recruit pregnant women to clinical trials when there is potential benefit to mother or offspring and preclinical work has not raised major concerns [48]. Like neonates and children, pregnant women need to be protected with research not protected from research. Pregnant and lactating women are not inherently vulnerable, and their involvement in trials should be considered on a case-by-case basis rather than being ruled out in general.

Vaccines offer many benefits to pregnant women and their offspring and have been studied during the COVID-19 pandemic in pregnancy-specific and general studies, but research has been insufficient for the needs of perinatal health [49]. Vaccine hesitancy remains a challenge but should not be promoted by hesitancy to recruit pregnant women to trials [50]. Inequitable access to vaccines is a prominent feature of the COVID-19 pandemic and has disproportionate effect on pregnant women. The COVAX collaboration is developing ways to increase access to COVID-19 vaccines by integrating diverse existing partnerships [51].

14.4 Discussion

Many perinatal collaborations for research about the COVID-19 pandemic followed an accelerated pathway. However, most of these studies, and by extension the perinatal community, were not well prepared for the pandemic, met well-established criteria for high-quality research during a pandemic incompletely, and are not well positioned for the next pandemic.

14.4.1 Ways of Working

It can be argued that rigorous collaboration comes at a price: that the bureaucracy of setting up formal collaborations is a distraction from doing the work. On the other hand, avoiding biases, e.g. with population-based studies, makes coordinated studies more useful. Replication of results is always useful in science, but we need to avoid unproductive duplication of effort. A sceptic might argue that the large number of studies in the perinatal aspects of the COVID-19 pandemic was driven by the wish for individuals and institutions to be seen as research leaders. On the contrary, the advantages of team science are well recognised [52]. Realists will argue that individuals and institutions need to take credit in the current environment. There is enough work to do, and sufficient ways of approaching the field, that ownership and 'territoriality' of data and results can be accommodated when necessary.

Unfortunately, the urge among multiple groups to lead studies reduces the efficiency and effectiveness of research. The public good will be served by sharing data and techniques to pool data. It is important to recognise sharing of data in appointment and promotion procedures. Systematic review and meta-analysis do not completely overcome the challenges of comparing multiple studies, particularly if the studies included in the reviews are not aligned with respect to terminology, covariates, and outcomes. Experience with multiple protocols can inform the 'ideal' protocol that can be adapted to the needs of future epidemics/pandemics and aligned with other master protocols such as ISARIC.

An alternative explanation for the patchwork of studies is that interested groups were not aware of each other, except through informal networks. It is now possible to build a global perinatal research community. The systematic reviews of the perinatal implications of SARS-CoV-2 mean that skilled investigators who authored reports have been identified. A network of those investigators would have access to many experienced sites across the globe. A network of investigators and sites would allow training that promotes research quality and rapid inception of studies. It is important that research activity is democratised and that sites can showcase their work. Individuals can proactively manage their own research profile to stimulate involvement in networks [53].

There have been calls for international research governance [54], and this is needed for perinatal health research about outbreaks. A top-down approach led by investigators and infrastructures—e.g. much of the UK response to emerging infections—has benefits but can miss out perinatal considerations. A bottom-up approach driven by patients, advocates, and clinicians has benefits, but to date perinatal medicine has not taken this route. Some clinical areas have well-developed advocacy groups that have substantial influence on policy and research, e.g. rare diseases through Rare Diseases Europe, EURORDIS [55]. The perinatal research community needs to develop top-down and bottom-up approaches so that good science and effective organisation is backed up by political influence and parental voices. A strong voice for women and families is an essential part of an effective research agenda for perinatal health but is poorly developed.

Planning and preparedness increase the value of research, but flexibility is still needed. Each epidemic or pandemic is different. SARS-CoV-2 has relatively less impact on pregnancy and perinatal outcomes than some other infections so that planning for future public health emergencies needs to account for the likelihood that other outbreaks will lead to significant needs for perinatal health research.

Partnerships are necessary but not sufficient. Collaboration within the perinatal community needs to be supplemented by proportionate approaches to ethics, information governance (including data linkage and transfer), and regulation for research involving medicines. While these processes can act as barriers to researchers, societal buy-in to research requires these frameworks to build trust. These processes have specific perinatal considerations that can be reviewed in the light of experience during the COVID-19 pandemic. The proactive voice of the perinatal community is needed to ensure that societal discussions take account of the specific features of research that addresses the needs of the mother/offspring dyad. Hopefully, ethics, information governance, and the regulation of medicines research will be streamlined for future public health emergencies. There is a risk that advances will not reflect the needs of perinatal health if the perinatal community does not act in a coordinated manner.

14.4.2 Ways Forward

A clear, consensus-driven research agenda is needed to target effort effectively within the perinatal health community and to persuade other communities to give perinatal health the attention it deserves; for example, see Fig. 14.2. The urgency of these needs will depend on the cell and tissue tropism of the virus that causes the outbreak. However, it is important to develop a comprehensive understanding of the perinatal implications of an outbreak because the consequences of an infection may not be obvious at first.

The agenda for perinatal health research needs to be matched with a global network of sites and an integrated, core set of protocols for key questions in perinatal health. It is important that this work is not done in isolation. The perinatal community needs to work with more general, global initiatives. Attracting attention and resource from global initiatives to support the sustainability of perinatal research into outbreaks of infectious disease will be easier with a coherent agenda, a network of sites, and well-constructed protocols that benefit from the experience during the COVID-19 pandemic. Sustainability of perinatal research will benefit from learning from, and partnership with, other elements of the outbreak research landscape.

Information
The timing and nature of:
    Maternal infection
    Neonatal infection
    Congenital malformations
    Vertical transmission
    Long-term effects of infection in pregnant women and neonates (e.g. long COVID)
    Effects of the infection on the placenta

Long-term follow-up of babies exposed to the infection before and after birth, including relevant imaging, developmental testing, other relevant phenotyping, and resource usage (health care, social care, education, family out of pocket expenses) with adequate control data

Methods
Population coverage of pregnant and non-pregnant women with complete ascertainment of outcomes of infection, pregnancy, neonatal progress, and childhood development. Adequate controls are needed to develop information for treatment and public health.

Shared terminologies including concepts and definitions

Protocols developed before an outbreak starts that address key uncertainties in the light of experience with previous outbreaks and which are amended at the start of each new outbreal

Shared data collection instruments that are streamlined for busy sites

Purposeful replication and minimal unnecessary duplication

Place
Comprehensive range of settings

Equitable access to research and the benefits of research

Process
Research agreements in place locally, nationally, internationally in advance

Timely approvals that include pregnant women and neonates for ethics, information governance, and medicines research, ideally prospectively with rapid amendments as an outbreak starts

Existing initiatives and sites in perinatal health are linked to allow optimisation of research methods and efficiency of research conduct

Clear, fair data sharing that is recognized by institutions for promotion for mothers and babies

Biosamples
Maternal samples of blood
Amniotic fluid when available
Neonatal blood
Respiratory fluid from mother and / or neonate
Samples of placenta
Other samples relevant to the outbreak

Clear, fair sample sharing that is recognized by institutions for promotion including samples from pregnancy and the placenta

Diagnostic and biomarker assays that are validated for perinatal samples and matrices.

Collaboration
International governance of perinatal health research that specifies and coordinates:
    Goals
    Aims
    Policies
    Variables
    Data collection
    Analysis
    Interpretation
    Authorship
    Recognition of investigators and site staff

Links with global, regional, and national research initiatives beyond perinatal health.

Fig. 14.2 The ideal situation for research about perinatal health during outbreaks of infectious disease

14.4.3 Global Initiatives

The WHO R&D Blueprint for ending the COVID-19 pandemic and tackling future pandemics [56] recognises that important knowledge gaps exist in maternal, pregnancy, and neonatal outcomes for women and neonates infected with SARS-CoV-2 and that rapid publication of Case Report Forms for pregnant women is essential. In general, several research activities should take place in any outbreak. Outbreaks should be detected quickly. It is essential to recognise early when an outbreak has a specific impact on pregnancy, vertical transmission, and neonates. Generic issues should be addressed including regulatory convergence, developing the global trust that is needed to underpin global research, equitable access to research and its benefits, and long-term investment in pandemic preparedness. WHO has a well-established and effective capability in perinatal health that needs to be at the centre of all perinatal collaborations [57]. WHO has convening power that is particularly relevant to low- and middle-income countries [16, 36, 58]. International collaborations need to be rooted in approaches that are inclusive and multidisciplinary. National collaborations need to reflect international approaches to research to allow comparisons across locations, benchmarking of clinical care, and pooling of results.

The Global Research Collaboration for Infectious Disease Preparedness (GloPID-R) is a global consortium of research funders [59]. GLOPID-R provides global coordination of funding in order to meet the need for effective and efficient research that is resourced in a timely way. GLOPID-R has reviewed the needs for epidemic/pandemic research [60]. Each research study should be designed to inform implementation and impact of the study findings. Implementation can be facilitated through the Access to COVID-19 Tools Accelerator for vaccines, therapeutics, diagnostics, and global surveillance [61] and the Coalition for Epidemic Preparedness Innovations (CEPI) [62]. Research may be useful but not commercially exploitable and may spill over into other topics. Some global and regional coordination is possible, but this needs to be complemented at national level, where the real control lies. In the future, the budget for epidemic and pandemic research may not be as generous as it was for COVID-19. Prioritisation is needed. Additionally, there are global initiatives for proportionate and streamlined approaches to intellectual property, information governance, and data rights. Capacity building is important for research funders. In the main report and recommendations by the advisory group co-chairs for GLOPID-R, there is no mention of perinatal research [60, 63]. Thus, there is a risk that the global, regional, and national coordination for funding of infectious disease research does not recognise the needs for perinatal health research and does not prioritise perinatal research, unless there is an integrated voice from the perinatal community.

The Organisation for Economic Cooperation and Development (OECD) has identified some improvements in the science, technology, and innovation (STI) environment that should result from the COVID-19 pandemic [2]. Policy should guide innovation towards needs. Transdisciplinary research is essential. Emerging technologies need to be explicitly linked to health resilience through government action. Training of scientists needs to be extended and broadened. Policy does not develop in a vacuum. Perinatal health will be left behind unless it makes explicit contributions to policy formation. This means that it is important to develop political will that supports perinatal health research at governmental level and within scientific community. Political will requires family advocates [64] such as a perinatal equivalent of EURORDIS [55].

Perinatal health research should not be conducted in isolation but needs to be integrated into the research landscape at global, regional, and international levels. This integration will promote the preparedness and sustainability of perinatal health research.

14.5 Conclusions

During the COVID-19 pandemic, perinatal medicine developed research networks that conducted research rapidly. This strong foundation for collaboration indicates an ability to provide good return on research investment and can be developed to prepare for future pandemics. The perinatal community can make a compelling case about the importance of its work. The perinatal community, including women and their families, needs to contribute more coherently to global efforts including the preparation of research about future outbreaks.

Acknowledgements I am grateful for insights into their work from the following people: Dominique Badr (Brussels), Andy Carlin (Brussels), Chris Gale (London), Pia Hardelid (London), Jenny Kurinczuk (Oxford), Claire Thorne (London), and particularly Calum Semple (Liverpool).

Figure 14.1 was designed by the research midwives at Liverpool Women's NHS Foundation Trust to support their work.

References

1. Ioannidis JP, et al. Increasing value and reducing waste in research design, conduct, and analysis. Lancet. 2014;383:166–75.
2. OECD. OECD science, technology and innovation outlook 2021: times of crisis and opportunity. Paris: OECD Publishing; 2021.
3. Cunningham E, Smyth B, Greene D. Correction: collaboration in the time of covid: a scientometric analysis of multidisciplinary SARS-Cov-2 research. Humanit Soc Sci Commun. 2021;8:264.
4. Research Collaborations. Bring big rewards: the world needs more. Nature. 2021;594:301–2.
5. ICC. Covid-19 pandemic: lessons for international research collaboration and information exchange. 2020. https://iccwbo.org/content/uploads/sites/3/2020/04/icc-statement-rd-collaboration.pdf.
6. Bump JB, Friberg P, Harper DR. International collaboration and Covid-19: what are we doing and where are we going? BMJ. 2021;372:180.

7. Goossens H, Derde L, Horby P, Bonten M. The European Clinical Research response to optimise treatment of patients with Covid-19: lessons learned, future perspective, and recommendations. Lancet Infect Dis. 2022;22:e153–8.
8. Tennyson R. The partnering tool book The Partnering Initiative (IBLF). 2011.
9. EC. Coronavirus global R&I collaboration portal: effective collaborations. 2022. https://coronavirus-global-collaboration.ec.europa.eu/effective-collaborations.
10. Maher B, Van Noorden R. How the covid pandemic is changing global science collaborations. Nature. 2021;594:316–9.
11. EC. European civil protection and humanitarian aid operations: disaster preparedness. 2021. https://ec.europa.eu/echo/what/humanitarian-aid/disaster-preparedness_en.
12. Lurie N, Manolio T, Patterson AP, Collins F, Frieden T. Research as a part of public health emergency response. N Engl J Med. 2013;368:1251–5.
13. Gale C, et al. National active surveillance to understand and inform neonatal care in Covid-19. Arch Dis Child Fetal Neonatal Ed. 2020;105:346–7.
14. Gale C, et al. Characteristics and outcomes of neonatal SARS-Cov-2 infection in the UK: a prospective national cohort study using active surveillance. Lancet Child Adolesc Health. 2021;5:113–21.
15. Knight M, et al. Characteristics and outcomes of pregnant women admitted to hospital with confirmed SARS-Cov-2 Infection in UK: national population based cohort study. BMJ. 2020;369:m2107.
16. Allotey J, et al. SARS-Cov-2 positivity in offspring and timing of mother-to-child transmission: living systematic review and meta-analysis. BMJ. 2022;376:e067696.
17. Badr DA, et al. Severe acute respiratory syndrome coronavirus 2 and pregnancy outcomes according to gestational age at time of infection. Emerg Infect Dis. 2021;27:2535–43.
18. Badr DA, et al. Are clinical outcomes worse for pregnant women at ≥20 weeks' gestation infected with coronavirus disease 2019? A multicenter case-control study with propensity score matching. Am J Obstet Gynecol. 2020;223:764–8.
19. CDC. Persons evaluated for 2019 novel coronavirus — United States. Atlanta, GA: CDC; 2020. https://www.cdc.gov/mmwr/volumes/69/wr/mm6906e1.htm?s_cid=mm6906e1_w.
20. Ellington S, et al. Characteristics of women of reproductive age with laboratory-confirmed Sars-Cov-2 infection by pregnancy status - United States, January 22-June 7, 2020. MMWR Morb Mortal Wkly Rep. 2020;69:769–75.
21. CDC. MMWR Covid-19 reports. Atlanta, GA: CDC; 2022. https://www.cdc.gov/mmwr/Novel_Coronavirus_Reports.html.
22. NPEU. UK Obstetric Surveillance System (UKOSS): a national system to study rare disorders of pregnancy. 2022. https://www.npeu.ox.ac.uk/ukoss.
23. Knight M. Pregnancy outcomes and Covid-19: benefits of a nine year gestation. 2020. https://blogs.bmj.com/bmj/2020/06/08/pregnancy-outcomes-and-covid-19-benefits-of-a-nine-year-gestation/.
24. NPEU. Mbrrace-UK: mothers and babies: reducing risk through audits and confidential enquiries across the UK. 2022. https://www.npeu.ox.ac.uk/mbrrace-uk.
25. Knight M, et al. Saving lives, improving mothers' care rapid report 2021: learning from Sars-Cov-2-related and associated maternal deaths in the UK June 2020 - March 2021. Oxford: Healthcare Quality Improvement Partnership and National Perinatal Epidemiology Unit, University of Oxford; 2021.
26. Banerjee J, et al. Pregnancy and neonatal outcomes in Covid-19: study protocol for a global registry of women with suspected or confirmed Sars-Cov-2 infection in pregnancy and their neonates, understanding natural history to guide treatment and prevention. BMJ Open. 2021;11:e041247.
27. Mullins E, et al. Pregnancy and neonatal outcomes of Covid-19: coreporting of common outcomes from Pan-Covid and AAP-Sonpm registries. Ultrasound Obstet Gynecol. 2021;57:573–81.

28. Gurol-Urganci I, et al. Obstetric interventions and pregnancy outcomes during the Covid-19 pandemic in England: a nationwide cohort study. PLoS Med. 2022;19:e1003884.
29. UCL. Virus watch: help stop the spread. 2022. http://ucl-virus-watch.net.
30. VERDI. The Verdi Project. 2022. https://verdiproject.org/the-project/.
31. Di Mascio D, et al. Risk factors associated with adverse fetal outcomes in pregnancies affected by coronavirus disease 2019 (Covid-19): a secondary analysis of the WAPM study on Covid-19. J Perinat Med. 2020;49:111–5.
32. WAPM. Maternal and perinatal outcomes of pregnant women with Sars-Cov-2 infection. Ultrasound Obstet Gynecol. 2021;57:232–41.
33. D'Antonio F, et al. Maternal and perinatal outcomes in high compared to low risk pregnancies complicated by severe acute respiratory syndrome coronavirus 2 infection (phase 2): the World Association of Perinatal Medicine Working Group on Coronavirus Disease 2019. Am J Obstet Gynecol MFM. 2021;3:100329.
34. Api O, et al. Clinical management of coronavirus disease 2019 (Covid-19) in pregnancy: recommendations of WAPM-World Association of Perinatal Medicine. J Perinat Med. 2020;48:857–66.
35. WHO. Generic protocol. A prospective cohort study investigating maternal, pregnancy and neonatal outcomes for women and neonates infected with Sars-Cov-2 V2.6. Geneva: WHO; 2020. https://www.who.int/publications/i/item/WHO-2019-nCoV-pregnancy-and-neonates-2020.1.
36. Yap M, et al. Clinical manifestations, prevalence, risk factors, outcomes, transmission, diagnosis and treatment of Covid-19 in pregnancy and postpartum: a living systematic review protocol. BMJ Open. 2020;10:e041868.
37. Allotey J, et al. Clinical manifestations, risk factors, and maternal and perinatal outcomes of coronavirus disease 2019 in pregnancy: living systematic review and meta-analysis. BMJ. 2020;370:m3320.
38. ISARIC. International Severe Acute Respiratory and Emerging Infection Consortium. 2022. https://isaric.org.
39. ISARIC. Isaric Covid-19 timeline 2019–2021. 2022. https://isaric.org/covid-19-pandemic-response-timeline/.
40. PREPARE. Prepare, Platform for European Preparedness against (Re-)Emerging Epidemics. 2021. https://www.prepare-europe.eu/index.html.
41. PREPARE. Multi-centre European Study of major infectious disease syndromes acute respiratory infections in adults protocol version 4.0. 2016. https://prepare.ersnet.org/lrmedia/2016/pdf/292.pdf.
42. COMBACTE. Combacte: combatting bacterial resistance in Europe. 2022. https://www.combacte.com.
43. ECRAID. Ecraid-Base. 2022. https://www.ecraid.eu/ecraid-base.
44. Giesbers S, et al. Treatment of Covid-19 in pregnant women: a systematic review and meta-analysis. Eur J Obstet Gynecol Reprod Biol. 2021;267:120–8.
45. WHO. Who Covid-19 solidarity therapeutics trial. Geneva: WHO; 2022. https://www.who.int/emergencies/diseases/novel-coronavirus-2019/global-research-on-novel-coronavirus-2019-ncov/solidarity-clinical-trial-for-covid-19-treatments.
46. RECOVERY. Recovery trial: randomised evaluation of Covid-19 therapy. 2022. https://www.recoverytrial.net.
47. REMAP-CAP. Remap-cap trial: all the information you need is right here at your fingertips. 2022. https://www.remapcap.eu/information-for-sites/.
48. Taylor MM, et al. Inclusion of pregnant women in Covid-19 treatment trials: a review and global call to action. Lancet Glob Health. 2021;9:e366–71.
49. De Rose DU, Salvatori G, Dotta A, Auriti C. Sars-Cov-2 vaccines during pregnancy and breastfeeding: a systematic review of maternal and neonatal outcomes. Viruses. 2022;14:539.
50. Costantine MM, Landon MB, Saade GR. Protection by exclusion: another missed opportunity to include pregnant women in research during the coronavirus disease 2019 (Covid-19) pandemic. Obstet Gynecol. 2020;136:26–8.

51. CEPI. Covax: Cepi's response to Covid-19. 2022. https://cepi.net/covax/.
52. Committee on the Science of Team, S, et al. Enhancing the effectiveness of team science. Washington, DC: National Academies Press; 2015.
53. Stroll J. Empowering collaboration and research visibility in a post covid-19 world. 2020. https://clarivate.com/blog/empowering-collaboration-and-research-visibility-in-a-post-covid-19-world/.
54. Peters DH, et al. In search of global governance for research in epidemics. Lancet. 2017;390:1632–3.
55. EURORDIS. Eurordis rare disease Europe: the voice of rare disease patients in Europe. 2022. https://www.eurordis.org.
56. WHO. How global research can end this pandemic and tackle future ones: building a resilient research architecture and capability to protect us all. 2022. https://cdn.who.int/media/docs/default-source/blue-print/final-report-of-the-global-research-and-innovation-forum-2022.pdf?sfvrsn=4a59021f_5&download=true.
57. WHO. Sexual and reproductive health and research (SRH): maternal and perinatal health. 2022. https://www.who.int/teams/sexual-and-reproductive-health-and-research-(srh)/areas-of-work/maternal-and-perinatal-health.
58. Adanu R, et al. Strengthening research capacity through regional partners: the HRP Alliance at the World Health Organization. Reprod Health. 2020;17:131.
59. GLOPID-R. Global research collaboration for infectious disease preparedness. 2022. https://www.glopid-r.org.
60. GLOPID-R. Covid-19 research recommendations and considerations for Glopid-R 2021–2023. 2021. https://www.glopid-r.org/wp-content/uploads/2021/09/glopid-r-sag-report.pdf.
61. WHO. The access to Covid-19 tools (act) accelerator. Geneva: WHO; 2022. https://www.who.int/initiatives/act-accelerator.
62. CEPI. Preparing for future pandemics. 2022. https://cepi.net.
63. GLOPID-R. Glopid-R co-chairs recommendations following the 2021 Glopid-R Scientific Advisory Group Report. 2021. https://www.glopid-r.org/wp-content/uploads/2021/09/glopid-r-sag-report-co-chairs-recommendations.pdf.
64. Turner MA, Kenny L, Alfirevic Z. Challenges in designing clinical trials to test new drugs in the pregnant woman and fetus. Clin Perinatol. 2019;46:399–416.

Chapter 15
Impact of COVID-19 Lockdowns on Maternal and Perinatal Health

Jasper V. Been, Marijn J. Vermeulen, and Brenda M. Kazemier

15.1 Introduction

15.1.1 Spread of the Pandemic and Initial Policy Responses

The first quarter of 2020 marked the global spread of the novel coronavirus SARS-CoV-2 and of its key clinical manifestation, coronavirus disease 2019 (COVID-19). By the end of January 2020, the World Health Organization (WHO) had declared the outbreak a 'public health emergency of international concern', with 98 confirmed cases in 18 countries outside China [1]. Six weeks later, the global number of cases had surpassed 100,000, and the situation was formally marked a pandemic on 11 March 2020 [1]. Governments across the globe instituted—and quickly escalated—a range of unprecedented public health measures to mitigate further spread of the pandemic and to curb its impact on healthcare resources (i.e. to 'flatten the curve') [2].

J. V. Been (✉)
Division of Neonatology, Department of Paediatrics and Department of Obstetrics and Gynaecology, Erasmus MC Sophia Children's Hospital, University Medical Centre Rotterdam, Rotterdam, The Netherlands
e-mail: j.been@erasmusmc.nl

M. J. Vermeulen
Division of Neonatology, Department of Paediatrics and Department of Obstetrics and Gynaecology, Erasmus MC Sophia Children's Hospital, University Medical Centre Rotterdam, Rotterdam, The Netherlands

Care4Neo, Dutch Neonatal Patient and Parent Organisation, Rotterdam The Netherlands
e-mail: m.j.vermeulen@erasmusmc.nl

B. M. Kazemier
Department of Obstetrics, Amsterdam Reproduction and Development Research Institute, Amsterdam UMC, Amsterdam, The Netherlands
e-mail: b.m.kazemier@amsterdamumc.nl

© The Author(s), under exclusive license to Springer Nature Switzerland AG 2023
D. De Luca, A. Benachi (eds.), *COVID-19 and Perinatology*,
https://doi.org/10.1007/978-3-031-29135-4_15

Initial measures included mass media campaigns to advise strict hygiene measures, isolation upon development of suggestive symptoms, social distancing, prohibition of mass gatherings, and contact tracing of established cases. In response to further intensification of the pandemic, additional approaches were implemented, including stay-at-home orders, travel restrictions, closing of 'non-essential' services and of public places, school closures, and curfews. Adding to the impact of the pandemic itself, such 'lockdowns' caused a substantial disruption of virtually any aspect previously considered a normal feature of society. Whereas this situation was soon recognised to represent a unique natural experiment [3, 4], very few would have anticipated its highly unusual impact on birth outcomes soon to be observed.

15.1.2 Drop in Preterm Births Following Lockdowns

Two months into the first lockdown era, preprints from Ireland and Denmark independently reported a substantial and unexpected drop in preterm births [5, 6]. In Ireland, Prof. Roy Philip and colleagues from Limerick Hospital noted that very few preterm babies had been admitted to their unit in the first quarter of 2020. In fact, not a single extremely low-birth-weight infant (ELBWI; i.e. birth weight < 1000 g) had been born during that period. Comparison of the rates among over 90,000 livebirths across a 20-year period confirmed that the low numbers were indeed exceptional. Philip and colleagues published their findings in a preprint on 5 June 2020 [5], demonstrating a 73% reduction in very-low-birth-weight infants (VLBWIs; i.e. birth weight < 1500 g) in January to April 2020 as compared to the corresponding calendar periods across the preceding 19 years. Two weeks earlier, a team from Denmark led by Gitte Hedermann had posted a preprint describing their nationwide cohort study on over 30,000 newborns which assessed the link between lockdown and preterm birth incidence [6]. During their first month of lockdown, rates of extremely preterm birth (i.e. gestational age < 28 weeks) were an astonishing 90% lower than in the corresponding calendar periods across the previous 5 years.

These intriguing findings soon went viral following coverage by *The New York Times* [7]. Various perinatal care providers from across the globe were interviewed, with several sharing similar experiences of 'nearly empty' neonatal intensive care units (NICUs) [7], although the anecdotal reductions were generally estimated to be less pronounced than in the Irish and Danish studies [5, 6]. These observations sparked enthusiasm among the perinatal health care community: Could this unusual phenomenon be the starting point for identification of novel preventive measures for preterm birth? A possible implication with huge potential for impact, given that worldwide over 1 in 10 babies are born preterm, contributing substantially to global child mortality and causing long-term adverse consequences among survivors [8]. At the same time, many questions emerged: Was this reproducible elsewhere? Was the reduction specific to either spontaneous or provider-initiated preterm deliveries? Was there a change in other pregnancy outcomes? Could an increase in stillbirths partly explain the observed reduction in babies born preterm? And perhaps most importantly, if these observations were causal, which mechanisms explained the findings?

15.1.3 Chapter Overview

Two years into the pandemic, several studies have addressed these and other questions regarding the indirect effects of the pandemic and its associated lockdowns on perinatal and maternal health, and many others are underway. In this chapter, we provide an overview of evidence from across the globe on this topic published up until Spring 2022. Systematic reviews and meta-analyses will be our starting points, and we will selectively discuss individual studies as relevant. We highlight common methodological drawbacks of published studies as well as preliminary evidence pointing towards specific mechanisms that may explain the observed impact. Implications for practice, policy, and future research will be briefly considered.

15.2 Impact of Lockdown Measures on Perinatal Outcomes

15.2.1 Impact of Lockdown on Preterm Birth

Following the preliminary evidence from Denmark and Ireland, several studies were conducted elsewhere to assess the link between lockdowns and perinatal outcomes, in particular preterm birth. This yielded a much more diverse picture: While several early studies also found a reduced incidence of preterm birth following lockdowns [9–11], this reduction was usually much more moderate than in the Danish and Irish studies. Also, a number of studies found no evidence of a reduction [12, 13]. A Nepalese study even noted a rise in the proportion of institutional births that were preterm [14]. Interpretation of this study is, however, complicated by the fact that institutional deliveries dropped substantially overall. This likely introduced bias as women delivering preterm were probably more inclined to deliver institutionally.

Early into 2021, Barbara Chmielewska and colleagues were the first to systematically review published evidence on the topic [15]. They identified 18 reports assessing the link between lockdowns and preterm birth. In a pooled analysis of 15 of these studies, no statistically significant overall impact of lockdown on preterm birth was identified: odds ratio (OR), 0.94; 95% confidence interval (CI), 0.87–1.02. A reduction was, however, observed when restricting the analysis to 12 studies undertaken in high-income countries (HICs): OR, 0.91; 95% CI, 0.84–0.99. Although a Dutch national quasi-experimental study on over 1.5 million newborns—the largest study conducted at the time—was not included in the meta-analysis [9], a post-hoc analysis showed that this did not have a major bearing on the findings [16]. Subgroup analyses suggested that the observed reduction in preterm births was primarily seen among spontaneous deliveries, although interpretation was limited by the small number of studies assessing this [15].

Additional systematic reviews and meta-analyses have been published since [17, 18]. Vaccaro and colleagues pooled data from 11 studies, yielding findings very similar to those reported by Chmielewska et al. regarding the association between lockdown and preterm birth: risk ratio (RR), 0.93; 95% CI, 0.84–1.03 [17]. A living systematic review by Yang and colleagues, which recently received its second update, is currently the most comprehensive assessment on the topic [18]. Their meta-analysis of 43 studies demonstrated an overall reduction in preterm birth incidence following lockdowns: OR, 0.95; 95% CI 0.93–0.98. Subgroup analyses showed that the reduction was mainly driven by studies from single centres and by drops in spontaneous rather than induced preterm births. Again, both systematic reviews excluded the study from the Netherlands because this report provided multiple estimates for the link between lockdown and preterm birth (i.e. for various starting points of lockdown and for varying time windows around these points) [9]. The Dutch study showed a 15%–23% reduction in preterm births across the first 2–4 months of lockdown, when defined by timing of implementation of the first set of mitigation measures [9].

Overall, the current evidence base indicates that there was indeed a reduction in preterm births following lockdowns. The reduction was, however, more moderate than suggested by the initial Irish and Danish reports [19, 20]. Follow-on studies from Ireland and Denmark also yielded much smaller effect estimates for the association between lockdown and preterm birth [21, 22]. A three-country comparison including Danish national registry data did not find a significant reduction in preterm births or in those born before 32 weeks of gestation [21]. An analysis of births from a Dublin hospital showed that preterm births were indeed lower in the first 7 months of 2020 as compared to the same calendar period in 2021, but the reduction was relatively small (7.4% vs. 8.6%; $p = 0.03$) [22].

Many aspects influence interpretation of the overall evidence base, including methodological issues, which we will discuss later. In addition, there has been substantial variation in the timing and comprehensiveness of lockdown measures between countries and subnational regions [2]. Similarly, there were stark geographical differences in the baseline incidence of preterm birth [8]. Healthcare system responses to the pandemic have also varied considerably across the globe. Several regions reallocated maternal and perinatal care resources to address COVID-19, while others were able to sustain pre-pandemic levels of care provision. These and other sources of variation likely contributed to the observed heterogeneity between studies. In addition, selective publication of studies with positive findings may have caused publication bias in this field. The international Perinatal Outcomes in the Pandemic (iPOP) study seeks to address some of these issues via international data integration using a standardised approach to data reporting and analysis [23]. Findings from a first pooled analysis of population-level data from 18 countries (including 51 million births) and of data from healthcare facilities from another eight countries (including 700,000 births) are expected soon.

15.2.2 Impact of Lockdown on Other Perinatal Outcomes

The reduction in preterm births following lockdown has generally been welcomed as a possible silver lining to the pandemic's dark cloud. However, a key concern has been that this positive outcome could be offset by an increase in stillbirths as a result of reduced care seeking or suboptimal care provision [12]. Clearly, appreciation of the overall impact of COVID-19 lockdowns on perinatal health requires assessment of a wider range of birth outcomes than preterm birth alone.

In their meta-analysis, Chmielewska and colleagues indeed observed an increase in stillbirths across 12 studies: OR, 1.28; 95% CI, 1.07–1.54 [15]. Again, similar findings were reported from the meta-analysis by Vaccaro et al.: RR, 1.33; 95% CI 1.04–1.69 (8 studies) [17]. However, the meta-analysis from the latest update of the living systematic review found no increased incidence of stillbirth following lockdowns across 31 studies: OR, 1.07; 95% CI 0.97–1.18 [18]. No statistically significant changes in neonatal mortality [15, 18], NICU admission [15], or low Apgar scores [15] were observed in any of the meta-analyses. These observations should be interpreted with care given the low number of studies assessing these outcomes. Reductions in the incidence of low birth weight have been observed [15, 17, 18], likely at least in part reflecting lower occurrence of preterm birth. In addition to these systematic reviews, the iPCP study will also be providing estimates of the association of lockdown with stillbirth and low birth weight across participating countries [23].

15.3 Impact of Lockdown Measures on Maternal Outcomes

In order to correctly interpret a change in preterm births, it is necessary to also take into account the impact of the lockdown on maternal outcomes. Restricted access to care, women's reluctance to visit health facilities, and quarantine measures may have contributed to delays in diagnosis and management of pregnancy-related complications, thus potentially impacting maternal and perinatal outcomes.

15.3.1 Impact of Lockdown on Hypertensive Disorders of Pregnancy

Pre-eclampsia is an important driver of iatrogenic preterm birth contributing to approximately 38% of iatrogenic preterm births between 28 and 31 weeks and approximately 22% of iatrogenic preterm births between 32 and 36 weeks [24]. In addition, pregnancy-induced hypertension is associated with an increased risk of stillbirth and neonatal mortality [25]. Therefore, changes in perinatal outcomes cannot be interpreted without evaluating possible changes in maternal outcomes as well.

Hypertensive disorders in pregnancy were found not to be statistically different in the pandemic compared to pre-pandemic period in HICs: OR, 0.99; 95% CI, 0.67–1.46 (5 studies) [15]. One single-centre study from China did report an increase in hypertensive disorders of pregnancy (OR, 5.59; 95% CI, 1.59–19.7) [26]. Incidence of pre-eclampsia was reported in studies from China [27], Zimbabwe [28], Australia [29], and England [30], all reporting no statistical difference in the pandemic compared to the pre-pandemic period.

15.3.2 *Impact of Lockdown on Other Maternal Outcomes*

Maternal death was reported to be increased with an OR of 1.37 (95% CI, 1.22–1.53), based on two studies from Mexico and India in the meta-analysis by Chmielewska and colleagues [15]. This increase was mainly driven by the study from Mexico which showed a stark increase in maternal deaths due to respiratory diseases in 2020. They reported that COVID-19 was the leading cause of maternal mortality in their country in 2020 [31]. As such, this increase in maternal deaths in Mexico more likely reflects a direct impact of the pandemic itself rather than an indirect impact mediated via lockdown measures.

Maternal death is a rare outcome in HICs; therefore, a possible impact of lockdown on maternal mortality in HICs is much more difficult to assess. Other outcomes such as maternal morbidity that can lead to maternal death could help to get a grasp of possible impact in HICs. For instance, surgical treatment of ectopic pregnancies was reported to be increased during lockdown (OR, 5.81; 95% CI, 2.16–15.6), based on a meta-analysis of three studies from the USA and two from Italy. This increase was found to be primarily due to an increased risk of ruptured ectopic pregnancies during lockdown [15], which could be the result of delays in presentation [32]. Obstetric postpartum haemorrhage is another cause of maternal death both in HICs and low-and-middle-income countries (LMICs). A meta-analysis of two HIC studies found no association between lockdown and the incidence of postpartum haemorrhage (OR, 1.02; 95% CI, 0.87–1.19) [15]. A single study from Israel found an increased risk of pregnancy-related venous thromboembolism events [33]. This higher rate was evident specifically during the two post-lockdown periods, suggesting a possible lag effect of population immobility resulting from the national lockdown restrictions. Whether this is a true effect due to, for instance, decreased physical activity during pregnancy, needs further investigation.

No impact of lockdown on the incidence of gestational diabetes was found in the meta-analysis by Chmielewska and colleagues in either HICs (OR, 1.02; 95% CI, 0.85–1.22; 5 studies) or in LMICs (OR, 1.01; 95% CI, 0.60–1.71; 1 study) [15]. However, impaired glycaemic control in women with gestational diabetes has been reported, possibly due to reduced physical activity and changes in dietary patterns during lockdown [34].

The impact of lockdown on maternal mental health and changes on care provision will be described later in this chapter.

15.3.3 Impact of Lockdown on Start and Mode of Delivery

Not only maternal outcomes can influence perinatal outcomes, but also possible changes in birth processes such as start and mode of delivery are important to take into account. Neither start of delivery nor mode of delivery were found to be impacted by the pandemic or the lockdown. Induction of labour in HICs remained stable (OR, 1.03; 95% CI, 0.90–1.19; 6 studies) as did the number of caesarean deliveries (OR, 1.03; 95% CI, 0.99–1.07; 17 studies) and instrumental vaginal deliveries (OR, 1.06; 95% CI, 0.97–1.15; 7 studies) [15]. However, maternal length of stay was reduced after both vaginal births and caesarean sections during the pandemic [32].

15.4 Impact of Lockdown on Postnatal Care and Breastfeeding

For those who experienced preterm birth during the COVID-19 lockdowns, special and intensive neonatal care provision and parent support varied widely [35, 36]. Institutions and caregivers struggled to find a balance between limiting the risks of viral spread, on the one hand, and providing patient and family-centred care, on the other. This was a particular challenge as family-centred care requires intense emotional and physical contact (including skin-to-skin care) of newborns with their parents and carers [35, 37]. Variation in containment strategies at national, regional, and hospital level, and across the different stages of lockdowns, led to stark differences in companion support during labour, family visiting policies, and peripartum and neonatal caregiver support [38]. In an international survey covering 12 countries, support reported by parents ranged from full allowance to be present with their newborn, to only maternal access, time-limited access, or complete parental visiting restriction [36]. Large variation was also seen in kangaroo mother care, breastfeeding support, and accessibility of follow-up clinics [35, 36]. The most restricted policies were generally associated with worse pregnancy outcomes, poorer maternal mental health, and less favourable neonatal outcomes, although long-term data are lacking [38].

Based on the advantages of breastfeeding and the unlikely risk of vertical transmission [39], the WHO and United Nations International Children's Emergency Fund (UNICEF) soon recommended protecting, promoting, and supporting direct breastfeeding and rooming-in with basic preventive measures [40, 41]. In many countries, however, the safety of this policy was being questioned, and some hospitals started routinely separating mothers and newborns and discouraged direct breastfeeding [42]. Even if mothers were expressing milk for their preterm infant, some hospitals restricted them from bringing the milk into the hospital [43]. Meanwhile, access to pasteurised human donor milk, which is recommended by the WHO as the first alternative if own mother's milk is unavailable, was also vulnerable [44]. Although global breastfeeding data during the pandemic are lacking [45], declined rates during lockdown were observed in hospitalised infants [46].

At the same time, positive experiences were also reported. Among South-African parents of preterm infants and those with mental health issues, strong senses of resilience were reported [47]. In a survey among over 1,200 breastfeeding mothers in the UK, 42% felt that breastfeeding was protected due to lockdown, because of increased time at home, less pressure, and fewer visitors [48]. Over 90% of 6,000 women surveyed in Belgium refuted that the pandemic affected their breastfeeding practices, with half of them even considering giving breastfeeding for a longer period because of COVID-19 [49].

15.5 Inequalities in Impact of Lockdown on Maternal and Perinatal Health

While the COVID-19 pandemic and associated lockdowns affected virtually every individual across the globe in one way or another, the distribution of this impact has been far from equal. Via impacting certain subgroups of the population more prominently than others, the pandemic has clearly aggravated existing inequalities in society, including with regard to health [50]. As such, COVID-19 may be considered a 'syndemic': 'a co-occurring, synergistic pandemic which interacts with and exacerbates existing chronic health and social conditions' [50]. In addition to the effects of the pandemic itself, lockdown measures also disproportionately affected deprived groups via increased economic losses, key worker roles, overcrowding, gender-based violence, and other mechanisms [50]. Disparities in the effect of COVID-19 on obstetric care have been observed across racial and ethnic categories, across socioeconomic indicators (e.g. household income, household size, area of residence, neighbourhood density, unemployment rates), and across various markers of access to care such as insurance status, primary language, and immigration status [51]. In addition, inequalities in the uptake of care provision alternatives such as telemedicine can influence how the pandemic affected population subgroups across countries as well as within countries [52]. It is, therefore, important to consider such inequalities when assessing the impact of lockdowns on maternal and perinatal health.

At the country level, the pandemic and lockdowns appear to have inadvertently affected women and newborns in LMICs as compared to those living in HICs. The meta-analysis by Chmielewska and colleagues showed that reductions in preterm birth were confined to HICs and not observed in LMICs (OR, 1.05; 95% CI, 0.81–1.35; 3 studies). Also, increases in stillbirth were statistically significant only for LMICs (OR, 1.29; 95% CI, 1.06–1.58; 4 studies), although the point estimate was comparable for HICs [15]. An increase in maternal mortality was observed across two LMIC studies [15], albeit largely driven by the study from Mexico which likely included many deaths due to COVID-19 [31]. While maternal mortality data in relation to lockdowns from HICs were lacking at the time, a study combining experiences from three maternity hospitals in Melbourne later found no change in maternal deaths following lockdown [29]. While none of the subsequent meta-analyses reported subgroup analyses according to country income level [17, 18], the iPOP study will include this comparison [23].

Inconsistency exists in findings from studies assessing variation in the impact of lockdown on maternal and perinatal health according to socioeconomic status (SES) or ethnic background. In the Netherlands, the observed reduction in preterm births following lockdown appeared to have been confined to women living in the most affluent neighbourhoods [9]. These findings are in line with those from a single-centre study from Pittsburgh, where preterm birth reductions also tended to favour women from advantaged neighbourhoods [53]. In contrast, data from a single institution in Chicago indicate that following lockdown, preterm birth rates decreased only among women in deprived neighbourhoods [54]. Inequalities in the occurrence of low birth weight also diminished between women delivering in private versus public facilities in Argentina following lockdown [55]. Changes in perinatal outcomes or obstetric interventions following lockdown did not vary according to SES in a nationwide study in England [30]. An interaction with ethnicity was, however, present: white women experienced a decrease in preterm birth following lockdown, while rates increased for women with a minority ethnic background [30]. A similar pattern was observed in the Pittsburgh study [53], whereas ethnic disparities in preterm birth did not materially change following lockdown in California and across two New York hospitals [56, 57].

Regarding breastfeeding, low SES mothers also faced more barriers, as data from nutritional support programmes in various countries show [48, 58, 59]. Given the recognised long-term health, societal, and economic benefits of breastfeeding for mother and child, this is an additional factor increasing health disparities.

Taken together, while the positive effects of lockdowns on preterm birth rates appear confined to HICs, LMICs experienced increased rates of stillbirth and perhaps also of maternal mortality. Evidence regarding differential patterning of the impact of lockdown on perinatal health within populations according to SES and ethnic background is conflicting, and this area requires further study.

15.6 Methodological Considerations

Appropriately evaluating natural experiments is a complex undertaking. Many methodological pitfalls apply, and a range of approaches to addressing these exist, each with their pros and cons. Key drawbacks of the current evidence base underlying our understanding of the link between lockdowns and maternal and perinatal health are that there is substantial variation in the robustness of methodological approaches applied and that meta-analyses did not take this variation into account. We highlight some of these issues to aid interpretation of the available evidence and help guide future studies.

15.6.1 Methodological Considerations: Original Studies

Many original studies assessing the link between lockdowns and maternal and perinatal health used an uncontrolled before-after design, where the mean rate of the outcome of interest was compared between the pre-lockdown and the lockdown period. A key drawback of this approach is that underlying temporal trends in the outcome of interest are not taken into account. Such temporal variation includes long-term underlying time trends as well as seasonal variation in the incidence of the outcome. Both aspects are commonly present regarding health outcomes and are well established for preterm birth [8, 60]. Not taking into account such underlying trends runs a substantial risk of misinterpretation of the findings.

Clear descriptions of the study population and outcome definition and assessment are of utmost importance, especially in preterm birth research. Preterm birth is not a uniform clinical entity but rather a syndrome with different underlying mechanisms of disease [61]. Stratifying analyses by iatrogenic versus spontaneous preterm birth is important to gain at least some insight into the underlying pathological processes. In practice, this can be challenging. For instance, induction of labour in case of premature prelabour rupture of membranes with signs of infection can be regarded by one as spontaneous preterm birth, whereas another regards this as an iatrogenic preterm birth. Clearly defining the study population is important in terms of composition of the pregnancies (e.g. multiple versus singleton births) and regarding in- or exclusion of stillbirths and/or major congenital anomalies among the preterm births.

Given the reliance of evaluation of natural experiments on observational approaches, confounding is a key issue to address. One important situation where this may influence the findings is when important demographic changes over time occur in population composition that are associated with the outcome of interest. This can be partially addressed by adjusting for such demographic characteristics in the analyses. Another approach is to focus on very narrow time windows (i.e. months) around the event—in this case the lockdown—whereby it can reasonably be assumed that no important demographic changes occurred in the population. This approach was applied when evaluating changes in preterm birth incidence following the Dutch lockdown using a difference-in-discontinuity approach [9]. A range of quasi-experimental approaches are available to address limitations of uncontrolled designs [62], and these should be more widely applied in future studies to solidify the current evidence base.

Another important source of confounding is co-intervention, i.e. another important change that may affect the outcome co-occurs with the event of interest [63]. In case of evaluating lockdowns, the obvious co-intervention—or perhaps more appropriately, 'co-exposure'—is the pandemic itself, although there may be others. Separating out the effects of the pandemic from those of the lockdowns is virtually impossible, although excluding confirmed COVID-19 cases from the study population where possible is a good start.

Because the pandemic and lockdowns were unanticipated, the vast majority of studies assessing their impact on maternal and perinatal outcomes rely on retrospective data, often from routinely collected data sources such as national birth registries. A risk of relying on institutional data (rather than population-based data) is that following lockdown, women may have changed institutions to receive their care or may have chosen to deliver at home, introducing bias via selective data missingness [14]. Population-based data may be expected to provide less biased estimates. It is furthermore important to note that in order to enable rapid analyses of the link between lockdown and preterm birth, researchers have sometimes had to rely on suboptimal data sources. These include neonatal screening databases, in which stillbirths and early neonatal deaths are missing [9, 20]. Changes in registration are another important potential source of bias. Before embarking on data analysis, it is therefore essential to check that registration of pregnancies and deliveries did not materially change as a result of the pandemic or lockdowns.

Finally, appropriately defining lockdown is a challenge. The initial Irish study, for example, evaluated changes in very-low-birth-weight babies from January 2020 onwards [5], although the first confirmed COVID-19 case in Ireland occurred only by the end of February, and true lockdown measures were introduced no earlier than March [64]. The quasi-experimental study in the Netherlands found reductions in preterm birth incidence when lockdown was defined by the first day that mitigation measures were introduced, but not when later lockdown intensifications were considered as the starting point [9]. This is another aspect complicating comparison of findings across studies. In the iPOP study, this is pragmatically addressed by defining the start of lockdown by the day that the Oxford Stringency Index, a composite measure of lockdown stringency [2], first topped 50 points out of 100, allowing uniformisation across participating countries [23].

15.6.2 *Methodological Considerations: Meta-Analyses*

The reliability of estimates from meta-analyses depends largely on the robustness of the underlying studies. Systematic reviews, therefore, typically include a risk-of-bias assessment of individual reports that are included. The vastly expanding number of studies that assessed the impact of lockdown on maternal and perinatal health allows future meta-analyses to focus on the highest quality evidence by restricting to low-risk-of-bias studies. In addition, the Cochrane Effective Practice and Organisation of Care guidelines can be helpful in defining the types of studies that typically provide the highest level of evidence [65, 66]. Whereas meta-analyses in this field so far have generally focused on pooling unadjusted data [15, 17, 18], for the reasons outlined above, it would be important in future meta-analyses to rely more on pooled adjusted effect estimates.

15.7 Exploring the Underlying Mechanisms

As outlined, there are clear indications that the COVID-19 pandemic and associated lockdowns impacted maternal and perinatal outcomes, including to some degree reducing the incidence of preterm birth. Determining the mechanisms behind the observed changes is essential to derive potential lessons on how these outcomes may be improved in the future, both within and outside the setting of a pandemic. Here, we briefly highlight the potential contribution of some of these mechanisms to the patterns observed, in particular in relation to a reduction in preterm birth incidence, and focus on those that are potentially modifiable.

15.7.1 Changes in Healthcare Seeking and Delivery

The COVID-19 pandemic affected care processes to various degrees across time and geographical location. In many places, maternal healthcare services were disrupted because routine non-emergency services were not provided, care processes changed to reduce spread of the virus by minimising contact, and shortages of proper protection materials for healthcare workers were an issue [67]. Travel restrictions and reduced availability of public transport limited some women from accessing essential maternity care services [68]. Studies from Nepal and India reported reductions in the number of institutionalised births of up to 52% [14, 69]. These and other changes are likely to have resulted in suboptimal care provision for many women during the antenatal, perinatal, and postpartum stages, in particular in low-resource settings.

Also in HICs, antenatal care changed for women, as many face-to-face consultations were replaced by teleconsultations [15] and as attendance restrictions were imposed for partners and other supporters during check-ups, delivery [70], and postpartum care [71], for example. A meta-analysis showed an overall drop of 39% in care appointments during the pandemic period across seven studies [32]. One in five women reported having voluntarily postponed or foregone at least one consultation [71]. Increased fear of contracting COVID-19 during pregnancy was found to be associated with postponing or cancelling routine obstetric appointments [72]. A study from Melbourne showed that teleconsultations can safely replace a substantial proportion of antenatal consultations [73]. If replicated across various settings, such observations can provide important guidance for future pregnancy care.

In a meta-analysis of seven studies, a drop was noted in unscheduled care attendance at maternity triage, urgent care, or obstetric emergency departments: incidence rate ratio (IRR), 0.74; 95% CI, 0.60–0.91 [32]. Among those women who did present to emergency care, the proportion of hospital admissions was higher [32]. Taken together, this suggests that women avoided or delayed seeking obstetric care in many circumstances, but that when they did seek care, their presentations were generally more severe. It is well imaginable that a general tendency to delay or avoid care has limited the detection of foetal distress and of maternal complications, hence contributing to an increased risk of adverse pregnancy outcomes such as stillbirth. Perhaps somewhat counterintuitively, reduced care-seeking may also have contributed to a reduction in iatrogenic preterm delivery, as foetal distress and pre-eclampsia which would otherwise have been an indication for iatrogenic preterm delivery went unnoticed as women stayed at home. This may in part explain the observed reduction in iatrogenic preterm deliveries in several countries [74], including across the USA [75]. In-depth and cross-country analyses of stakeholder experiences during the pandemic, including those of healthcare professionals and women receiving care at the time, can provide valuable lessons to guide future pandemic responses [76].

15.7.2 Maternal Stress and Working Conditions

Mothers experiencing high levels of stress or depressive symptoms are known to be at increased risk of adverse pregnancy outcomes, including preterm birth [77]. Maternal mental health was affected considerably by the lockdown and by the fear of contracting COVID-19 [78]. In a systematic review of the 11 studies reporting on maternal mental health, seven reported a statistically significant increase in postnatal depression, maternal anxiety, or both [15]. In a meta-analysis of three studies, the pooled mean increase on Edinburgh Perinatal/Postnatal Depression Scale (scale range: 0–30) was 0.42, 95% CI 0.02–0.81 [15]. A more recent meta-analysis suggested that antenatal anxiety was particularly high, with 40% of pregnant women overall and 56% in Europe, experiencing anxiety while pregnant during the COVID-19 crisis [79]. Overall rates of depression were also considerable: 27% in the antenatal period and 17% in the postnatal period [79]. Given the differential strain of the COVID-19 crisis on individuals depending on their socioeconomic circumstances, the adverse impact on maternal mental health also likely affected women in vulnerable situations disproportionally.

The COVID-19 crisis and associated lockdowns caused marked changes in work and working conditions. For some women, working conditions might have deteriorated due to increased stress or hazardous working conditions, but for others, working from home or working less might have improved conditions for their pregnant bodies. Given the recognised link between maternal working conditions and adverse pregnancy outcomes [80, 81], such changes may have contributed to the observed changes in perinatal outcomes during the pandemic. Job insecurity is likely to have increased stress for many, and marked increases in unemployment have been reported during and after the lockdown [82], impacting socioeconomic position as well as emotional stress and well-being. The exact contribution of these changing conditions to the observed changes in perinatal outcomes needs to be further investigated, with specific focus on exploring differences across socioeconomic subgroups and according to type of work.

15.7.3 Maternal Infections

The measures introduced following spread of the SARS-CoV-2 coronavirus pandemic, including consecutive lockdowns, have had an unprecedented impact on the prevalence and seasonality of many other infections worldwide. A marked decrease in respiratory syncytial virus infection in the 2020 winter season [83], a shorter and much less pronounced influenza season [84], and a lower prevalence of congenital cytomegalovirus infection in the year 2020 are just a few examples [85]. The introduction of measures such as social distancing, quarantine measures, mask wearing in public places, and regular handwashing also likely impacted the incidence of bacterial infections, including genitourinary infections and sexually transmitted diseases. In children, the incidence of cystitis and pyelonephritis was found to be lower during a period of social restrictions in the lockdown [86].

Infection and inflammation are major contributors to preterm birth, either directly through intrauterine infection or indirectly via infectious disease in the mother such as pyelonephritis, appendicitis, or for instance severe pneumonia [87]. It is therefore plausible that a change in the prevalence of maternal infections due to COVID-19 and lockdown measures may have impacted the incidence of preterm birth.

15.7.4 Air Pollution

The mitigation measures during the COVID-19 pandemic have substantially reduced commuting by car, air travel, and, to a more limited extent, industrial activities, which has resulted in substantial improvements of air quality all over the world. In the Netherlands, for example, the spring 2020 lockdown resulted in reductions of 18%–30% for nitrogen dioxide (NO_2) and 20% for particulate matter 2.5 (PM2.5), with a large contribution of reduced traffic-related exposure [88]. Reductions of similar magnitude were observed during lockdown across South and Southeast Asian cities [89]. Given the established link between air pollution and adverse pregnancy outcomes [90], these reductions may well have translated into benefits to perinatal health. A modelling study estimated that if the 23% reduction in PM2.5 levels observed following lockdown in New York City would be sustained, more than 900 preterm births could be avoided over the next 5 years [91]. More work is needed to quantify the contribution of improved ambient air quality to the observed changes in perinatal outcomes following lockdown.

15.7.5 Other Mechanisms

Given the wide-ranging disruptive impact of the COVID-19 crisis and associated lockdowns, many more mechanisms might be implicated in the fluctuations in adverse pregnancy outcomes. These include changes in physical activity [92], in access to essential medicines [89], in smoking prevalence, and in dietary patterns, including in intake of supplements [82]. Disentangling the contribution of these and other pathways to the variation in pregnancy outcomes observed following lockdowns will be a key challenge for future research.

15.8 Future Research Needs and Implications

The COVID-19 pandemic and associated lockdowns constitute a natural experiment of unequalled impact in recent history, both in terms of geographical spread and regarding the wide range of aspects of everyday life affected within a very short time frame. Natural experiments provide a robust opportunity to establish causal mechanisms under circumstances were randomised controlled trials are not feasible [93]. There is, thus, substantial current momentum to quantify and help understand its impact on maternal and perinatal health and inequalities in these outcomes in order to disentangle the underlying mechanisms of the observed link between the COVID-19 lockdown and perinatal outcomes, in particular preterm birth.

At present, and as highlighted earlier, the overall picture is complicated by limitations of the underlying data and lack of robustness of the analytic approaches from individual studies [16]. There is, thus, a clear need for additional methodologically sound approaches to assess the impact of lockdowns on a broad range of maternal and perinatal health outcomes using high-quality population-based datasets. These insights can be based on epidemiological (i.e. quasi-experimental) evaluations, supplemented with information from mixed-methods approaches (including qualitative research) and cohort studies.

Research focused on the maternal and perinatal effects of the COVID-19 pandemic and associated lockdowns can also help us to be better prepared in the likely event of a future pandemic. Together with patient and professional organisations, an action plan aimed at optimising pregnancy and perinatal care during future pandemics should be created, while minimising infection risk. Such efforts should be undertaken at (sub)national and international level. Pandemic preparedness plans should include detailed scripts describing appropriate and balanced adaptations to regular care across the various tiers (i.e. primary, secondary, and tertiary care) during different phases of a pandemic and lockdown. Particular attention is needed to adequately support parents in vulnerable situations, optimise contact between parents and their newborns, and stimulate safe breastfeeding.

Output of ongoing research should be reflected on by relevant stakeholders, including patient and public representatives, healthcare professionals, and policymakers, in order to identify targets for future prevention—both within and outside the setting of a pandemic—via changing practice (e.g. guidelines) and policy. In addition, future initiatives should work closely together with patient and public representatives to formulate and disseminate recommendations towards the general public. Pregnant women and their families need to be informed on the mechanisms that they themselves can influence directly, with particular attention to enabling adequate information transfer and support to women in vulnerable circumstances.

Such efforts have the potential to benefit maternal and perinatal health for future generations and reduce health inequalities at their earliest origins and as such help achieve a lasting benefit of the global COVID-19 tragedy [3, 94].

15.9 Conclusion

Pregnancy and childbirth are highly intriguing events that—willingly or unwillingly—impact on every single member of society. Despite their universal relevance and despite substantial research efforts to understand the underlying complexities, many unknowns remain. Tremendous advances in maternal and perinatal survival have been achieved over the last century [95, 96]. Whereas significant progress is possible and still being made in many low-resource settings, improvements in perinatal and maternal health outcomes have plateaued in HICs. The observed reductions in preterm births following COVID-19 lockdowns in several settings suggest that modifiable factors exist that carry potential for prevention which is not currently optimally employed. In similar ways, we may learn from disruptions that occurred during lockdown that affected other maternal and perinatal outcomes in order to help optimise future practice and policy. Filling these knowledge gaps can open up novel opportunities for improving maternal and perinatal health in the future.

References

1. World Health Organization. Timeline: WHO's COVID-19 response: World Health Organization. 2022. https://www.who.int/emergencies/diseases/novel-coronavirus-2019/interactive-timeline/#!. Accessed 28 Apr 2022.
2. Hale T, Angrist N, Cameron-Blake E, Hallas L, Kira B, Majumdar S, et al. Oxford COVID-19 government response tracker. Blavatnik School of Government. 2020. https://www.bsg.ox.ac.uk/research/research-projects/coronavirus-government-response-tracker. Accessed 28 Apr 2022.
3. Been JV, Sheikh A. COVID-19 must catalyse key global natural experiments. J Glob Health. 2020;10(1):010104.
4. Rosen J. Pandemic upheaval offers a huge natural experiment. Nature. 2021;596(7870):149–51.
5. Philip RK, Purtill H, Reidy E, Daly M, Imcha M, McGrath D, et al. Reduction in preterm births during the COVID-19 lockdown in Ireland: a natural experiment allowing analysis of data from the prior two decades. medRxiv. 2020:2020.06.03.20121442.
6. Hedermann G, Hedley PL, Baekvad-Hansen M, Hjalgrim H, Rostgaard K, Poorisrisak P, et al. Changes in premature birth rates during the Danish nationwide COVID-19 lockdown: a nationwide register-based prevalence proportion study. medRxiv. 2020:2020.05.22.20109793.
7. Preston E. During coronavirus lockdowns, some doctors wondered: where are the preemies? The New York Times. 2020.
8. Chawanpaiboon S, Vogel JP, Moller AB, Lumbiganon P, Petzold M, Hogan D, et al. Global, regional, and national estimates of levels of preterm birth in 2014: a systematic review and modelling analysis. Lancet Glob Health. 2019;7(1):e37–46.

9. Been JV, Burgos Ochoa L, Bertens LCM, Schoenmakers S, Steegers EAP, Reiss IKM. Impact of COVID-19 mitigation measures on the incidence of preterm birth: a national quasi-experimental study. Lancet Public Health. 2020;5(11):e604–e11.
10. Kasuga Y, Tanaka M, Ochiai D. Preterm delivery and hypertensive disorder of pregnancy were reduced during the COVID-19 pandemic: a single hospital-based study. J Obstet Gynaecol Res. 2020;46:2703. https://doi.org/10.1111/jog.14518.
11. Berghella V, Boelig R, Roman A, Burd J, Anderson K. Decreased incidence of preterm birth during coronavirus disease 2019 pandemic. Am J Obstet Gynecol MFM. 2020;2(4):100258.
12. Khalil A, von Dadelszen P, Draycott T, Ugwumadu A, O'Brien P, Magee L. Change in the incidence of stillbirth and preterm delivery during the COVID-19 pandemic. JAMA. 2020;324(7):705–6.
13. Justman N, Shahak G, Gutzeit O, Ben Zvi D, Ginsberg Y, Solt I, et al. Lockdown with a price: the impact of the COVID-19 pandemic on prenatal care and perinatal outcomes in a tertiary care center. Isr Med Assoc J. 2020;22(9):533–7.
14. Kc A, Gurung R, Kinney MV, Sunny AK, Moinuddin M, Basnet O, et al. Effect of the COVID-19 pandemic response on intrapartum care, stillbirth, and neonatal mortality outcomes in Nepal: a prospective observational study. Lancet Glob Health. 2020;8(10):e1273–e81.
15. Chmielewska B, Barratt I, Townsend R, Kalafat E, van der Meulen J, Gurol-Urganci I, et al. Effects of the COVID-19 pandemic on maternal and perinatal outcomes: a systematic review and meta-analysis. Lancet Glob Health. 2021;9(6):e759–e72.
16. Ochoa LB, Brockway M, Stock SJ, Been JV. COVID-19 and maternal and perinatal outcomes. Lancet Glob Health. 2021;9(8):e1063–e4.
17. Vaccaro C, Mahmoud F, Aboulatta L, Aloud B, Eltonsy S. The impact of COVID-19 first wave national lockdowns on perinatal outcomes: a rapid review and meta-analysis. BMC Pregnancy Childbirth. 2021;21(1):676.
18. Yang J, D'Souza R, Kharrat A, Fell DB, Snelgrove JW, Shah PS. COVID-19 pandemic and population-level pregnancy and neonatal outcomes in general population: a living systematic review and meta-analysis (update#2: November 20, 2021). Acta Obstet Gynecol Scand. 2022;101(3):273–92.
19. Philip RK, Purtill H, Reidy E, Daly M, Imcha M, McGrath D, et al. Unprecedented reduction in births of very low birthweight (VLBW) and extremely low birthweight (ELBW) infants during the COVID-19 lockdown in Ireland: a 'natural experiment' allowing analysis of data from the prior two decades. BMJ Glob Health 2020;5(9):e003075.
20. Hedermann G, Hedley PL, Bækvad-Hansen M, Hjalgrim H, Rostgaard K, Poorisrisak P, et al. Danish premature birth rates during the COVID-19 lockdown. Arch Dis Child Fetal Neonatal Ed. 2021;106(1):93–5.
21. Oakley LL, Örtqvist AK, Kinge J, Hansen AV, Petersen TG, Södering J, et al. Preterm birth after the introduction of COVID-19 mitigation measures in Norway, Sweden, and Denmark: a registry-based difference-in-differences study. Am J Obstet Gynecol. 2021;226(4):550.e1–550.e22.
22. McDonnell S, McNamee E, Lindow SW, O'Connell MP. The impact of the Covid-19 pandemic on maternity services: a review of maternal and neonatal outcomes before, during and after the pandemic. Eur J Obstet Gynecol Reprod Biol. 2020;255:172–6.
23. Stock SJ, Zoega H, Brockway M, Mulholland RH, Miller JE, Been JV, et al. The international perinatal outcomes in the pandemic (iPOP) study: protocol. Wellcome Open Res. 2021;6:21.
24. Auger N, Le TU, Park AL, Luo ZC. Association between maternal comorbidity and preterm birth by severity and clinical subtype: retrospective cohort study. BMC Pregnancy Childbirth. 2011;11:67.
25. Ananth CV, Basso O. Impact of pregnancy-induced hypertension on stillbirth and neonatal mortality. Epidemiology. 2010;21(1):118–23.
26. Gu XX, Chen K, Yu H, Liang GY, Chen H, Shen Y. How to prevent in-hospital COVID-19 infection and reassure women about the safety of pregnancy: experience from an obstetric center in China. J Int Med Res. 2020;48(7):300060520939337.

27. Dong M, Qian R, Wang J, Fan J, Ye Y, Zhou H, et al. Associations of COVID-19 lockdown with gestational length and preterm birth in China. BMC Pregnancy Childbirth. 2021;21(1):795.
28. Shakespeare C, Dube H, Moyo S, Ngwenya S. Resilience and vulnerability of maternity services in Zimbabwe: a comparative analysis of the effect of Covid-19 and lockdown control measures on maternal and perinatal outcomes, a single-centre cross-sectional study at Mpilo Central Hospital. BMC Pregnancy Childbirth. 2021;21(1):416.
29. Rolnik DL, Matheson A, Liu Y, Chu S, McGannon C, Mulcahy B, et al. Impact of COVID-19 pandemic restrictions on pregnancy duration and outcome in Melbourne, Australia. Ultrasound Obstet Gynecol. 2021;58(5):677–87.
30. Gurol-Urganci I, Waite L, Webster K, Jardine J, Carroll F, Dunn G, et al. Obstetric interventions and pregnancy outcomes during the COVID-19 pandemic in England: a nationwide cohort study. PLoS Med. 2022;19(1):e1003884.
31. Lumbreras-Marquez MI, Campos-Zamora M, Seifert SM, Kim J, Lumbreras-Marquez J, Vazquez-Alaniz F, et al. Excess maternal deaths associated with coronavirus disease 2019 (COVID-19) in Mexico. Obstet Gynecol. 2020;136(6):1114–6.
32. Townsend R, Chmielewska B, Barratt I, Kalafat E, van der Meulen J, Gurol-Urganci I, et al. Global changes in maternity care provision during the COVID-19 pandemic: a systematic review and meta-analysis. EClinicalMedicine. 2021;37:100947.
33. Gabrieli D, Cahen-Peretz A, Shimonovitz T, Marks-Garber K, Amsalem H, Kalish Y, et al. Thromboembolic events in pregnant and puerperal women after COVID-19 lockdowns: a retrospective cohort study. Int J Gynaecol Obstet. 2021;155(1):95–100.
34. Ghesquiere L, Garabedian C, Drumez E, Lemaitre M, Cazaubiel M, Bengler C, et al. Effects of COVID-19 pandemic lockdown on gestational diabetes mellitus: a retrospective study. Diabetes Metab. 2021;47(2):101201.
35. Rao SPN, Minckas N, Medvedev MM, Gathara D, Prashantha YN, Seifu Estifanos A, et al. Small and sick newborn care during the COVID-19 pandemic: global survey and thematic analysis of healthcare providers' voices and experiences. BMJ Glob Health. 2021;6(3):e004347.
36. Kostenzer J, von Rosenstiel-Pulver C, Hoffmann J, Walsh A, Mader S, Zimmermann LJI, et al. Parents' experiences regarding neonatal care during the COVID-19 pandemic: country-specific findings of a multinational survey. BMJ Open. 2022;12(4):e056856.
37. Carter BS, Willis T, Knackstedt A. Neonatal family-centered care in a pandemic. J Perinatol. 2021;41(5):1177–9.
38. Mok YK, Cheung KW, Wang W, Li RHW, Shek NWM, Yu Ng EH. The effects of not having continuous companion support during labour on pregnancy and neonatal outcomes during the COVID-19 pandemic. Midwifery. 2022;108:103293.
39. Salvatore CM, Han JY, Acker KP, Tiwari P, Jin J, Brandler M, et al. Neonatal management and outcomes during the COVID-19 pandemic: an observation cohort study. Lancet Child Adolesc Health. 2020;4(10):721–7.
40. World Health Organization. WHO frequently asked questions: breastfeeding and COVID-19 for health care workers. J Hum Lact. 2020;36(3):392–6.
41. UNICEF. Supporting baby friendly assessments: supporting health professionals during COVID-19. 2021. https://www.unicef.org.uk/babyfriendly/infant-feeding-during-the-covid-19-outbreak. Accessed 28 Apr 2022.
42. Vu Hoang D, Cashin J, Gribble K, Marinelli K, Mathisen R. Misalignment of global COVID-19 breastfeeding and newborn care guidelines with World Health Organization recommendations. BMJ Nutr Prev Health. 2020;3(2):339–50.
43. Gunes AO, Dincer E, Karadag N, Topcuoglu S, Karatekin G. Effects of COVID-19 pandemic on breastfeeding rates in a neonatal intensive care unit. J Perinat Med. 2021;49(4):500–5.
44. Shenker N, Staff M, Vickers A, Aprigio J, Tiwari S, Nangia S, et al. Maintaining human milk bank services throughout the COVID-19 pandemic: a global response. Matern Child Nutr. 2021;17(3):e13131.
45. Global Breastfeeding Collective, UNICEF, World Health Organization. Global Breastfeeding Scorecard 2021: protecting breastfeeding through bold national actions during the COVID-19

pandemic and beyond. 2021. https://www.who.int/publications/i/item/WHO-HEP-NFS-21.45. Accessed 28 Apr 2022.
46. Zanardo V, Tortora D, Guerrini P, Garani G, Severino L, Soldera G, et al. Infant feeding initiation practices in the context of COVID-19 lockdown. Early Hum Dev. 2021;152:105286.
47. Farley E, Edwards A, Numanoglu E, Phillips TK. Lockdown babies: birth and new parenting experiences during the 2020 Covid-19 lockdown in South Africa, a cross-sectional study. Women Birth. 2022;35(4):394–402.
48. Brown A, Shenker N. Experiences of breastfeeding during COVID-19: lessons for future practical and emotional support. Matern Child Nutr. 2021;17(1):e13088.
49. Ceulemans M, Verbakel JY, Van Calsteren K, Eerdekens A, Allegaert K, Foulon V. SARS-CoV-2 infections and impact of the COVID-19 pandemic in pregnancy and breastfeeding: results from an observational study in primary care in Belgium. Int J Environ Res Public Health. 2020;17(18):6766.
50. Bambra C, Lynch J, Smith KE. The unequal pandemic: COVID-19 and health inequalities. 1st ed. Bristol: University Press; 2021.
51. Emeruwa UN, Gyamfi-Bannerman C, Miller RS. Health care disparities in the COVID-19 pandemic in the United States: a focus on obstetrics. Clin Obstet Gynecol. 2022;65(1):123–33.
52. Potenza S, Marzan MB, Rolnik DL, Palmer K, Said J, Whitehead C, et al. Business as usual during the COVID-19 pandemic? Reflections on state-wide trends in maternity telehealth consultations during lockdown in Victoria and New South Wales. Aust N Z J Obstet Gynaecol. 2021;61(6):982–5.
53. Lemon L, Edwards RP, Simhan HN. What is driving the decreased incidence of preterm birth during the coronavirus disease 2019 pandemic? Am J Obstet Gynecol MFM. 2021;3(3):100330.
54. Fisher SA, Sakowicz A, Barnard C, Kidder S, Miller ES. Neighborhood deprivation and preterm delivery during the coronavirus 2019 pandemic. Am J Obstet Gynecol MFM. 2022;4(1):100493.
55. Cuestas E, Gómez-Flores ME, Charras MD, Peyrano AJ, Montenegro C, Sosa-Boye I, et al. Socioeconomic inequalities in low birth weight risk before and during the COVID-19 pandemic in Argentina: a cross-sectional study. Lancet Reg Health Am 2021;2:100049.
56. Janevic T, Glazer KB, Vieira L, Weber E, Stone J, Stern T, et al. Racial/ethnic disparities in very preterm birth and preterm birth before and during the COVID-19 pandemic. JAMA Netw Open. 2021;4(3):e211816.
57. Main EK, Chang SC, Carpenter AM, Wise PH, Stevenson DK, Shaw GM, et al. Singleton preterm birth rates for racial and ethnic groups during the coronavirus disease 2019 pandemic in California. Am J Obstet Gynecol. 2021;224(2):239–41.
58. Koleilat M, Whaley SE, Clapp C. The impact of COVID-19 on breastfeeding rates in a low-income population. Breastfeed Med 2022;17(1):33–7.
59. Sayed N, Burger R, Harper A, Swart EC. Lockdown-associated hunger may be affecting breastfeeding: findings from a large SMS survey in South Africa. Int J Environ Res Public Health. 2021;19(1):351.
60. Hviid A, Laksafoss A, Hedley P, Lausten-Thomsen U, Hjalgrim H, Christiansen M, et al. Assessment of seasonality and extremely preterm birth in Denmark. JAMA Netw Open. 2022;5(2):e2145800.
61. Romero R, Dey SK, Fisher SJ. Preterm labor: one syndrome, many causes. Science. 2014;345(6198):760–5.
62. Craig P, Katikireddi SV, Leyland A, Popham F. Natural experiments: an overview of methods, approaches, and contributions to public health intervention research. Annu Rev Public Health. 2017;38:39–56.
63. Mikus M, Sokol Karadjole V, Kalafatic D, Oreskovic S, Sarcevic A. Increase of stillbirths and unplanned out-of-hospital births during coronavirus disease 2019 lockdown and the Zagreb earthquake. Acta Obstet Gynecol Scand. 2021;100(11):2119–20.
64. Perumal V, Curran T, Hunter M. First case of COVID-19 in Ireland. Ulster Med J. 2020;89(2):128.

65. Cochrane Effective Practice and Organisation of Care. What study designs can be considered for inclusion in an EPOC review and what should they be called? 2017. https://epoc.cochrane.org/sites/epoc.cochrane.org/files/public/uploads/EPOC%20Study%20Designs%20About.pdf. Accessed 28 Apr 2022.
66. Faber T, Kumar A, Mackenbach JP, Millett C, Basu S, Sheikh A, et al. Effect of tobacco control policies on perinatal and child health: a systematic review and meta-analysis. Lancet Public Health. 2017;2(9):e420–e37.
67. Mackworth-Young CR, Chingono R, Mavodza C, McHugh G, Tembo M, Chikwari CD, et al. Community perspectives on the COVID-19 response, Zimbabwe. Bull World Health Organ. 2021;99(2):85–91.
68. Murewanhema G, Makurumidze R. Essential health services delivery in Zimbabwe during the COVID-19 pandemic: perspectives and recommendations. Pan Afr Med J. 2020;35(Suppl 2):143.
69. Goyal M, Singh P, Singh K, Shekhar S, Agrawal N, Misra S. The effect of the COVID-19 pandemic on maternal health due to delay in seeking health care: experience from a tertiary center. Int J Gynaecol Obstet. 2021;152(2):231–5.
70. Morniroli D, Consales A, Colombo L, Bezze EN, Zanotta L, Plevani L, et al. Exploring the impact of restricted partners' visiting policies on non-infected mothers' mental health and breastfeeding rates during the COVID-19 pandemic. Int J Environ Res Public Health. 2021;18(12):6347.
71. Doncarli A, Araujo-Chaveron L, Crenn-Hebert C, Demiguel V, Boudet-Berquier J, Barry Y, et al. Impact of the SARS-CoV-2 pandemic and first lockdown on pregnancy monitoring in France: the COVIMATER cross-sectional study. BMC Pregnancy Childbirth. 2021;21(1):799.
72. Shayganfard M, Mahdavi F, Haghighi M, Sadeghi Bahmani D, Brand S. Health anxiety predicts postponing or cancelling routine medical health care appointments among women in perinatal stage during the Covid-19 lockdown. Int J Environ Res Public Health. 2020;17(21):8272.
73. Palmer KR, Tanner M, Davies-Tuck M, Rindt A, Papacostas K, Giles ML, et al. Widespread implementation of a low-cost telehealth service in the delivery of antenatal care during the COVID-19 pandemic: an interrupted time-series analysis. Lancet. 2021;398(10294):41–52.
74. Klumper J, Kazemier BM, Been JV, Bloemenkamp KWM, de Boer MA, Erwich J, et al. Association between COVID-19 lockdown measures and the incidence of iatrogenic versus spontaneous very preterm births in The Netherlands: a retrospective study. BMC Pregnancy Childbirth. 2021;21(1):767.
75. Dench D, Joyce T, Minkoff H. United States preterm birth rate and COVID-19. Pediatrics. 2022;149:e2021055495.
76. van den Berg L, Balaam MC, Nowland R, Moncrieff G, Topalidou A, Thompson S, et al. The United Kingdom and The Netherlands maternity care responses to COVID-19: a comparative study. Women Birth. 2022;36(1):127–35.
77. Staneva A, Bogossian F, Pritchard M, Wittkowski A. The effects of maternal depression, anxiety, and perceived stress during pregnancy on preterm birth: a systematic review. Women Birth. 2015;28(3):179–93.
78. Schoenmakers S, Verweij EJJ, Beijers R, Bijma HH, Been JV, Steegers-Theunissen RPM, et al. The impact of maternal prenatal stress related to the COVID-19 pandemic during the first 1000 days: a historical perspective. Int J Environ Res Public Health. 2022;19(8):4710.
79. Shorey SY, Ng ED, Chee CYI. Anxiety and depressive symptoms of women in the perinatal period during the COVID-19 pandemic: a systematic review and meta-analysis. Scand J Public Health. 2021;49(7):730–40.
80. van Beukering MD, van Melick MJ, Mol BW, Frings-Dresen MH, Hulshof CT. Physically demanding work and preterm delivery: a systematic review and meta-analysis. Int Arch Occup Environ Health. 2014;87(8):809–34.
81. van Melick MJ, van Beukering MD, Mol BW, Frings-Dresen MH, Hulshof CT. Shift work, long working hours and preterm birth: a systematic review and meta-analysis. Int Arch Occup Environ Health. 2014;87(8):835–49.

82. Muhaidat N, Fram K, Thekrallah F, Qatawneh A, Al-Btoush A. Pregnancy during COVID-19 outbreak: the impact of lockdown in a middle-income country on antenatal healthcare and wellbeing. Int J Women's Health. 2020;12:1065–73.
83. Torres-Fernandez D, Casellas A, Mellado MJ, Calvo C, Bassat Q. Acute bronchiolitis and respiratory syncytial virus seasonal transmission during the COVID-19 pandemic in Spain: a national perspective from the pediatric Spanish Society (AEP). J Clin Virol. 2021;145:105027.
84. Kuitunen I, Artama M, Makela L, Backman K, Heiskanen-Kosma T, Renko M. Effect of social distancing due to the COVID-19 pandemic on the incidence of viral respiratory tract infections in children in Finland during early 2020. Pediatr Infect Dis J. 2020;39(12):e423–7.
85. Fernandez C, Chasqueira MJ, Marques A, Rodrigues L, Marcal M, Tuna M, et al. Lower prevalence of congenital cytomegalovirus infection in Portugal: possible impact of COVID-19 lockdown? Eur J Pediatr. 2022;181(3):1259–62.
86. Kuitunen I, Artama M, Haapanen M, Renko M. Urinary tract infections decreased in Finnish children during the COVID-19 pandemic. Eur J Pediatr. 2022;181:1979. https://doi.org/10.1007/s00431-022-04389-9.
87. Goldenberg RL, Culhane JF, Iams JD, Romero R. Epidemiology and causes of preterm birth. Lancet. 2008;371(9606):75–84.
88. Velders GJM, Willers SM, Wesselink J, van den Elshout S, van der Swaluw E, Mooibroek D, et al. Improvements in air quality in The Netherlands during the corona lockdown based on observations and model simulations. Atmos Environ. 2021;247:118158.
89. Roy S, Saha M, Dhar B, Pandit S, Nasrin R. Geospatial analysis of COVID-19 lockdown effects on air quality in the South and Southeast Asian region. Sci Total Environ. 2021;756:144009.
90. Ghosh R, Causey K, Burkart K, Wozniak S, Cohen A, Brauer M. Ambient and household PM2.5 pollution and adverse perinatal outcomes: a meta-regression and analysis of attributable global burden for 204 countries and territories. PLoS Med. 2021;18(9):e1003718.
91. Perera F, Berberian A, Cooley D, Shenaut E, Olmstead H, Ross Z, et al. Potential health benefits of sustained air quality improvements in New York City: a simulation based on air pollution levels during the COVID-19 shutdown. Environ Res. 2020;193:110555.
92. Hegaard HK, Rom AL, Christensen KB, Broberg L, Hogh S, Christiansen CH, et al. Lifestyle habits among pregnant women in Denmark during the first COVID-19 lockdown compared with a historical period–a hospital-based cross-sectional study. Int J Environ Res Public Health. 2021;18(13):7128.
93. de Vocht F, Katikireddi SV, McQuire C, Tilling K, Hickman M, Craig P. Conceptualising natural and quasi experiments in public health. BMC Med Res Methodol. 2021;21(1):32.
94. Jacob CM, Briana DD, Di Renzo GC, Modi N, Bustreo F, Conti G, et al. Building resilient societies after COVID-19: the case for investing in maternal, neonatal, and child health. Lancet Public Health. 2020;5(11):e624–e7.
95. GBD 2015 Maternal Mortality Collaborators. Global, regional, and national levels of maternal mortality, 1990–2015: a systematic analysis for the Global Burden of Disease Study 2015. Lancet. 2016;388(10053):1775–812
96. GBD 2019 Under-5 Mortality Collaborators. Global, regional, and national progress towards Sustainable Development Goal 3.2 for neonatal and child health: all-cause and cause-specific mortality findings from the Global Burden of Disease Study 2019. Lancet. 2021;398(10303):870–905.

Chapter 16
Prevention of Future Pandemics and Impact on Perinatology

Fidelia Cascini, Alberto Lontano, Giovanna Failla, Valeria Puleo, and Walter Ricciardi

16.1 Background

The COVID-19 pandemic has placed a major stress test on healthcare services because there have been a huge number of requests, questions, and doubts from both patients and the general population directed to healthcare professionals and scientists that each required prompt and critical health information [1]. Further, the pandemic has undoubtedly had a major impact on all of humankind, including pregnant women and newborns. Based on current scientific evidence, it is established that pregnant women or women who recently got pregnant are more likely to get severely ill with COVID-19 compared to the general population [2]. In addition, they are at higher risk of severe pregnancy outcomes (such as preeclampsia, preterm birth, etc.) compared with pregnant women who were not confirmed with COVID-19 [2, 3], implying that the best prevention strategy is vaccination.

Getting a COVID-19 vaccine and then a booster shot can help protect these people from severe outcomes caused by COVID-19 [4]. COVID-19 vaccination is recommended for people who are pregnant, breastfeeding, trying to conceive at the moment, or in the future [5, 6]. Research and evidence about the safety and effectiveness of COVID-19 vaccination during pregnancy has been established and benefits of receiving a COVID-19 vaccine exceed any occurred or potential risks of vaccination during pregnancy [4].

Nevertheless, since vaccines entered the battlefield as one of the main successful weapons against SARS-CoV-2, scientists in the field of perinatology unfortunately expressed contrasting opinions initially. Numerous public concerns about the safety

---

F. Cascini (✉) · A. Lontano · G. Failla · V. Puleo · W. Ricciardi
Section of Hygiene and Public Health, Department of Life Sciences and Public Health, Università Cattolica del Sacro Cuore, Rome, Italy
e-mail: fidelia.cascini1@unicatt.it; alberto.lontano01@icatt.it; walter.ricciardi@unicatt.it

of COVID-19 vaccination during pregnancy have emerged [7]. This was confusing for the population; thus, pregnant women found themselves unarmed against a flood of fake news, misinformation, and disinformation.

The difference between misinformation and disinformation should be clarified upfront: misinformation includes false information, initially considered to be true, therefore without the intent to mislead [8]. On the other hand, disinformation can be defined as the intention to share and spread "deliberately misleading or biased information; manipulated narrative or facts; propaganda" [9].

In this chapter, we present an overview of the online content related to COVID-19 vaccines and pregnancy that is identified as inaccurate. More specifically, it analyzes what are the most engaging/popular categories of fake news, along with some of its examples, and how the national and international legislative bodies have addressed the problem of inaccurate information regarding COVID-19 vaccines and perinatology.

16.2 Prevention and Communication

A clear communication during an emergency is important and essential for a successful response and recovery: A structured governance of communication is required in public health [10], especially when dealing with crises such as pandemic emergencies and the related occurrence of infodemics [11]. Peoples' reactions to the crisis can be complicated by new communication channels, such as social media, which force people to cope with massive amounts of information that aren't always expressed by relevant experts. At the same time, public health experts and institutions are responsible for the timely sharing of official and evidence-based recommendations [12].

New disciplines have thus emerged that aim to study the phenomenon of infodemics in order to propose useful tools for combating fake news, misinformation, and disinformation. The most significant new discipline is that of infodemiology and infoveillance [13]. The term "infodemiology" was coined by Eysenbach in 2002 [14], while the World Health Organization (WHO) promoted the first Infodemiology Conference in 2020 [15]. It is clear that a growing interest in these new disciplines has been expressed.

An interesting aspect of the infodemic that has emerged during the pandemic has been the race to censor misinformation. Some experts from the UK Royal Society point out that this is not the best approach, as it would be preferable to track misinformation and fight it with the power of truthful information, fact-checking labels, regulating recommendation algorithms, and demonetization [16].

In order to analyze the problem of misinformation and disinformation in COVID-19-related perinatology, a search was conducted directly on three of the most frequently used social media channels in Italy, namely, Facebook, Instagram, and Twitter [17]. The results of this analysis show how dangerous social media can be when they transmit inaccurate, false, and harmful information. Subsequently, examples of fake news disseminated by newspapers, journals, and magazines will be presented. A review of European institutional websites dealing with COVID-19 vaccine during pregnancy will then be showed.

16.2.1 Facebook and Fake News

The analysis of Facebook groups considered all Italian public groups about pregnancy. Their names are listed in Table 16.1:

Each group was analyzed by searching for the key word '*vaccino*" (vaccine). In Table 16.2, the main topics in which the highest misinformation and fake news were identified are listed:

In addition to citing news without its source, group members quoted online magazines or newspapers, such as The Daily Expose, an online sensationalist and misinformation magazine [18].

One of the most frequent objections to COVID-19 vaccines during pregnancy was the unsafety of vaccines because they were not supported by sufficient scientific data and developed too rapidly.

Table 16.1 Facebook groups considered in the search

Facebook group
Gravidanza ai tempi del Covid-19
Gruppo Donne e Mamme
Mamme
Community Diventare Mamma –STORIE DI DONNE
Mamme e pancine
noi mamme
Gravidanza e Allattamento
Il Club delle mamme
Mamme Networker

Table 16.2 Main topics found in the Facebook groups

Main topic
Unsafety of vaccines
Types of vaccine
Lack of efficacy against new variants
Vaccine-induced immediate and long-term effects
Augmented risk of adverse events in patients with cardiological or hematological problems
Trimester suitable for vaccination
Infertility
Illness-induced antibodies better than vaccine-induced ones
Menstrual period modifications

Moreover, some patients quoted only an extract of the webpage of the Italian National Institute of Health [19], referring to the fact that up to date, there are no sufficient data to fully state the safety of COVID-19 vaccines during pregnancy. However, they omitted to cite that the ISS advised the administration of the vaccine because the benefits outweigh the risks.

Other doubts expressed included the possibility that the vaccine may act as a DNA modifier, either of the patient or of the future child, and the potential immediate and long-term side effects.

On the other hand, COVID-19 vaccination was attributed with an augmented risk of adverse events in patients with cardiological or hematological problems. What is more, it was associated with menstrual period modifications in terms of duration and quantity.

Finally, the analysis showed that women were skeptical about the best period to administer the vaccine during pregnancy (most doubts were about vaccine safety during the first trimester), the type of vaccine (some patients didn't trust Spikevax), the efficacy against new variants, and the fact that vaccine-induced antibodies might be better than illness-induced ones.

16.2.2 Twitter and Fake News About Pregnancy and the COVID-19 Vaccination

The content of fake news about the COVID-19 vaccine and prenatal care was investigated on Twitter as well.

Also on Twitter, the information about the atrocious damage is devastating, even to the point of mentioning the risk of death in vaccinated people compared to unvaccinated people.

"New England Journal of Medicine finds that women who got v4x3d - within 30 days of becoming pregnant and up to 20 weeks pregnant - had a miscarriage rate of 82%." pointed a July 5, 2021 tweet, referring to the COVID-19 vaccine [20]. The tweet relates to a study published on June 17, 2021, by The New England Journal of Medicine but reported a completely inaccurate information referring to that study. Similar rumors about the same study also appeared on other social media (i.e., Instagram). The study presents data from the Vaccine Adverse Event Reporting System (VAERS), the V-safe After Vaccination Health Checker surveillance system, and the V-safe COVID-19 Vaccine Pregnancy Registry and provides preliminary information about COVID-19 vaccine safety among pregnant people. It found no clear safety risks among pregnant people who received mRNA COVID-19 vaccines but recognized that "more longitudinal follow-up, including follow-up of large numbers of women vaccinated earlier in pregnancy, is necessary to inform maternal, pregnancy, and infant outcomes"[21]. Contrary to the study's findings, social media posts assert that vaccines represent a serious threat to pregnancies. It is worth pointing out that a single post has been able to trigger a hurricane of misinformation that has made many pregnant people reluctant to receive vaccines, even though almost all recent US deaths from the disease (occurred between April 4 and December 25, 2021) were among unvaccinated people [22].

Such a misinterpretation of the results of the study is related to an incomplete interpretation of the scientific results by those who do not have the skills to evaluate the scientific evidence properly and correctly. Similar incidents have occurred frequently around the world during the current health emergency.

16.2.3 YouTube and Fake News About Pregnancy and the COVID-19 Vaccination Abortion

Fake news about the COVID-19 vaccine was investigated on YouTube as well.

One of the most alarming and concerning false information found online is that vaccinations are the cause of a 366% increase in spontaneous abortions in the COVID era [18]. These figures come from a well-known misinformation website and have spread exponentially on all social networks, echoing on YouTube.

Most of the fake news can be found in the comments on the videos, while many doctors try to counteract them with correct, scientific information on vaccine safety.

Here are two examples:

> I received my first dose 10 days before I became pregnant. A week after the positive test, I had a massive haemorrhage with clots and bruising. I have not experienced such problems in other pregnancies. Now I am pregnant again and have not and will not do the second dose and I am fine. I received a lot of pressure to do it, both from family members and institutions, I will protect my baby and I will not do it.
>
> Two doctors in Vancouver tried to raise the alarm after having 13 stillbirths in 24 hours in vaccinated mothers. Usually for that hospital it's 1 stillbirth a month.

Scientific evidence suggests that the administration of mRNA COVID-19 vaccine during pregnancy is not associated with an increased risk of miscarriage, compared to the general population. This is what emerges from a study, still in progress, conducted in the USA by a group of researchers from the Centers for Disease Control and Prevention (CDC) and published on the "Research Square" platform. The survey involved a sample of about 2,456 pregnant women who had received the mRNA vaccine in the preconception phase or within the first 20 weeks of gestation [23, 24].

Another popular piece of fake news on YouTube is that the adverse effects of vaccines are kept hidden by pharmaceutical companies, authorities, and policy makers.

In Italy, this fake news can soon be disproved: the pharmacovigilance data is public and has the same system for Sars-CoV-2 vaccines and all other drugs. In Italy, the All Is Fine Association [25] publishes a report of suspected adverse event reports (www.aifa.gov.it/farmacovigilanza-vaccini-covid-19) in addition to the European Medicines Agency (EMA), the European Union regulatory body. In the case of adverse events that did not occur in the authorization studies, if after investigation a causal relationship with the vaccination is suspected or demonstrated, they are added to the list of adverse reactions. In addition, studies have been carried out to support vaccine efficacy and safety. In particular, a study conducted on a total of 913 women vaccinated during the second or third trimester that compared the outcomes with unvaccinated women showed that "prenatal maternal COVID-19 vaccine has no adverse effects on pregnancy course and outcomes. These findings may help pregnant women and health care providers to make informed decision regarding vaccination" [26].

16.2.4 Instagram and Fake News

On Instagram, it only takes a second for the fake news that has just been inoculated to start producing its negative effects. All it takes is a catchy or alarming title for it to be immediately interacted with and the exponential sharing can begin. From there, it can quickly go viral and citizens lose the ability to understand whether it is true or false, with very high social and economic costs.

One of the most common "hoaxes" spread on Instagram is that the COVID-19 vaccine changes DNA and are used in experimental purposes.

COVID-19 vaccines do not change or interact in any way with the nucleus of the cell where the DNA resides, so there is no possibility of changing the genetic code. Both mRNA and viral vector vaccines, which have been approved by the EMA, provide instructions to our cells to activate an immune response in order to develop protection against Sars-CoV-2.

The ISS says that this "hoax" is completely wrong and is trying to ensure that people have the correct information [27].

Moreover, the vaccines are in no way used for experimental purposes. The clinical use of the COVID-19 vaccines used in Italy has been duly authorized by the EMA and the world's major regulatory bodies. The development process has accelerated at an unprecedented global level but, as the EMA states, "conditional authorisation ensures that the approved vaccine meets the strict EU criteria of safety, efficacy and quality, and that it is produced and controlled in certified facilities," in line with the highest pharmaceutical standards. Nevertheless, the RNA technology has been under study for at least a decade and is not unknown to the scientific community [28].

16.2.5 Newspapers, Journals, and Magazines

Newspapers have also dealt with the phenomenon of pregnancy-related fake news.

Both national and international newspapers have been scoured and various types of fake news have been detected that appeal to the most diverse psychological mechanisms of pregnant women.

The types found are as follows:

1. False context: e.g., photos attributed to false events and therefore decontextualized, such as photos of children with malformations falsely attributed to the Sars-Cov-2 vaccine.
2. Instrumental/ideological content: can be shared to attack a defined target using one of the other meanings.
3. Engineered content: typically deep fakes, but also photomontages, etc. One of the most easily implemented manipulations is the falsification of scientific study tables.
4. Outdated content: outdated information disseminated as current. For example, old false information on smallpox attributed to the Sars-Cov-2 vaccine.

The BBC's health section represents the phenomenon of social media and fake news.

Posts with erroneous content suggested that the Pfizer vaccine could cause infertility in women. But claims on social media that the COVID-19 vaccine could affect female fertility are unfounded, experts have said. There is no "plausible biological mechanism" to explain such a phenomenon, said Professor Lucy Chappell, professor of obstetrics at King's College London and spokeswoman for the Royal College of Obstetricians and Gynecologists. Some people deliberately pointed to an earlier version of the UK government's published guidance, saying it was "unknown" whether the Pfizer vaccine had an impact on fertility. This has since been updated to clarify that animal studies indicate no harmful effect on the reproductive system (2021).

In addition to the circulation of fake news, confusion is generated by the way scientists describe or tweet about the phenomenon compared to how most citizens would understand them.

When scientists say or write in tweets that "there is no evidence," they mean that there has not yet been a long-term study on this specific vaccine but that does not mean that there are no facts here. Professor Chappell pointed out that there is plenty of evidence from other vaccines with nonliving viruses, including the flu vaccine, and that they have no impact on fertility and are completely safe and recommended for use during pregnancy [29].

Some rumors have suggested that the vaccine could threaten fertility because it contains proteins that are also used to produce the placenta. Posts on social media have claimed that this could lead to the body attacking the placenta. This is not true. After vaccination, our organism recognizes the coronavirus based on its typical spike protein and can fight it in a targeted manner. This protein remotely resembles a human placental development protein, but the similarity is too remote to confuse the organism; it is impossible for antibodies developed against the coronavirus' spike protein to also attack the organism's protein responsible for placental development.

Currently, disinformation content is censored, articles and posts are deleted, and groups are closed. But according to a report published today by the UK's Royal

Society, the solution to online scientific misinformation is not to delete it from the Internet. Instead of censoring this content, the report's authors recommend tackling misinformation by supporting diverse media and sustainably funding independent fact-checking organizations, monitoring sources of scientific misinformation, and limiting their reach, as well as investing in information literacy.

Some articles are still present on the web and give false reports about the number of miscarriages due to the administration of the Sars-CoV-2 vaccine.

The newspaper Exposé reported on March 21, 2021: "Number of women to lose their unborn child after having the Covid Vaccine increases by 366% in just six weeks" [18].

A false report was included that shows that four miscarriages could be attributed to the administration of the Pfizer-BionTechmRNA according to the data obtained by the Medicines and Healthcare products Regulatory Agency (MHRA) Yellow Card Scheme up to January 24, 2021.

Similar to the falsification of the report on the previous vaccine, the report on the AstraZeneca vaccination claims that two women lost their unborn babies after the administration of the Oxford/AstraZeneca vaccine. It is also claimed that vaccinations are administered by doctors and nurses against government advice [18].

In such a scenario, it is understandable that there is an erosion of trust among the general population.

16.3 European Institutional Websites Dealing with COVID-19 Vaccine During Pregnancy

The institutional websites of all the European Union members plus the UK were analyzed (see Table 16.3). Information related to COVID-19-related risks, trimester suitable for vaccination, vaccine safety during pregnancy, advisable type of vaccine, and fake news was searched for each of them.

The research was carried out in English, and only the pages written in English were considered, as to guarantee the reproducibility of the research.

For 11 out of 28 countries, it wasn't possible to find any institutional website with information about COVID-19 vaccines and pregnancy: Those countries were mainly located in Eastern or Southern Europe, as can be seen in the map below (Fig. 16.1a).

Except for Cyprus and Germany, all countries with institutional websites, dealt with the risks of COVID-19 infection during pregnancy in unvaccinated women, as seen in Fig. 16.1b.

On the contrary, no agreement could be found on the trimester most suitable to administer the first dose: Belgium, Ireland, Finland, Netherlands, and the UK preferred to quickly reach a widespread coverage among pregnant women, while the other countries opted for a more cautious approach, postponing the administration of the first dose until after the second trimester (Fig. 16.1c).

Table 16.3 Information related to COVID-19-related risks, trimester suitable for vaccination, vaccine safety during pregnancy, advisable type of vaccine, and fake news for each European country

Country	Institution	COVID-19-related risks for pregnant women	Trimesters suitable for vaccination	Vaccine safety during pregnancy	Type of vaccine	Fake news
World	World Health Organization	+	−	+	−	−
USA	Centers for Disease Control and Prevention	−	+	+	+	+
Europe	European Medicines Agency	+	+	+	+	+
Austria	The Austrian Ministry of Social Affairs, Health, Care and Consumer Protection	+	+	+	+	+
Belgium	Conseil Supérieur de la Santé	+	+	+	+	−
Bulgaria	−	−	−	−	−	−
Cyprus	Ministry of Interior Press and Information Office	−	−	+	−	+
Croatia	−	−	−	−	−	−
Denmark	Danish Health Authority	+	+	+	+	+
Estonia	Government Office of Estonia	+	−	+	−	+
Finland	Finnish Institute for Health and Welfare	+	+	+	−	−
France	Académie Nationale de Médecine	+	−	+	−	+
Germany	Federal Ministry of Health	−	+	+	−	+
Greece	−	−	−	−	−	−
Ireland	Health Service Executive	+	+	+	+	+
Italy	Istituto Superiore di Sanità [xiv]	+	+	+	+	+
Latvia	−	−	−	−	−	−
Lithuania	−	−	−	−	−	−
Luxembourg	The Luxembourg Government	+	+	+	+	−
Malta	Government of Malta	+	+	+	+	−

(continued)

Table 16.3 (continued)

Country	Institution	COVID-19-related risks for pregnant women	Trimesters suitable for vaccination	Vaccine safety during pregnancy	Type of vaccine	Fake news
Netherlands	The National Institute for Public Health and the Environment	+	+	+	+	+
Poland	–	–	–	–	–	–
Portugal	–	–	–	–	–	–
Czech rep.	Ministry of Health of Czech Republic	+	+	+	–	–
Romania	–	–	–	–	–	–
Slovak Republic	Ministry of Health of the Slovak Republic	–	–	+	–	–
Slovenia	–	–	–	–	–	–
Spain	–	–	–	–	–	–
Sweden	Public Health Agency of Sweden	+	+	+	+	+
Hungary	–	–	–	–	–	–
UK	National Health Service, Government Digital Service, British Society for Immunology	+	+	+	+	+

In some cases, like Italy or Cyprus, the administration of the first dose was possible also during the first trimester, deferring the decision to the physician.

American and international public health organizations didn't agree on this topic either. The WHO didn't express a clear opinion on the issue, while the CDC was in favor of vaccination starting from the first trimester and the EMA recommended vaccination starting from the second trimester or, otherwise, in line with national guidelines.

Regarding the safety of the vaccination during pregnancy, the WHO advised vaccination only when the benefits outweighed the potential risks since pregnant women were not included in the initial clinical trials of COVID-19 vaccines.

The same position was shared by France, Germany, and Slovakia, whereas other countries agreed on the need to prevent serious COVID-19 consequences during pregnancy and on the general safety of the vaccine, even if stronger data was needed (Fig. 16.1d).

With the exception of the WHO, international organizations and all countries with an institutional website showed a preference for mRNA vaccines (Comirnaty and Spikevax produced by Pfizer and Moderna), but more evidence is currently available from Israel and the USA about their use in pregnant women.

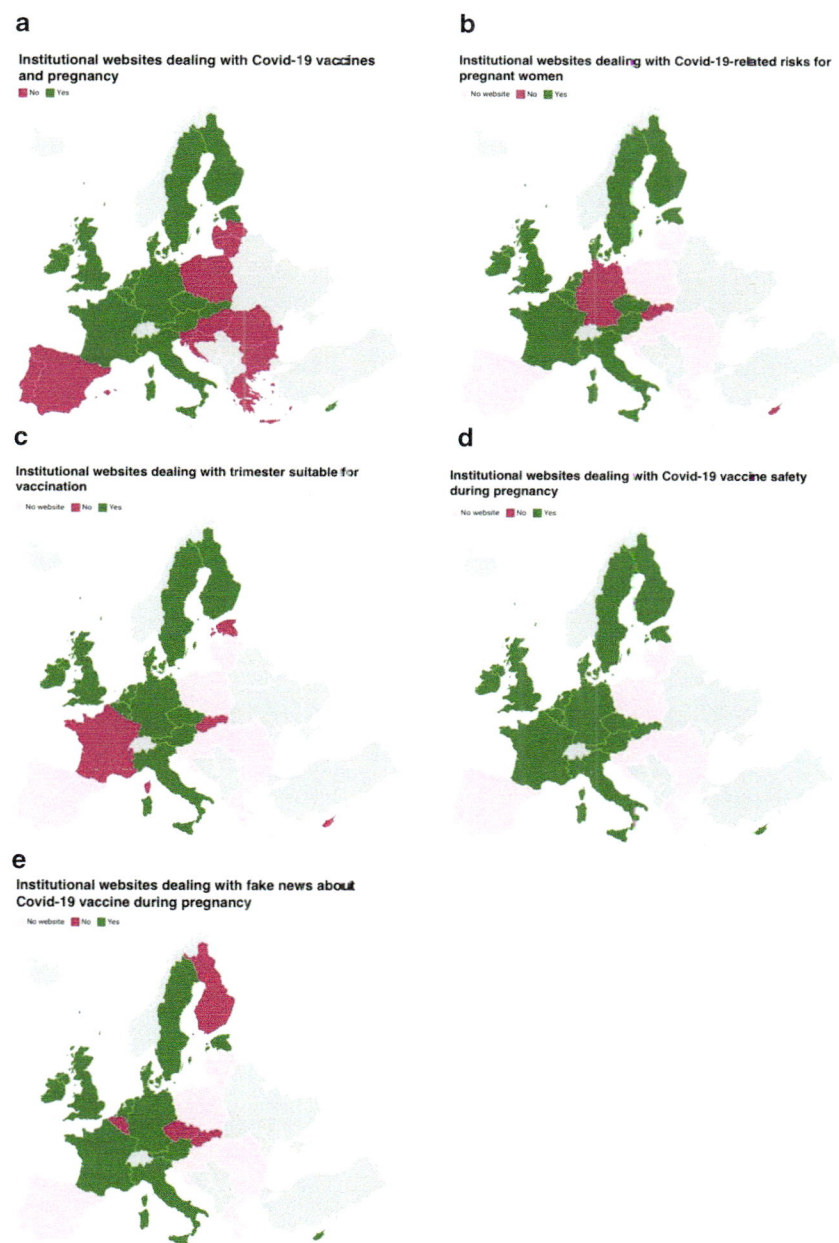

Fig. 16.1 Institutional websites across the world that reported information regarding COVID-19 and pregnancy: (**a**) Institutional websites dealing with COVID-19 vaccines and pregnancy; (**b**) Institutional websites dealing with COVID-19-related risks for pregnant women; (**c**) Institutional websites dealing with trimester suitable for vaccination; (**d**) Institutional websites dealing with COVID-19 vaccine safety during pregnancy; (**e**) Institutional websites dealing with fake news about COVID-19

Belgium, Malta, and the UK admitted Vaxzevria (produced by Oxford, AstraZeneca) for the second dose just in case it was used for the first dose, while the other countries used an mRNA vaccine for the recall; in all of Europe, only Sweden allowed vaccines other than Comirnaty, Spikevax, and Vaxzevria (Janssen and Nuvaxovid, produced by Jonson and Jonson and Novavax).

Regarding fake news and COVID-19 vaccination, no countries but Austria had a clear paragraph aimed at counteracting fake news on its webpage.

As a consequence of fake news spread on social networks or online sensationalist journals claiming that COVID-19 vaccination causes an augmented risk of infertility, miscarriage, or premature birth [29, 30], all countries with an institutional webpage debunked fake news about infertility (Fig. 16.1e). The CDC, the EMA, Estonia, and Sweden also exposed fake news about miscarriages, and France and Estonia stated that there were no risks for the future development of the child.

16.4 Conclusions and Recommendations

The COVID-19 pandemic has shown to be a major public health concern, and the further pandemic, the infodemic has spread in the meantime as well. In fact, fake news can spread as fast as viruses and can become viral very quickly. We live in the era where social media have gained great popularity as a source of seeking information even with the aim to bring health-related conclusions, and the current pandemic has shown how great their potential and impact actually is. The problem of vaccine hesitancy is tightly connected and exaggerated specifically because of social media influence, and numerous studies conducted in the last 2 years have showed that not only are social media users more vaccine hesitant but also that anti-vaxx clusters are better connected (than their opponents) and that vaccine hesitant topics are more prevalent on social media (than pro-vaccine ones) [31]. Given that a large percent of the general population is reluctant to receiving the vaccine and that social media reliance is recognized as a potential important cofactor, it is not of surprise that this delicate population of women has fears of receiving the jab as well. Although several high-quality studies concluded that COVID-19 can have more serious manifestations in pregnant than in nonpregnant women, this population still has concerns regarding vaccination.

The experiences accumulated over the months during the vaccination campaign, combined with preclinical data, clearly show that mRNA vaccines are safe for both pregnant and breastfeeding women. In some reference centers around the world (e.g., Paris, Israel, Belgium, Ireland, USA), vaccination during pregnancy is offered routinely. There are no different contraindications to vaccination from the rest of the population nor does the vaccine affect a woman's fertility. However, the community is still facing the problem of vaccine rejection in this population of women.

Andrew Satin, M.D., director of gynecology and obstetrics at Johns Hopkins, and Jeanne Sheffield, M.D., director of maternal-fetal medicine, elaborated on this: "Confusion around this issue arose when a false report surfaced on social media, saying that the spike protein on this coronavirus was the same as another spike protein called syncitin-1 that is involved in the growth and attachment of placenta during pregnancy. The false report said that getting the COVID-19 vaccine would cause a woman's body to fight this different spike protein and affect her fertility. The two spike proteins are completely different and getting the COVID-19 vaccine will not affect the fertility of women who are seeking to become pregnant, including through in vitro fertilization methods. During the Pfizer vaccine tests, 23 women volunteers involved in the study became pregnant, and the only one in the trial who suffered a pregnancy loss had not received the actual vaccine, but a placebo" [32].

Therefore, it is of great importance to promote relevant, scientifically proven information regarding immunization of pregnant and lactating women and address the issue of inaccurate information that has been spreading on the web and affecting their health-related decisions. To do this, science-guided and effective communication is vital and can be used as a valuable tool to address vaccine hesitancy in currently/future pregnant and breastfeeding women. A great deal of work, therefore, needs to be done to ensure that information on these issues is delivered in a scientifically effective manner, with the appropriate expertise and in a way that is comprehensible to the general population, to practice prevention and limit avoidable impacts of pandemics on perinatology.

References

1. Johansen T, Ackerman E, Curfman A, et al. The impact of digital transformation on patient experience: reflections on patient-centred care from around the world. Digital and technology driven transformations in healthcare, Work Group 1; 2021.
2. Allotey J, Stallings E, Bonet M, et al. Clinical manifestations, risk factors, and maternal and perinatal outcomes of coronavirus disease 2019 in pregnancy: living systematic review and meta-analysis. BMJ. 2020;370:m3320. https://doi.org/10.1136/BMJ.M3320.
3. Wei SQ, Bilodeau-Bertrand M, Liu S, Auger N. The impact of COVID-19 on pregnancy outcomes: a systematic review and meta-analysis. CMAJ. 2021;193:E540–8. https://doi.org/10.1503/CMAJ.202604.
4. Prasad S, Kalafat E, Blakeway H, et al. Systematic review and meta-analysis of the effectiveness and perinatal outcomes of COVID-19 vaccination in pregnancy. Nat Commun. 2022;13(1):2414. https://doi.org/10.1038/s41467-022-30052-w.
5. American College of Obstetricians and Gynecologists. COVID-19 vaccines and pregnancy: conversation guide; 2022.
6. Centre for Disease Control and Prevention. COVID-19 vaccines while pregnant or breastfeeding; 2022.
7. Zauche LH, Wallace B, Smoots AN, et al. Receipt of mRNA CCVID-19 vaccines preconception and during pregnancy and risk of self-reported spontaneous abortions, CDC v-safe COVID-19 Vaccine Pregnancy Registry 2020-21. Res Sq. 2021;rs.3.rs-798175. https://doi.org/10.21203/RS.3.RS-798175/V1.
8. CSI Library. Definitions of terms - misinformation and disinformation: thinking critically about information sources. In: CUNY College of Staten Island Library. 2021. https://library.csi.cuny.edu/misinformation. Accessed 31 May 2022.
9. Brown E. Fake news, Misinformation & Disinformation. In: Central Washington University Libraries. 2022. https://guides.lib.uw.edu/c.php?g=345925&p=7772376. Accessed 31 May 2022.

10. World Health Organization. Drawing light from the pandemic: a new strategy for health and sustainable development (2021). World Health Organization; 2021.
11. ISS COVID-19 Training Working Group. Training for preparedness in the COVID-19 emergency: the case report of the Istituto Superiore di Sanità; 2020.
12. National Institute of Disaster Management ND. Disaster communication. In: East Asia Summit; 2021.
13. Eysenbach G. Infodemiology and infoveillance: framework for an emerging set of public health informatics methods to analyze search, communication and publication behavior on the Internet. J Med Internet Res. 2009;11:e11. https://doi.org/10.2196/JMIR.1157.
14. Eysenbach G. Infodemiology: the epidemiology of (mis)information. Am J Med. 2002;113:763–5. https://doi.org/10.1016/S0002-9343(02)01473-0.
15. 1st WHO Infodemiology Conference. 2020. https://www.who.int/teams/risk-communication/infodemic-management/1st-who-infodemiology-conference. Accessed 31 May 2022.
16. Bencharif S-T. Tackle scientific misinformation, but don't delete it, says UK Royal Society report. In: POLITICO. 2022. https://www.politico.eu/article/tackle-scientific-misinformation-but-dont-delete-it-says-u-k-royal-society-report/. Accessed 31 May 2022.
17. Redazione Online. Quali sono stati i social più usati nel 2021? In: Business Intelligence Group. 2021. https://www.businessintelligencegroup.it/social-piu-usati/. Accessed 8 June 2022.
18. The Expose. Number of women to lose their unborn child after having the Covid vaccine increases by 366% in just six weeks. In: The Expose. 2021. https://expose-news.com/2021/03/21/miscarriages-after-having-covid-vaccine-increases-by-366-percent/. Accessed 31 May 2022.
19. Donati S. COVID-19 vaccination in pregnancy and breastfeeding. In: Epidemiology for public health, Istituto Superiore di Sanità. 2021. https://www.epicentro.iss.it/en/vaccines/covid-19-pregnancy-breastfeeding. Accessed 31 May 2022.
20. AFP. Study on COVID-19 vaccines misleadingly linked to miscarriages. In: BOOM. 2021. https://www.boomlive.in/world/fake-news-covid-19-vaccine-us-cdc-study-miscarriages-pregnant-women-13948. Accessed 31 May 2022.
21. Shimabukuro TT, Kim SY, Myers TR, et al. Preliminary findings of mRNA Covid-19 vaccine safety in pregnant persons. N Engl J Med. 2021;384:2273–82. https://doi.org/10.1056/NEJMOA2104983.
22. Johnson AG, Amin AB, Ali AR, et al. COVID-19 incidence and death rates among unvaccinated and fully vaccinated adults with and without booster doses during periods of delta and omicron variant emergence — 25 U.S. Jurisdictions, April 4–December 25, 2021. Centers for Disease Control MMWR Office; 2022.
23. Dagan N, Barda N, Biron-Shental T, et al. Effectiveness of the BNT162b2 mRNA COVID-19 vaccine in pregnancy. Nat Med. 2021;27(10):1693–5. https://doi.org/10.1038/s41591-021-01490-8.
24. Kharbanda EO, Haapala J, Desilva M, et al. Spontaneous abortion following COVID-19 vaccination during pregnancy. JAMA. 2021;326:1629–31. https://doi.org/10.1001/JAMA.2021.15494.
25. Agenzia Italiana del Farmaco. 2022. https://www.aifa.gov.it/. Accessed 31 May 2022.
26. Wainstock T, Yoles I, Sergienko R, Sheiner E. Prenatal maternal COVID-19 vaccination and pregnancy outcomes. Vaccine. 2021;39:6037–40. https://doi.org/10.1016/J.VACCINE.2021.09.012.
27. Instituto Superiore di Sanita. Covid: dall'Iss un vademecum contro le fake news sui vaccini. 2021. https://www.iss.it/covid19-fake-news/-/asset_publisher/qgZFrRLpL1jG/content/id/5814462. Accessed 31 May 2022.
28. European Medicine Agency. COVID-19 vaccines: development, evaluation, approval and monitoring. In: EMA. 2020. https://www.ema.europa.eu/en/human-regulatory/overview/public-health-threats/coronavirus-disease-covid-19/treatments-vaccines/vaccines-covid-19/covid-19-vaccines-development-evaluation-approval-monitoring#scientific-evaluation-and-approval-section. Accessed 31 May 2022.

29. Schraer R. Covid: claims vaccinations harm fertility unfounded. In BBC News. 2021. https://www.bbc.com/news/health-56012529. Accessed 31 May 2022.
30. Medaris A. Anti-vaxxers falsely link a doctor's miscarriage to COVID-19 vaccine. In: Insider. 2021. https://www.businessinsider.com/coronavirus-vaccine-does-not-cause-miscarriage-pregnancy-loss-evidence-2021-2?r=US&IR=T. Accessed 31 May 2022.
31. Cascini F, Pantovic A, Al-Ajlouni YA, et al. Social media and attitudes towards a COVID-19 vaccination: a systematic review of the literature. eClinicalMedicine. 2022;48:101454. https://doi.org/10.1016/J.ECLINM.2022.101454.
32. Satin A, Sheffield J. The COVID-19 vaccine and pregnancy: what you need to know. In: Johns Hopkins Medicine. 2022. https://www.hopkinsmedicine.org/health/conditions-and-diseases/coronavirus/the-covid19-vaccine-and-pregnancy-what-you-need-to-know. Accessed 31 May 2022.

Part V
Psychology and Ethics

Chapter 17
Perinatal Psychological and Psychiatric Impact of the SARS-CoV-2 Pandemic Health Crisis

Alexandra Doncarli, Catherine Crenn-Hebert, Sarah Tebeka, and Nolwenn Regnault

Highlights
- The COVID-19 pandemic has had a major impact on the perinatal period in mothers, with an increase in the prevalence of major psychiatric symptoms, including anxiety, depression, acute stress, post-traumatic stress disorder, dissociation, and thoughts about self-harming.
- Its impact is stronger in women with a history of psychiatric disorders, leading to a deterioration in pre-existing clinical symptoms and the development of psychiatric co-morbidities.
- We suggest the following targeted measures to detect and prevent mental health deterioration: (a) providing comprehensive, consensual, and updated information to pregnant women about the impact of the pandemic on their pregnancy and childbirth in order to reassure them; (b) facilitating/strengthening access to psychological/psychiatric care (including teleconsultation); and (c) reducing social isolation by setting up specific support groups, systematic screening for psychiatric disorders, and proactive support for vulnerable women.

A. Doncarli · N. Regnault (✉)
Direction of Non-Communicable Diseases and Trauma, Santé Publique France, Saint-Maurice, France
e-mail: Nolwenn.REGNAULT@santepubliquefrance.fr

C. Crenn-Hebert
Department of Gynecology and Obstetrics, Louis Mourier University Hospital, AP-HP, Colombes, France

S. Tebeka
Direction of Non-Communicable Diseases and Trauma, Santé Publique France, Saint-Maurice, France

Université Paris Cité, INSERM U1266, Paris, France

Department of Psychiatry, AP-HP, Louis Mourier Hospital, Colombes, France

© The Author(s), under exclusive license to Springer Nature Switzerland AG 2023
D. De Luca, A. Benachi (eds.), *COVID-19 and Perinatology*,
https://doi.org/10.1007/978-3-031-29136-4_17

17.1 Introduction

The perinatal period, which includes pregnancy, birth, and the first-year postpartum, is a time of profound biological, physiological, social, and emotional changes that can make women more vulnerable to the onset or worsening of psychiatric symptoms and disorders such as anxiety and anxiety disorders [1]. Perinatal psychiatric disorders are sometimes very serious and can lead to suicide. According to the most recent data available, suicides are the second and fourth leading causes of maternal death in, respectively, France and the United Kingdom and Ireland taken together [2–4].

As observed for previous pandemics, the SARS-CoV-2 pandemic and associated lockdowns may have exacerbated this vulnerability to mental health problems and increased their prevalence in women during the perinatal period [5]. Based on international data, we review the impact of the SARS-CoV-2 pandemic on perinatal mental health and psychiatric disorders and suggest interventions for women during this crucial period in their lives.

17.2 Mental Health of Pregnant Versus Non-pregnant Women during the SARS-CoV-2 Pandemic

To our knowledge, few studies to date have compared the differential impact of the SARS-CoV-2 pandemic on the mental health of pregnant and non-pregnant women. Moreover, these studies have reported conflicting results. Specifically, Zhou et al. in China found that pregnant women ($n = 544$) reported significantly fewer symptoms of depression, anxiety, insomnia, and post-traumatic stress disorder (PTSD) than non-pregnant counterparts ($n = 315$) interviewed between February and March 2020 [6]. In line with this finding, the Covimater survey, conducted by Santé Publique France in July 2020 on 500 pregnant women during France's first lockdown (March 17 to May 11, 2020), found a significantly lower frequency of anxiety in participants than that found in non-pregnant women of childbearing age (18–49 years) in another French survey conducted in the general population using the same self-diagnostic tool (HAD scale) over the same period (14.2% vs. 24.8%) (article in press). In contrast, a longitudinal Argentinean study found a significantly higher increase in the mean scores of depressive symptoms (BDI-II scale), anxiety (STAI scale), and negative effect (PANAS scale) in pregnant women ($n = 102$) than in non-pregnant women ($n = 102$), 47 days after the country's first lockdown started. In addition, pregnant women had a larger decrease in their mean positive affect score (PANAS scale) [7].

The discrepancy observed between the first two studies (i.e. Zhou et al. and Covimater) and the Argentinean study could be linked to the fact that they were conducted at different times during the epidemic. More specifically, the first two studies were conducted after peak contamination during the first wave in China and after the first lockdown ended in France. It is therefore probable that pregnant and non-pregnant women were less psychologically stressed at these time points. Interestingly, in both studies, pregnant women were less psychiatrically affected than their non-pregnant counterparts. To explain this, we hypothesise that pregnant women may have arrived at a state of reduced stress more quickly than non-pregnant women because they were able to discuss their concerns more easily and frequently with health professionals during the monitoring of their pregnancy. In the third study, which showed higher psychological distress in pregnant women, data were collected during the first lockdown in Argentina, which was a time of uncertainty in economic, medical, and educational terms for the whole population. Pregnant women – a population already in a situation of profound emotional change – may consequently have been even more psychologically or psychiatrically affected during the pandemic than non-pregnant women.

Few longitudinal studies were conducted internationally during the beginning of the SARS-CoV-2 pandemic and during the first related lockdowns. A study in the United Kingdom of 11 pregnant women infected with SARS-CoV-2 before and at different times during the country's first strict lockdown suggested parabolic kinetics for anxiety (GAD-7 scale) and depressive (PHQ-9 scale) scores [8]. The authors observed a peak in anxiety and depression scores coinciding with a peak in pandemic-related deaths in the first few weeks of this lockdown. Both scores then lowered as reassuring information from the Royal Colleges of Obstetrics and Gynaecology was disseminated. In particular, the anxiety score returned to a level similar to that observed before the lockdown [8].

To conclude, pregnant and non-pregnant women may, therefore, have followed the same psychological and psychiatric disorder kinetics but with different intensities depending on the timeframe considered. More specifically, at the beginning of the pandemic and at the start of the first strict lockdown, pregnant women may have presented psychiatric symptoms more frequently than non-pregnant women. On the contrary, once the lockdown was over and follow-up markers were more reassuring, pregnant women may have been less affected by psychological manifestations than their non-pregnant counterparts thanks to reassuring consultations with doctors during follow-up visits for their pregnancy.

Despite these hypotheses, the very small number of studies and the conflicting results observed do not allow us to conclude that the SARS-CoV-2 pandemic led to excess risk of psychological problems or psychiatric disorders in pregnant women compared to non-pregnant women of childbearing age.

17.3 Mental Health of Pregnant Women During the Pandemic Versus Before the Pandemic

Several literature reviews show that pregnant women and new mothers may have experienced an increase in psychiatric symptoms during the SARS-CoV-2 pandemic.

For example, in their systematic review of the literature in June 2021, Chmielewska et al. reported that of the 11 studies they analysed measuring maternal mental health, seven showed a significant increase in postnatal depression, maternal anxiety, or both [9]. In their meta-analysis, Yan et al. sought to quantify observed increases in psychiatric symptoms and estimated that the pandemic increased the relative risk of perinatal anxiety and depressive symptomatology by 1.65 (95% CI [1.25–2.19]) and 1.08 (95% CI [0.80–1.46]), respectively, [10] compared with pre-pandemic pregnant women and recent mothers. Similarly, in Tomfohr-Madsen et al.'s literature review followed by a meta-analysis in 2021 [11], symptoms of depression (meta-analysis of 37 studies) and anxiety (meta-analysis of 34 studies) were reported by over 25.6% (95% CI [21.8–29.9]) and 30.5% (95% CI [22.6–39.8]) of the pregnant women surveyed during the pandemic period, respectively, compared with 11.9% (95% CI [11.4–12.5]) and 22.4% (95% CI [19.6–25.1]) in two pre-pandemic meta-analyses [1, 12]. These increases in depressive and anxiety symptomatology varied across geographical areas, but only anxiety rates were significantly different between the areas studied. Specifically, rates of anxiety in pregnant women were significantly lower in East Asia than in Europe and North America [11]. To our knowledge, the only data currently available for France come from the Covimater survey which only looked at anxiety in pregnant women. It found that the rate of anxiety in this population was of the same order of magnitude as that observed before the pandemic both internationally [1] and in France [13]. One explanatory hypothesis for this is that in France, just as was observed in the United Kingdom, peaks in anxiety were observed in the first month of the pandemic and in the first month of the lockdown, followed by a decrease and a return to pre-pandemic levels (i.e. when the Covimater survey was conducted). At the beginning of the summer of 2020, the pandemic monitoring indicators may have been perceived as reassuring by pregnant women and a phenomenon of adaptation or habituation to the risk of COVID-19—something observed in the general population of women of childbearing age—may also have existed in this population [14].

In addition to anxiety and depression, the prevalence of other psychiatric disorders also significantly increased during the SARS-CoV-2 pandemic. For example, in the USA, severe clinical stress was more frequent in mothers who gave birth during this period than in those who delivered beforehand (OR = 1.38; 95% CI [1.01–1.89]). The consequences of this stress are an increase in post-traumatic symptoms related to childbirth, attachment difficulties, and breastfeeding initiation problems [15]. Similarly, in Canada, post-traumatic stress and dissociation symptoms were more frequent in women who were pregnant during the SARS-CoV-2 pandemic period than in pregnant women in the preceding years [16].

Finally, in China, the relative risk of a pregnant woman to have had thoughts about self-harming almost tripled after the global pandemic was declared (adjusted RR: 2.85; 95% CI [1.70–8.85]) [17].

17.4 Impact of the Pandemic on Pregnant Women with Pre-existing Psychiatric Disorders

Outside of any epidemic context, lockdowns and social isolation are described as risk factors for psychiatric disorders in the general population, and especially in vulnerable populations such as children, adolescents, the elderly, women, and people with psychiatric disorders [18, 19]. The global SARS-CoV-2 pandemic had added an additional complicating factor. For example, pregnant women with pre-existing psychiatric disorders were found to be at particular risk of psychiatric comorbidities [16]. During the pandemic and the first month of Italy's first lockdown, pregnant women who reported a history of depression and/or anxiety disorders had significantly higher levels of anxiety (STAI-Y scale) and significantly more post-traumatic stress symptoms (NSESSS) than pregnant women with no reported psychiatric history [20]. Similarly, a US study conducted during the pandemic showed that independently of age, ethnicity, education, income level, and parity, perinatal women with a history of depression had almost twice the risk of clinically proven depressive symptoms (CES-D score $> =16$; OR = 1.91; $p < 0.01$) compared to women without a history of depression. Moreover, women in that study with a history of post-traumatic stress disorder (PTSD) were 3.73 times more likely to experience recurrence of PTSD symptoms (PCL-C score $> =45$; $p < 0.01$) than those women with no history of PTSD. Finally, women with pre-existing generalised anxiety disorder in the same study were significantly more likely to have recurrent anxiety symptoms (GAD-7 $> =10$; OR = 2.74; $p < 0.001$) but also to report depressive symptoms (OR = 1.58; $p < 0.01$) or PTSD (OR = 1.73; $p < 0.05$) than those women with no history of anxiety disorder [21].

In addition, in Italy, women with a psychiatric history were significantly more concerned about the health status of their child, their relatives, and the future of society in general than those pregnant women with no previous psychopathological diagnosis [20]. Overall, these results observed in perinatal women are in line with those found in the general population [22].

17.5 Risk of the Development of Perinatal Psychiatric Disorders During the SARS-CoV-2 Pandemic and Protective Factors

According to a recent review of the literature based on 81 studies, the women most at risk of depression or anxiety during the SARS-CoV-2 pandemic were those most demographically or socio-economically disadvantaged (i.e. younger age; low level of education; full-time employment; lots of professional stress; low income/difficult financial situation), socially disadvantaged women, and those with no family support (i.e., in charge of a large family, marital or family difficulties, conflict in general) [23]. Furthermore, women who felt isolated or unsupported in general, those with a documented history of psychiatric problems prior to the pandemic, those who had experienced COVID-19-like symptoms, those with overweight or obesity, and multiparous women, were all independently at higher risk of depression or anxiety [10, 23]. Elsewhere, reduced antenatal care during the pandemic was associated with an increase in symptoms of depression and anxiety [23].

Protective factors against poor mental health during the pandemic included good sleep quality, physical exercise, access to information about antenatal care during the pandemic, and good patient-perceived medical support [23, 24].

These results are in line with those presented above in the French Covimater survey which found that pregnant women were more likely to present anxiety symptoms when they (a) had a pregnancy-related pathology (gestational diabetes, preeclampsia, hypertension, etc.), (b) overweight/obesity, (c) a friend or family member who had been diagnosed with COVID-19 or who presented symptoms suggestive of the disease, (d) perceived little or no social support during the lockdown, (e) had one or more children under the age of six in the household, (f) reported unsuccessful attempts to have an exchange with a healthcare professional about their pregnancy or about the hospitalisation process for childbirth, and (g) had no access to medication to treat mood disorders or sleep disorders. In the same study, the authors also examined factors influencing a deterioration of self-perceived mental health during the period of the first French lockdown (21.1% of the participants self-reported that their pre-lockdown mental health state was good/quite good but was quite poor/poor during the lockdown). Specifically, women who perceived little or no social support (i.e. family, friends, etc.) and those who reported a heavier workload during the lockdown were significantly more likely to suffer psychological deterioration. In contrast, a good level of knowledge about the modes of transmission of the SARS-CoV-2 virus was a protective factor.

17.6 Intervention Options to Prevent Deterioration of Perinatal Mental Health During a Pandemic

In terms of future pandemics in general, it seems essential to facilitate access to up-to-date consensus-based training on the impact of the pandemic during the perinatal period. This kind of training should not only target pregnant women but the public in general. With regard to the SARS-CoV-2 pandemic, several studies have shown that a good level of knowledge about the modes of transmission of the virus and access to information delivered by organisations who pregnant women perceive to be competent are protective factors against stress, anxiety, and depressive symptoms in this population [24].

In addition, easier access to existing resources on the subject of mental health in general (e.g. the NHS website[1]) can enable pregnant women to better understand their emotions and empower them to call for support from mental health professionals if necessary during their pregnancy and after childbirth.

Virtual support groups for pregnant women such as those set up by peer associations like Maternal Mental Health Alliance[2] can be very useful at the beginning of a pandemic and during related lockdowns. Developing such initiatives would help to ease feelings of isolation—a recurrent factor in perinatal depression and anxiety—and encourage women to seek medical follow-up when necessary.

In the context of pandemic-related lockdowns, access to remote psychological/psychiatric and perinatal care (teleconsultations or telephone consultations) should be facilitated for all pregnant and postpartum women and in particular for those with a history of psychological or psychiatric care. This requires a rethinking of the organisation of care, taking into account the links between gynaecology, obstetrics, psychiatry, paediatrics, and general medical services in inpatient and outpatient settings. The coordination of all professionals around one contact person in order to ensure the successful management of the perinatal process is envisaged in France as part of the country's 'first 1000 days' action plan and could provide a response to this need.

Early detection of women who are psychologically vulnerable and/or have other risk factors (e.g. social precarity, problems with their partner) is also essential, especially in the event of a pandemic. This could be done at the time of registration at the maternity hospital or during perinatal visits. In France, early prenatal and postnatal visits have been mandatory since May 2020 and July 2022, respectively. Their goal is to identify women at risk of or already experiencing psychological distress at two points in the perinatal period. However, the latest French National Confidential Enquiry of Maternal Mortality report (2013–2015) showed that the median time of occurrence of maternal suicides is approximately 4 months after delivery, which suggests the need to remain vigilant even when women have no complaints until at least 1 year post-partum [4, 25]. If necessary, targeted and graduated proactive support for suicide or psychological deterioration prevention could be provided, ranging from relatively simple tools to improve well-being (mindfulness meditation, sophrology, adapted sports practices, etc.)[3] to support from peer associations and psychotherapy, until a relationship is established with a specialised perinatal psychiatry unit.

---

[1] https://www.nhs.uk/pregnancy/keeping-well/mental-health/

[2] https://maternalmentalhealthalliance.org/about/

[3] https://www.nhs.uk/pregnancy/keeping-well/mental-health/

17.7 Conclusion

The current SARS-CoV-2 pandemic has led to an increase in the frequency of psychiatric symptoms and disorders in women in the perinatal period. Particular attention must, therefore, be paid to this vulnerable population, especially those with a history of psychiatric disorder. This could be achieved by providing the following support measures to pregnant women during this period:

- Increasing the availability of consensual and regularly updated information on the impact of SARS-CoV-2 on pregnancy and childbirth via one or more scientific reference sites and via a medical contact person
- Facilitating and strengthening exchanges with health professionals, providing remote psychological support (via access to teleconsultations), and prescribing of medication if necessary
- Supporting women through discussion and support groups in order to limit their sense of isolation

A screening and prevention strategy for pregnant women or women with young children is fundamental to limit the negative impacts of altered mental health on the course of their pregnancy, on the establishment of the mother-newborn bond, and on the development of the infant and child.

Acknowledgments Our thanks to Jude Sweeney (Milan, Italy) for the English revision and copy-editing of this chapter.

Declaration of Competing Interest The authors declare that they have no known competing inancial interests or personal relationships that could have influenced the work reported in this chapter.

References

1. Dennis CL, Falah-Hassani K, Shiri R. Prevalence of antenatal and postnatal anxiety: systematic review and meta-analysis. Br J Psychiatry. 2017;210(5):315–23.
2. Santé publique France. Les morts maternelles en France: mieux comprendre pour mieux prévenir. 6e rapport de l'Enquête Nationale Confidentielle sur les Morts Maternelles (ENCMM) [Internet]. 2021. p. 237. https://www.santepubliquefrance.fr/maladies-et-traumatismes/maladies-cardiovasculaires-et-accident-vasculaire-cerebral/maladies-vasculaires-de-la-grossesse/documents/enquetes-etudes/les-morts-maternelles-en-france-mieux-comprendre-pour-mieux-prevenir.-6e-rapport-de-l-enquete-nationale-confidentielle-sur-les-morts-maternelles.
3. National Perinatal Epidemiology Unit University of Oxford. Saving lives improving mothers' care - lessons learned to inform maternity care from the UK and Ireland Confidential Enquiries into Maternal Deaths and Morbidity 2015–17 [Internet]. 2019. https://www.npeu.ox.ac.uk/mbrrace-uk/presentations/saving-lives-improving-mothers-care.
4. Deneux-Tharaux C, Morau E, Dreyfus M. 6th report on maternal deaths in France 2013-2015, lessons learned to improve care. J Gynecol Obstet Hum Reprod. 2022;51(5):102367. https://doi.org/10.1016/j.jogoh.2022.102367.

5. Gardner PJ, Moallef P. Psychological impact on SARS survivors: critical review of the English language literature. Can Psychol. 2015;56(1):123–35.
6. Zhou Y, Shi H, Liu Z, Peng S, Wang R, Qi L, et al. The prevalence of psychiatric symptoms of pregnant and non-pregnant women during the COVID-19 epidemic. Transl Psychiatry. 2020;10(1):319. https://doi.org/10.1038/s41398-020-01006-x.
7. López-Morales H, Del Valle MV, Canet-Juric L, Andrés ML, Galli JI, Poó F, et al. Mental health of pregnant women during the COVID-19 pandemic: a longitudinal study. Psychiatry Res. 2021;295:113567.
8. Kotabagi P, Fortune L, Essien S, Nauta M, Yoong W. Anxiety and depression levels among pregnant women with COVID-19. Acta Obstet Gynecol Scand. 2020;99(7):953–4.
9. Chmielewska B, Barratt I, Townsend R, Kalafat E, van der Meulen J, Gurol-Urganci I, et al. Effects of the COVID-19 pandemic on maternal and perinatal outcomes: a systematic review and meta-analysis. Lancet Glob Health. 2021;9(6):e759–72.
10. Yan H, Ding Y, Guo W. Mental health of pregnant and postpartum women during the coronavirus disease 2019 pandemic: a systematic review and meta-analysis. Front Psychol. 2020;11:617001.
11. Tomfohr-Madsen LM, Racine N, Giesbrecht GF, Lebel C, Madigan S. Depression and anxiety in pregnancy during COVID-19: a rapid review and meta-analysis. Psychiatry Res. 2021;300:113912.
12. Woody CA, Ferrari AJ, Siskind DJ, Whiteford HA, Harris MG. A systematic review and meta-regression of the prevalence and incidence of perinatal depression. J Affect Disord. 2017;219:86–92.
13. Ibanez G, Charles M-A, Forhan A, Magnin G, Thiebaugeorges O, Kaminski M, et al. Depression and anxiety in women during pregnancy and neonatal outcome: data from the EDEN mother-child cohort. Early Hum Dev. 2012;88(8):643–9.
14. Christine C-C, Christophe L. La santé mentale des Français face au Covid-19: prévalences, évolutions et déterminants de l'anxiété au cours des deux premières semaines de confinement (Enquête CoviPrev, 23–25 mars et 30 mars-1er avril 2020). Bull Epidémiol Hebd. 2020;13:260–9. http://beh.santepubliquefrance.fr/beh/2020/13/2020_13_1.html
15. Mayopoulos GA, Ein-Dor T, Dishy GA, Nandru R, Chan SJ, Hanley LE, et al. COVID-19 is associated with traumatic childbirth and subsequent mother-infant bonding problems. J Affect Disord. 2021 Mar;1(282):122–5.
16. Berthelot N, Lemieux R, Garon-Bissonnette J, Drouin-Maziade C, Martel É, Maziade M. Uptrend in distress and psychiatric symptomatology in pregnant women during the coronavirus disease 2019 pandemic. Acta Obstet Gynecol Scand. 2020;99(7):848–55.
17. Wu Y, Zhang C, Liu H, Duan C, Li C, Fan J, et al. Perinatal depressive and anxiety symptoms of pregnant women during the coronavirus disease 2019 outbreak in China. Am J Obstet Gynecol. 2020;223(2):240.e1–9.
18. Perrin PC, McCabe OL, Everly GS, Links JM. Preparing for an influenza pandemic: mental health considerations. Prehosp Disaster Med. 2009;24(3):223–30.
19. Usher K, Bhullar N, Jackson D. Life in the pandemic: social isolation and mental health. J Clin Nurs. 2020;29(15–16):2756–7.
20. Ravaldi C, Ricca V, Wilson A, Homer C, Vannacci A. Previous psychopathology predicted severe COVID-19 concern, anxiety, and PTSD symptoms in pregnant women during 'lockdown' in Italy. Arch Womens Ment Health. 2020;23(6):783–6.
21. Liu CH, Erdei C, Mittal L. Risk factors for depression, anxiety, and PTSD symptoms in perinatal women during the COVID-19 pandemic. Psychiatry Res. 2021;295:113552.
22. Asmundson GJG, Paluszek MM, Landry CA, Rachor GS, McKay D, Taylor S. Do pre-existing anxiety-related and mood disorders differentially impact COVID-19 stress responses and coping? J Anxiety Disord. 2020;74:102271.
23. Iyengar U, Jaiprakash B, Haitsuka H, Kim S. One year into the pandemic: a systematic review of perinatal mental health outcomes during COVID-19. Front Psych. 2021;12:674194.

24. Jiang H, Jin L, Qian X, Xiong X, La X, Chen W, et al. Maternal mental health status and approaches for accessing antenatal care information during the COVID-19 epidemic in China: cross-sectional study. J Med Internet Res. 2021;23(1):e18722.
25. Vacheron M-N, Dugravier R, Tessier V, Deneux-tharaux C. Suicide maternel périnatal: comment prévenir? L'Encéphale [Internet]. 2022 Mar 21. https://www.sciencedirect.com/science/article/pii/S0013700622000446.

Chapter 18
Collateral Damage of the COVID-19 Pandemic for the Next Generation: A Call to Action

Sam Schoenmakers, Roseriet Beijers, and E. J. (Joanne) Verweij

18.1 Introduction

The several global waves of the COVID-19 pandemic and its associated international mitigation measurements have had devastating effects on social, financial, and professional lives. Vulnerable members of society, including pregnant women and the (un)born generation, were affected the most. Though there were also positive effects observed after the lockdowns, such as a reduction of air pollution and preterm birth [1, 2], many pregnant women reported negative aspects including social isolation and decreased access to perinatal health care. Accordingly, pregnant women's known vulnerability for mental health problems has become a concern during the COVID-19 pandemic, also because of the known effects of prenatal stress for the unborn child. The current chapter provides a historic overview of peer-reviewed research on the transgenerational effects of prenatal maternal stress caused by natural and man-made disasters during the last century. Hereby, we aim to draw

---

S. Schoenmakers (✉)
Division of Obstetrics and Fetal Medicine, Department of Obstetrics and Gynaecology, Erasmus MC, University Medical Center Rotterdam, Rotterdam, The Netherlands
e-mail: s.schoenmakers@erasmusmc.nl

R. Beijers
Social Development, Behavioural Science Institute, Radboud University, Nijmegen, The Netherlands

Cognitive Neuroscience, Donders Institute, Radboud University Medical Center, Nijmegen, The Netherlands
e-mail: roseriet.beijers@ru.nl

E. J. (J.)Verweij
Department of Obstetrics, Leiden University Medical Center, Leiden, The Netherlands
e-mail: e.j.t.verweij@lumc.nl

© The Author(s), under exclusive license to Springer Nature Switzerland AG 2023
D. De Luca, A. Benachi (eds.), *COVID-19 and Perinatology*, https://doi.org/10.1007/978-3-031-29136-4_18

attention to the psychological impact of the COVID-19 pandemic on women of reproductive age and its potential associated short-t and long-term consequences for the health of children who are conceived, carried, and born during this pandemic. We plea for prompt detection and effective intervention to reduce the repercussion of transgenerational effects of the COVID-19 pandemic.

18.2 COVID-19 Effects on Pregnant Women's Mental Health

Pregnancy involves profound physiological and psychological changes in women. As such, pregnancy is known to be a sensitive period for developing symptoms of anxiety, depression, and stress [3]. Before COVID-19, considerable numbers of pregnant women, ranging between 7% and 40%, suffered from mental health problems [4, 5]. These numbers increased considerably during the COVID-19 pandemic [6–8]. In the Netherlands, for example, more than 1 in 10 women experienced clinically relevant symptoms of depression, and nearly 1 in 2 women experienced clinically relevant symptoms of anxiety [8]. Also, up to 24% of the women reported having a probable anxiety disorder [9–11]. Pregnant women reported to have fear of infection, fear of vertical transmission, fear of adverse birth and child outcomes, social isolation, uncertainty about their partner's presence during medical appointments and delivery, increased domestic abuse, and other collateral damage, including vaccine hesitancy [6, 7] (see also Box 18.1).

> **Box 18.1 COVID-19 Guidelines for (Expecting) Parents**
> Based on experiences with influenza and previous coronaviruses, an open-access guideline Coronavirus (COVID-19) infection in pregnancy by the Royal College of Obstetricians and Gynaecologists (RCOG) was published [12]. This first guideline was quickly followed by daily to weekly revised national and international COVID-19 and pregnancy guidelines with country-specific recommendations, based on either historical or very limited current insight, knowledge, and expert opinions. The initial recommendations were aimed at complying and paralleling with COVID-19 mitigation measures to prevent or minimize the risk for transmission or infection of SARS-CoV-2. These recommendations were fueled by data from previous corona virus (SARS-CoV and MERS-CoV) outbreaks that showed impressive mortality rates, up to 20%, in infected pregnant women [13, 14]. The recommendations included minimizing hospital visits; physical distancing between physician and patient; restricting outpatient clinic consultations, hospital deliveries, and visits; remaining indoors and self-isolate when symptomatic for at least 7 days; delaying routine obstetrical care until after the self-isolation period, and when in labor, use of private transport and deliver in isolation (RCOG, NVOG).

The result of the COVID-19 pandemic and its associated recommendations for pregnant women was a triad of disruption of standard of medical care, delivery, and expectancy. The medical personal protective clothes, equipment, and obligatory physical distancing interfered with delivery of standard medical care, and a change in attitude of healthcare professionals toward an increasing fear of getting infected themselves. Pregnant women showed an increased hesitation to adhere to antenatal routine check-ups and a marked reduced attendance of fetal anomaly scans, interfering with, respectively, detection of gestational-related diseases and reproductive autonomy of women [15].

The restriction rules also applied to the visiting policies of the Neonatal Care Intensive Units, interfering with parental and neonatal bonding, especially in cases of maternal COVID-19-related iatrogenic preterm birth. In addition, while homebirth is a traditionally common practice in the Netherlands, most developed countries promote hospital-based deliveries based on safety and liability concerns. However, already in March 2020, shortly after the introduction of COVID-19 in the USA, hospital-based deliveries were quickly questioned due to fear of hospital-acquired COVID-19 infections, promoting homebirth deliveries without the presence of adequate experienced personnel or logistics (Gammon K, NYT, March 2020). Not only the COVID-19 pandemic itself but also the unprecedented long-term and repetitive mitigation measures have deeply impacted societies and healthcare worldwide [16–18].

Although aimed at reducing infection and risk of spreading, the negative effects of the mitigation measures resulted in decreased access to healthcare and increased mental health problems, domestic violence, and poverty [15, 19–21]. Importantly, the latter seem to effect groups of lower socioeconomic status harder, worsening current health and socioeconomic inequalities within populations [22, 23]. These initial restrictive rules of potentially delivering in solitude, isolation at home after discharge, and the uncertainty of the duration, continuation, or reinstating of temporary mitigation measures have only added to the unexpected levels of collateral damage of COVID-19 resulting in increased levels of psychological distress in pregnant women, their families, and future generations.

Over the course of the pandemic, it became evident that an actual COVID-19 infection during pregnancy can also cause placental infection, with massive placental necrosis [24], and an increased risk for fetal distress and stillbirth as a result [25, 26]. On top of all that, the availability of the COVID-19 vaccines provoked an additional psychological concern and hesitancy of vaccine uptake in pregnant women, since evidence of safety and efficacy of COVID-19 vaccination during pregnancy was lacking [27–29]. In general, vaccine uptake during pregnancy is confronted with a variety of barriers [30]. For example, pregnant women are traditionally excluded from clinical vaccination trails [31], as was the case with the COVID-19 vaccines. All of these consequences of the COVID-19 pandemic and its mitigation measures for pregnant women likely contributed to increased levels of psychological stress.

18.3 Fetal Programming

Fetal programming, or prenatal programming, is a concept that suggests certain events occurring during critical points of pregnancy may cause profound, long-term, or even permanent effects on the fetus and the infant long after birth [32, 33]. Moreover, some of these effects seem to be even transmitted from the offspring to the next generation [3, 34]. The concept of fetal programming is also described in the Developmental Origins of Health and Disease (DOHaD) paradigm [35], also known as Barker's hypothesis [36].

The DOHaD paradigm states that sensitive windows during fetal development exist, in which tissue development and function in utero and during early postnatal life can be modified by external environmental exposures. These modifications can result in increased risks for adverse health outcomes (i.e., non-communicable diseases such as heart and vascular diseases, cancer [37]), and (neuro)developmental outcomes (i.e., socioemotional problems, autism spectrum disorder (ASD), and attention deficit hyperactivity disorder (ADHD) [3, 32, 33]).

Researchers proposing the concept of fetal programming and DOHaD established a new area of research into the developmental causes of disease, pointing toward the in utero environment. These researchers have studied the effects of fetal programming with respect to many factors, such as maternal nutrition and stress during pregnancy. Indeed, exposure during pregnancy to stress has been associated with a range of poor outcomes for the child [34]. For example, effects of maternal stress are found on offspring neurodevelopment, cognitive development, negative affectivity, behavior problems, and psychiatric disorders [3, 38]. Offspring of both sexes are found susceptible to prenatal stress, but effects might differ. Moreover, there is not one specific vulnerable period of gestation; prenatal stress effects vary for different gestational ages possibly depending on the developmental stage of specific body and brain areas [3].

Maternal prenatal exposure to disasters have also been studied, as such unexpected situations provide a natural experiment to study maternal stress (reviewed in [38]). As the COVID-19 pandemic meets the United Nations 2009 definition of a disaster, which is defined as a serious disruption of the functioning of a community or society, causing widespread human, material, economic, or environmental losses which exceed the ability of the affected community or society to cope by using its own resources [39], we believe that the lessons learned from research on disasters should quickly be applied to the COVID-19 pandemic in order to prevent or timely detect long-term consequences.

18.4 Historical Lessons of Prenatal Maternal Stress

Transgenerational health and socioeconomic effects have been documented of in utero exposure to increased levels of prenatal maternal stress due to previous well-documented global disasters, such as the influenza pandemic of 1918, Quebec Ice Storm, and the 9/11 Terrorist Attacks in 2001 [39]. As an example of such transgenerational effects, the offspring of women who were pregnant and present in New York City during the terrorist attacks on the World Trade Center in 2001, and whom developed post-traumatic stress disorder (PTSD), showed lower levels of cortisol. Lower levels of cortisol might be a sign of a hyporeactive HPA axis and might put these offspring at a higher biological risk to develop PTSD themselves (see also Box 18.2) [40].

> **Box 18.2 Potential Mechanisms of Fetal Programming**
> While accumulating evidence indicates that maternal psychological stress during pregnancy adversely affects child outcomes, knowledge on the possible mechanisms underlying these relations is limited. In this box, we review the most often proposed mechanism, namely, the involvement of the hypothalamic-pituitary-adrenal (HPA) axis and cortisol, and highlight some other, less well-studied potential mechanisms. For a more elaborated review on potential mechanisms underlying the links between maternal prenatal stress and child outcomes, please see [34].
>
> *Hypothalamic-pituitary-adrenal (HPA) axis and cortisol*
> When the pregnant mother is exposed to stress, the hypothalamic-pituitary-adrenal (HPA) axis is activated, resulting in the release of multiple hormones, including cortisol [34]. Subsequently, there are multiple ways through which heightened maternal cortisol levels can result in heightened cortisol levels in the fetus, including direct transport and increased production of placental CRH [34]. While fetuses need cortisol for various aspects of brain development and late gestational lung maturation [41], exposure to high cortisol concentrations in utero is thought to compromise fetal behavioral, immunological, and brain development [42].
>
> Animal studies into the effects of fetal exposure to high concentrations of cortisol have shown prenatal and long-term postnatal effects on the offspring. Prenatal exposure to increased cortisol seems related to a reduction of neuronal cell proliferation and differentiation as well as a general inhibition of neurogenesis. Postnatal effects show pronounced thinning of the cerebral cortex and reduced cortical folding. Human studies found, for example, long-term adverse effects of maternal administered corticosteroids. Maternal administered corticosteroids are used as fetal therapy in cases of imminent preterm birth for accelerating fetal lung maturation. The protective mechanism of maternally administered antenatal corticosteroids for the fetus is based on a

combination of local physiological and biochemical effects resulting in increased production of surfactant, enhanced lung maturity, and accelerated clearance of lung fluids [43]. Dexamethasone and betamethasone are currently recommended dosing regimens of ACS, with dexamethasone phosphate having a biological half-life of 36–72 h, betamethasone sodium phosphate of 36–72 h, and betamethasone acetate a long biological half-life. Essential for their specific indication, both corticosteriods are able to transfer via the placenta to the fetal circulation in their active form [44]. A systematic review and meta-analyses of 30 studies of long-term outcomes after in utero ACS exposure concluded that even after one single course of administered antenatal corticosteroids, neonates being born late-preterm and term already have a significant increased risk for neurodevelopmental impairment later in life [45] .

Other potential mechanisms
Despite the clearly important role of cortisol in fetal programming, there are multiple indications that the associations between maternal prenatal psychological stress and offspring outcomes may be explained or complemented by other mechanisms than maternal HPA functioning and cortisol. For example, the number of studies that found evidence for associations between prenatal maternal cortisol and child outcomes is small [46]. Moreover, maternal reports of stress tend to be only weakly related, or even not at all related, to heightened maternal cortisol. These findings raise the possibility that other mechanisms might also be in play. Such mechanisms include compromised placental functioning, increased catecholamines, compromised maternal immune system and intestinal microbiota, and altered health behaviors including eating, sleep, and exercise. As such, it can be concluded that maternal prenatal psychological stress affects maternal emotions, behavior, and physiology in many ways and may influence the physiology and functioning of the fetus through a network of different pathways.

Disasters can be the result from natural causes, such as floodings or earthquakes, or can be the result of human intent, negligence, or error. The latter are so-called man-made disasters, including the Chernobyl meltdown, deepwater oil spilling, or plane crashes. The current COVID-19 pandemic is perceived as a combination between an initial natural disaster (ignited by the global spreading of SARS-CoV-2) and a secondary man-made disaster due to the establishment of the diverse national COVID-19 mitigation measures, and all are overarched by a general feeling of anxiety, uncertainty, unpredictability, and stress. Table 18.1 provides a historic overview of peer-reviewed research on the transgenerational effects of prenatal maternal stress caused by natural and man-made disasters during the last century.

Contrary to abovementioned disasters (Table 18.1), which were either regional, self-limiting, or, except for the famines, short term, the current COVID-19 disaster

Table 18.1 An overview of the effects of prenatal maternal stress caused by historical disasters (adapted from [38])

Disaster	Duration disaster	Type	Postpartum effects during the life course
1918 influenza pandemic (1918–1919)	1–2 years	Natural	• Exposure during mid and late gestation is associated with multiple morbidities later in life, such as depression, diabetes, renal disease, ischemic heart disease, higher mortality, and lower socioeconomic status (SES) [47–50]
The Dutch Famine, ("Dutch Hunger Winter") (1944–1945)	± 5 months	Natural and man-made	• Life-long effects on health, effects depending on the timing of exposure in gestation and the course of the catch-up period [51] • Exposure during early gestation is related to coronary heart disease, raised serum lipids, and more obesity, whereas midgestation exposure is associated with obstructive airway disease and microalbuminuria during the life course [52] • Twice more likely to develop schizophrenia [53–55]
Tangshan earthquake, China (1976)		Natural	• Higher serum uric-acid concentrations; 70% more likely to develop hyperuricemia approximately 33 years after the event, independent of traditional risk factors [56]
Quebec Ice Storm (1998)	± 6 h–5 weeks	Natural	• Negative impact on cognitive and language development of the unborn child, independent of maternal personality factors [57] • DNA methylation mediates the impact of exposure to prenatal maternal stress on BMI and central adiposity in children at age 13.5 years [58] • The level of prenatal maternal stress is associated with higher BMI levels and adiposity in children of ages 5.5, 8.5, 13.5, and 15.5 years [59]
9/11 terrorist attacks (2001)	± 1 day	Man-made	• Offspring at 1 year of age of mothers exposed to attacks on the World Trade Center during pregnancy show lower cortisol levels [40]
The QF2011 Queensland flood (Brisbane) (2011)	±36 h	Natural	• Association with prenatal maternal stress and alterations in placental glucocorticoid system [60] • Increased 4-year child anxiety symptoms [61]
Superstorm Sandy (2012)	±1 day	Natural	• Prenatal maternal depression amplified by Sandy; association with lower emotion regulation and greater distress at 6 months in neonates [62, 63]
Tailings dam breakage, Brazil (2015)	± hours (breakage itself)	Man-made	• Increased premature births [64]

has occurred unexpectedly, quickly, and globally and is long lasting. As such, COVID-19 effects of prenatal stress might be unique. While medical and financial consequences of the pandemic are already acknowledged, prevention and intervention protocols are also needed to address the psychological health of (expecting) new parents, since the effects of prenatal exposure to COVID-19 and associated maternal prenatal stress on the next generation may become visible long after the pandemic itself has resolved.

18.5 Lessons for Now and the Future

The current COVID-19 pandemic affects pregnant women all over the globe, independent of borders, culture, age, or socioeconomic or nutritional state. First of all, international consortia should be set up to investigate, monitor, and support pregnant and postpartum women and their offspring experiencing the pandemic and the different mitigation measures. Secondly, the previous lessons learned from scientific studies looking into fetal and transgenerational effects of prenatal maternal stress as a result from disasters (Table 18.1), combined with the current insights from DOHAD cohorts, can already be used as guidance to prevent or minimize effects on in utero development. Regional, national, and international maternal support programs should be prepared and set up to disrupt a vicious circle of intergenerational transmission of stress. Intervention programs for women early in pregnancy aimed at stress reduction have shown to be able to reduce perceived stress [65, 66], and high-risk pregnant women seem open to these interventions [67]. If a reduction in stress during pregnancy, due to intervention programs, will also lead to a decrease in prenatal-stress-related effects in the next generation is currently unknown [68].

Besides the (expecting) new parents, their offspring needs to be closely monitored to detect and effectively target vulnerable developmental windows to divert adverse outcomes later during the life course. This approach could allow for timely detection and treatment of cognitive, behavioral, and/or physical effects on the offspring and offers opportunities to evaluate the effects of treatment on both women and their offspring. To develop preventive and supportive programs for future pandemics and to interpret transgenerational effects of disaster exposure, international collaboration is mandatory.

In sum, we believe that the transgenerational lessons learned from historical experiences with disasters should quickly be applied to the current COVID-19 pandemic in order to prevent or timely detect similar long-term consequences on the offspring. As we need to make sure the ripples of COVID-19 do not evolve into unmanageable waves for the coming generation(s), special attention should be paid to potential, but currently less obvious, consequences of the COVID-19 pandemic, namely, those consequences on children conceived, carried, and born during the pandemic.

References

1. Been JV, et al. Impact of COVID-19 mitigation measures on the incidence of preterm birth: a national quasi-experimental study. Lancet Public Health. 2020;5:e604–11. https://doi.org/10.1016/S2468-2667(20)30223-1.
2. Son JY, et al. Reductions in mortality resulting from reduced air pollution levels due to COVID-19 mitigation measures. Sci Total Environ. 2020;744:141012. https://doi.org/10.1016/j.scitotenv.2020.141012.
3. Van den Bergh BRH, et al. Prenatal developmental origins of behavior and mental health: the influence of maternal stress in pregnancy. Neurosci Biobehav Rev. 2020;117:26–64. https://doi.org/10.1016/j.neubiorev.2017.07.003.
4. Browne PD, Bossenbroek R, Kluft A, van Tetering EMA, de Weerth C. Prenatal anxiety and depression: treatment uptake, barriers, and facilitators in midwifery care. J Womens Health (Larchmt). 2021;30:1116–26. https://doi.org/10.1089/jwh.2019.8198.
5. Missler M, van Straten A, Denissen J, Donker T, Beijers R. Effectiveness of a psycho-educational intervention for expecting parents to prevent postpartum parenting stress, depression and anxiety: a randomized controlled trial. BMC Pregnancy Childbirth. 2020;20:658. https://doi.org/10.1186/s12884-020-03341-9.
6. Barzilay R, et al. Resilience, COVID-19-related stress, anxiety and depression during the pandemic in a large population enriched for healthcare providers. Transl Psychiatry. 2020;10:291. https://doi.org/10.1038/s41398-020-00982-4.
7. Ghazanfarpour M, et al. Prevalence of anxiety and depression among pregnant women during the COVID-19 pandemic: a meta-analysis. J Psychosom Obstet Gynaecol. 2021;43:315–26. https://doi.org/10.1080/0167482X.2021.1929162.
8. Vacaru S, et al. The risk and protective factors of heightened prenatal anxiety and depression during the COVID-19 lockdown. Sci Rep. 2021;11:20261. https://doi.org/10.1038/s41598-021-99662-6.
9. Kwong ASF, et al. Mental health before and during the COVID-19 pandemic in two longitudinal UK population cohorts. Br J Psychiatry. 2021;218:334–43. https://doi.org/10.1192/bjp.2020.242.
10. Lebel C, MacKinnon A, Bagshawe M, Tomfohr-Madsen L, Giesbrecht G. Elevated depression and anxiety symptoms among pregnant individuals during the COVID-19 pandemic. J Affect Disord. 2020;277:5–13. https://doi.org/10.1016/j.jad.2020.07.126.
11. Saccone G, et al. Psychological impact of coronavirus disease 2019 in pregnant women. Am J Obstet Gynecol. 2020;223:293–5. https://doi.org/10.1016/j.ajog.2020.05.003.
12. Covid-19 and pregnancy. 2020;369:m1672. https://doi.org/10.1136/bmj.m1672.
13. Assiri AM, et al. Epidemiology of a novel recombinant Middle East respiratory syndrome coronavirus in humans in Saudi Arabia. J Infect Dis. 2016;214:712–21. https://doi.org/10.1093/infdis/jiw236.
14. Wong SF, Chow KM, de Swiet M. Severe acute respiratory syndrome and pregnancy. BJOG. 2003;110:641–2. https://doi.org/10.1046/j.1471-0528.2003.03008.x.
15. Verweij EJ, M'Hamdi HI, Steegers EAP, Reiss IKM, Schoenmakers S. Collateral damage of the covid-19 pandemic: a Dutch perinatal perspective. BMJ. 2020;369:m2326. https://doi.org/10.1136/bmj.m2326.
16. Ettman CK, et al. Prevalence of depression symptoms in US adults before and during the COVID-19 pandemic. JAMA Netw Open. 2020;3:e2019686. https://doi.org/10.1001/jamanetworkopen.2020.19686.
17. Josephson A, Kilic T, Michler JD. Socioeconomic impacts of COVID-19 in low-income countries. Nat Hum Behav. 2021;5:557. https://doi.org/10.1038/s41562-021-01096-7.
18. Wilke J, et al. Drastic reductions in mental well-being observed globally during the COVID-19 pandemic: results from the ASAP survey. Front Med (Lausanne). 2021;8:578959. https://doi.org/10.3389/fmed.2021.578959.

19. Boserup B, McKenney M, Elkbuli A. Alarming trends in US domestic violence during the COVID-19 pandemic. Am J Emerg Med. 2020;38:2753–5. https://doi.org/10.1016/j.ajem.2020.04.077.
20. Kwong ASF, et al. Mental health before and during the COVID-19 pandemic in two longitudinal UK population cohorts. Br J Psychiatry. 2020;218:334–43. https://doi.org/10.1192/bjp.2020.242.
21. Roberton T, et al. Early estimates of the indirect effects of the COVID-19 pandemic on maternal and child mortality in low-income and middle-income countries: a modelling study. Lancet Glob Health. 2020;8:e901–8. https://doi.org/10.1016/S2214-109X(20)30229-1.
22. Abrams EM, Szefler SJ. COVID-19 and the impact of social determinants of health. Lancet Respir Med. 2020;8:659–61. https://doi.org/10.1016/S2213-2600(20)30234-4.
23. Wiersinga WJ, Rhodes A, Cheng AC, Peacock SJ, Prescott HC. Pathophysiology, transmission, diagnosis, and treatment of coronavirus disease 2019 (COVID-19): a review. JAMA. 2020;24:782–93. https://doi.org/10.1001/jama.2020.12839.
24. Husen MF, et al. Unique severe COVID-19 placental signature independent of severity of clinical maternal symptoms. Viruses. 2021;13:1670. https://doi.org/10.3390/v13081670.
25. DeSisto CL, et al. Risk for stillbirth among women with and without COVID-19 at delivery hospitalization - United States, march 2020-September 2021. MMWR Morb Mortal Wkly Rep. 2021;70:1640–5. https://doi.org/10.15585/mmwr.mm7047e1.
26. Schwartz DA, et al. Placental tissue destruction and insufficiency from COVID-19 causes stillbirth and neonatal death from hypoxic-ischemic injury: a study of 68 cases with SARS-CoV-2 placentitis from 12 countries. Arch Pathol Lab Med. 2022;146:660. https://doi.org/10.5858/arpa.2022-0029-SA.
27. Goncu Ayhan S, et al. COVID-19 vaccine acceptance in pregnant women. Int J Gynaecol Obstet. 2021;154:291–6. https://doi.org/10.1002/ijgo.13713.
28. Riad A, et al. COVID-19 vaccine acceptance of pregnant and lactating women (PLW) in Czechia: an analytical cross-sectional study. Int J Environ Res Public Health. 2021;18:13373. https://doi.org/10.3390/ijerph182413373.
29. Skjefte M, et al. COVID-19 vaccine acceptance among pregnant women and mothers of young children: results of a survey in 16 countries. Eur J Epidemiol. 2021;36:197–211. https://doi.org/10.1007/s10654-021-00728-6.
30. Wilson RJ, Paterson P, Jarrett C, Larson HJ. Understanding factors influencing vaccination acceptance during pregnancy globally: a literature review. Vaccine. 2015;33:6420–9. https://doi.org/10.1016/j.vaccine.2015.08.046.
31. Van Spall HGC. Exclusion of pregnant and lactating women from COVID-19 vaccine trials: a missed opportunity. Eur Heart J. 2021;42:2724–6. https://doi.org/10.1093/eurheartj/ehab103.
32. Madigan S, et al. A meta-analysis of maternal prenatal depression and anxiety on child socioemotional development. J Am Acad Child Adolesc Psychiatry. 2018;57:645–657.e8. https://doi.org/10.1016/j.jaac.2018.06.012.
33. Manzari N, Matvienko-Sikar K, Baldoni F, O'Keeffe GW, Khashan AS. Prenatal maternal stress and risk of neurodevelopmental disorders in the offspring: a systematic review and meta-analysis. Soc Psychiatry Psychiatr Epidemiol. 2019;54:1299–309. https://doi.org/10.1007/s00127-019-01745-3.
34. Beijers R, Buitelaar JK, de Weerth C. Mechanisms underlying the effects of prenatal psychosocial stress on child outcomes: beyond the HPA axis. Eur Child Adolesc Psychiatry. 2014;23:943–56. https://doi.org/10.1007/s00787-014-0566-3.
35. Barker DJ. The developmental origins of adult disease. Eur J Epidemiol. 2003;18:733–6. https://doi.org/10.1023/a:1025388901248.
36. Barker DJ. The origins of the developmental origins theory. J Intern Med. 2007;261:412–7. https://doi.org/10.1111/j.1365-2796.2007.01809.x.
37. Barouki R, Gluckman PD, Grandjean P, Hanson M, Heindel JJ. Developmental origins of non-communicable disease: implications for research and public health. Environ Health. 2012;11:42. https://doi.org/10.1186/1476-069X-11-42.

38. Schoenmakers S, et al. The impact of maternal prenatal stress related to the COVID-19 pandemic during the first 1000 days: a historical perspective. Int J Environ Res Public Health. 2022;19:4710. https://doi.org/10.3390/ijerph19084710.
39. Reduction UNOfDR. Available online: https://www.unisdr.org/files/7817_UNISDRTerminologyEnglish.pdf. (accessed on 21 April 2023).
40. Yehuda R, et al. Transgenerational effects of posttraumatic stress disorder in babies of mothers exposed to the World Trade Center attacks during pregnancy. J Clin Endocrinol Metab. 2005;90:4115–8. https://doi.org/10.1210/jc.2005-0550.
41. Shapiro GD, Fraser WD, Frasch MG, Seguin JR. Psychosocial stress in pregnancy and preterm birth: associations and mechanisms. J Perinat Med. 2013;41:631–45. https://doi.org/10.1515/jpm-2012-0295.
42. Entringer S, et al. Influence of prenatal psychosocial stress on cytokine production in adult women. Dev Psychobiol. 2008;50:579–87. https://doi.org/10.1002/dev.20316.
43. Ballard PL, Ballard RA. Scientific basis and therapeutic regimens for use of antenatal glucocorticoids. Am J Obstet Gynecol. 1995;173:254–62. https://doi.org/10.1016/0002-9378(95)90210-4.
44. Hey E. Neonatal formulary: drug use in pregnancy and the first year of life. Wiley; 2011.
45. Ninan K, Liyanage SK, Murphy KE, Asztalos EV, McDonald SD. Evaluation of long-term outcomes associated with preterm exposure to antenatal corticosteroics: a systematic review and meta-analysis. JAMA Pediatr. 2022;176:e220483. https://doi.org/10.1001/jamapediatrics.2022.0483.
46. Zijlmans MA, Riksen-Walraven JM, de Weerth C. Associations between maternal prenatal cortisol concentrations and child outcomes: A systematic review Neurosci Biobehav Rev. 2015;53:1–24. https://doi.org/10.1016/j.neubiorev.2015.02.015.
47. Cook CJ, Fletcher JM, Forgues A. Multigenerational effects of early-life health shocks. Demography. 2019;56:1855–74. https://doi.org/10.1007/s13524-019-00804-3.
48. Helgertz J, Bengtsson T. The long-lasting influenza: the impact of fetal stress during the 1918 influenza pandemic on socioeconomic attainment and health in Sweden, 1968-2012. Demography. 2019;56:1389–425. https://doi.org/10.1007/s13524-019-00799-x.
49. Lin MJ, Liu EM. Does in utero exposure to illness matter? The 1918 influenza epidemic in Taiwan as a natural experiment. J Health Econ. 2014;37:152–63 https://doi.org/10.1016/j.jhealeco.2014.05.004.
50. Mazumder B, Almond D, Park K, Crimmins EM, Finch CE. Lingering prenatal effects of the 1918 influenza pandemic on cardiovascular disease. J Dev Orig Health Dis. 2010;1:26–34. https://doi.org/10.1017/S2040174409990031.
51. Kyle UG, Pichard C. The Dutch Famine of 1944-1945: a pathophysiological model of long-term consequences of wasting disease. Curr Opin Clin Nutr Metab Care. 2006;9:388–94. https://doi.org/10.1097/01.mco.0000232898.74415.42.
52. Painter RC, Roseboom TJ, Bleker OP. Prenatal exposure to the Dutch famine and disease in later life: an overview. Reprod Toxicol. 2005;20:345–52. https://doi.org/10.1016/j.reprotox.2005.04.005.
53. Neugebauer R, Hoek HW, Susser E. Prenatal exposure to wartime famine and development of antisocial personality disorder in early adulthood. JAMA. 1999;282:455–62. https://doi.org/10.1001/jama.282.5.455.
54. Susser E, et al. Schizophrenia after prenatal famine. Further evidence. Arch Gen Psychiatry. 1996;53:25–31. https://doi.org/10.1001/archpsyc.1996.01830010027005.
55. Susser ES, Lin SP. Schizophrenia after prenatal exposure to the Dutch Hunger Winter of 1944-1945. Arch Gen Psychiatry. 1992;49:983–8 https://doi.org/10.1001/archpsyc.1992.01820120071010.
56. Ji C, et al. Prenatal earthquake exposure and midlife uric acid levels among Chinese adults. Arthritis Care Res (Hoboken). 2017;69:703–8. https://doi.org/10.1002/acr.22973.

57. King S, Laplante DP. The effects of prenatal maternal stress on children's cognitive development: project ice storm. Stress. 2005;8:35–45. https://doi.org/10.1080/10253890500108391.
58. Cao-Lei L, et al. DNA methylation mediates the impact of exposure to prenatal maternal stress on BMI and central adiposity in children at age 13(1/2) years: project ice storm. Epigenetics. 2015;10:749–61. https://doi.org/10.1080/15592294.2015.1063771.
59. Liu GT, Dancause KN, Elgbeili G, Laplante DP, King S. Disaster-related prenatal maternal stress explains increasing amounts of variance in body composition through childhood and adolescence: project ice storm. Environ Res. 2016;150:1–7. https://doi.org/10.1016/j.envres.2016.04.039.
60. St-Pierre J, et al. Natural disaster-related prenatal maternal stress is associated with alterations in placental glucocorticoid system: the QF2011 Queensland flood study. Psychoneuroendocrinology. 2018;94:38–48. https://doi.org/10.1016/j.psyneuen.2018.04.027.
61. McLean MA, Cobham VE, Simcock G, Kildea S, King S. Toddler temperament mediates the effect of prenatal maternal stress on childhood anxiety symptomatology: the QF2011 Queensland flood study. Int J Environ Res Public Health. 2019;16:1998. https://doi.org/10.3390/ijerph16111998.
62. Nomura Y, et al. Influence of in utero exposure to maternal depression and natural disaster-related stress on infant temperament at 6 months: the children of superstorm Sandy. Infant Ment Health J. 2019;40:204–16. https://doi.org/10.1002/imhj.21766.
63. Zhang W, et al. Prenatal exposure to disaster-related traumatic stress and developmental trajectories of temperament in early childhood: superstorm Sandy pregnancy study. J Affect Disord. 2018;234:335–45. https://doi.org/10.1016/j.jad.2018.02.067.
64. Mrejen M, Perelman J, Machado DC. Environmental disasters and birth outcomes: impact of a tailings dam breakage in Brazil. Soc Sci Med. 2020;250:112868. https://doi.org/10.1016/j.socscimed.2020.112868.
65. Richter J, et al. Effects of an early intervention on perceived stress and diurnal cortisol in pregnant women with elevated stress, anxiety, and depressive symptomatology. J Psychosom Obstet Gynaecol. 2012;33:162–70. https://doi.org/10.3109/0167482X.2012.729111.
66. Zarenejad M, Yazdkhasti M, Rahimzadeh M, Mehdizadeh Tourzani Z, Esmaelzadeh-Saeieh S. The effect of mindfulness-based stress reduction on maternal anxiety and self-efficacy: a randomized controlled trial. Brain Behav. 2020;10:e01561. https://doi.org/10.1002/brb3.1561.
67. Thomas M, et al. Potential for a stress reduction intervention to promote healthy gestational weight gain: focus groups with low-income pregnant women. Womens Health Issues. 2014;24:e305–11. https://doi.org/10.1016/j.whi.2014.02.004.
68. Missler M, et al. Universal prevention of distress aimed at pregnant women: a systematic review and meta-analysis of psychological interventions. BMC Pregnancy Childbirth. 2021;21:276. https://doi.org/10.1186/s12884-021-03752-2.

Chapter 19
Management of Mental Health in Pregnant Women During COVID-19

Sara Molgora and Monica Accordini

19.1 Introduction: Mental Health in Pregnant Women

A growing body of studies has progressively investigated pregnant women's well-being, identifying pregnancy itself—as well as childbirth and postpartum—as a critical and potentially stressful event [1–4]. Indeed, during pregnancy, women are called to change their lifestyle and habits, while their self-image and identity undergo several major changes that may result in different forms of psychological distress [5]. Research has specifically studied the prevalence of anxiety, depression, and severe fear of childbirth (i.e., a clinical condition characterized by several physical symptoms, such as sleep disorders, panic attacks, etc.) reporting high rates of these conditions during pregnancy across countries [1, 2, 4, 6, 7].

In light of these studies, it is clear that pregnancy can be an extremely stressful event, capable of jeopardizing the mother's psychological stability as well as the stability of the couple [8, 9].

Furthermore, it is important to focus on expectant mothers' psychological well-being because psychological distress during pregnancy can influence not only the subjective experience of childbirth, by causing a negative, even traumatic, experience [10], but also the medical-obstetric aspects of labor and delivery, for example, in terms of prolonged labor and higher risk of operative deliveries or caesarean sections due to a reduced ability to cope with these events [11].

Several variables, both at an individual and interpersonal level, have been found to be associated with pregnant women's mental health, representing important risk or protective factors [9]. In particular, many studies have progressively highlighted the association between expectant mothers' psychological well-being and practical

---

S. Molgora (✉) · M. Accordini
Università Cattolica del Sacro Cuore di Milano, Milan, Italy
e-mail: sara.molgora@unicatt.it; monica.accordini@unicatt.it

© The Author(s), under exclusive license to Springer Nature Switzerland AG 2023
D. De Luca, A. Benachi (eds.), *COVID-19 and Perinatology*,
https://doi.org/10.1007/978-3-031-29136-4_19

and emotional social support, with lower levels of perceived social support or the absence of social support (from the partner, the extended formal or informal network) being among the most important predictors of antenatal anxiety, depression, and fear of childbirth [1, 12–14]. On the contrary, high perceived social support is an important protective factor for expectant mothers' mental health, and it is correlated with the good progress of pregnancy as well as with positive childbirth outcomes [15, 16]. Indeed, women who received support reported shorter labors, an overall better experience of birth, and even their newborn children had better health and were easier to bond with [17–19]. Furthermore, social support was found to discriminate among psychologically healthy and distressed expectant mothers [3]. Pregnant women who reported a gap between perceived (self-reported) support and "real" (coder-rated) support showed elevated PTSD symptoms and perceived stress during pregnancy [20]. Support, especially that received from the partner, was found to fully mediate the relation between women's concerns about pregnancy and childbirth and their psychological well-being [21].

Extensive research has found strong correlations between both perceived and received social support and constructs such as prenatal care, physical and emotional well-being, quality of life, life satisfaction, and happiness in pregnant women [22], thus confirming the buffering effect of social support on both environmental events and psychological stressors. Moreover, by providing mothers-to-be with better emotional tools to manage pregnancy and delivery, support also has an indirect benefit, potentially shielding the fetus from the negative effects of maternal distress, even in the long term [23].

With regard to support during pregnancy, an important role is played by antenatal classes: Some recent studies suggested that such an instrument may be beneficial for expectant mothers, although their access is restricted mostly to older, highly educated, and economically advantaged women [24]. Participation in antenatal classes was found to be associated with lower levels of fear of childbirth, especially in primiparous women [25]. Indeed, attending antenatal classes, focusing on childbirth preparation as well as parental education, allows prospective parents to express their concerns, better understand both the labor and delivery process, and master the first interactions with the newborn, facilitating the process of transitioning to parenthood [26]. Furthermore, besides providing useful information regarding the delivery process, fetal development, and newborn care, antenatal classes also allow women to build new acquaintances, meet other women sharing their joys and concerns, and find reassurances, thus increasing their sense of self-efficacy [27]. Finally, expectant mothers attending antenatal classes were found to have healthier nutritional behaviors and higher levels of physical activity compared to those who did not, suggesting the beneficial role of antenatal classes also in terms of promoting health-related behaviors [28].

Studies investigating the role of antenatal classes or interventions in reducing depression or anxiety symptoms have led to unsubstantial, often conflicting results [29]. A systematic review on the impact of psychological antenatal interventions on women's well-being found that such classes might have a beneficial role in normalizing women and couple's experiences and thus might provide them with reassurance and an increased sense of self-efficacy [30]. While conclusive evidence on the benefits of antenatal interventions cannot yet be drawn, an increasing body of research found beneficial effects in terms of increased awareness and resilience and reduction of symptoms among women with higher baseline distress [30, 31]. However, further investigation needs to be done on the topic, possibly distinguishing between the various form of interventions (e.g., psychological, educational, physical activity).

19.2 Expectant Mother's Mental Health During the COVID-19 Pandemic

The COVID-19 pandemic that has developed in 2019 and quickly spread throughout the entire globe led the World Health Organization to declare a global pandemic on March 20, 2020, and caused many countries to adopt mass quarantine and nationwide lockdowns to contain the virus spread. The forced isolation, limitation of movements, and lockdowns have had a significant impact on the general population's mental health. Several studies reported an increase of emotional distress and social disorders along with a decrease in psychological well-being following the pandemic outbreak, especially among young—younger than 50—women [e.g., 32, 33].

Literature focusing on the impact of the COVID-19 pandemic on expectant mothers found profound and severe effects on both pregnancy outcomes and on the mental health of such population [e.g., 34, 35]. Specifically, the pandemic outbreak increased the physiological vulnerability of an already fragile population while, at the same time, shrinking women's social and support networks and hindering their access to both pregnancy and mental healthcare facilities [36].

19.2.1 Care Provision and Care-Seeking Behaviors in the Time of COVID-19

With respect to pregnancy outcomes and the mothers' and babies' conditions, research is still inconclusive, and this may cause prospective mothers to be more anxious about pregnancy and delivery as they lack the necessary data to make an informed choice. One of the major stressors connected to the pandemic, especially in the initial phases of the outbreak, was not only the lack of information on the virus and its treatment but also the continuous changes in guidelines and behavioral prescriptions that made the lives of many increasingly wracked with uncertainty [37]. In general, the pandemic has imposed the need to rethink one's routine, while tasks once considered to be trivial or automatic have become a source of stress and mental load [38]. In a climate of constant change, no decision is routine, and this is especially true for expectant mothers who are already facing dramatic changes in several aspects of their lives. Specifically, the pandemic outbreak led to significant changes in women's expectations toward pregnancy and childbirth and caused increased feelings of uncertainty, fear, and concerns related to the risk of infection or complications for themselves and the fetus [39, 40].

While further studies on the effect of COVID-19 and lockdown measures are needed, some preliminary conclusions can be drawn: For example, a growing body of literature has found an increase in the number of C-sections and in preterm births among both infected and noninfected women [41, 42]. Despite that some of these interventions were required to guarantee a better and safer treatment of the COVID-19 symptoms, many others were thought to be iatrogenic [41]. Such interventions might guarantee the medical staff a certain degree of control over the patients, thus allowing them to plan their activities; however, they might, on the other side, cause women to feel they lack control over their delivery and believe they are incapable of taking good care of their babies [42]. Prior studies have, in fact, shown an association between C-sections and the occurrence of PTSD symptoms, mood disturbances, and negative self-perceptions among new mothers [43].

Not only the pandemic and the measures adopted to control the virus spread have been found to be responsible of adversarial delivery outcomes, they have also called for a reorganization of antenatal and obstetric care services and caused pregnant women health behavior to change [44]. For example, antenatal classes were stopped in most countries, and only a few hospitals and care facilities managed to provide online classes for expectant mothers; both nonurgent pre- and postnatal screenings and checkups were cancelled or postponed [45], potentially leading to complications and urgent hospital admissions; women had to attend visits unaccompanied; in many cases, prospective fathers were denied access during childbirth, delivery, and the immediate postpartum [9, 46], and this too has proven to negatively impact women's mental health in terms of increased anxiety and depressive symptoms [9]. Besides the difficulties on the healthcare providers' side, many expectant mothers autonomously decided to postpone screenings out of fear for themselves or their babies; moreover, the number of home births has increased in many countries, especially in North America [47].

These studies have proven that there have been significant changes in both care provision modes and care-seeking behaviors, such changes may result in additional risks for mothers-to-be and their babies and are possibly related to the observed worsening of pregnancy outcomes and to the increase of psychological symptoms among prospective mothers [48]. In this respect, several healthcare professionals have expressed their concern toward the restrictions limiting or forbidding the access to delivery rooms and maternity units to partners and other birth companions [9]. Birth companions provide women with continuous emotional and practical support and have proven to smooth women's birthing experience and even facilitate bonding with the newborn child [49].

These findings make pregnant women's mental health during the pandemic a public health issue [46, 50]. Indeed, there is consensus in the literature that the COVID-19 pandemic can be considered a specific contextual risk factor for pregnant women, adding another major stressor for these women and having particularly important detrimental effects on their mental health, quality of life, and overall well-being [35, 51].

19.2.2 Risk and Protective Factors

Specifically, an increasing number of studies are reporting higher levels of anxiety and depressive symptoms, severe fear of childbirth as well as more general stress, and reduced positive affectivity among expectant women during the pandemic in comparison to pre-pandemic similar cohorts of women (e.g., 9, 39, 52–55]. This is especially true for some categories of women; in particular, women with preexisting physical conditions have been shown to be at greater risk of developing mental health symptoms [56]. With regard to parity and preexisting psychological conditions, outcomes are controversial: While some studies have found primiparous women to be at greater risk of distress [36], others have found that women having more than one child are more prone to develop anxiety and depression [9]. This latter finding could be explained by the fact that women had to take care of their other child(ren) alone, while at the same time carrying on their pregnancy and balancing the other aspects of their lives. On the other hand, many primiparous women couldn't count on the presence of their partners or of a person of choice during medical appointments and screenings and had to go through the whole experience of pregnancy alone, without the emotional, practical, and informational support antenatal classes could have provided them with. With respect to preexisting mental health conditions, most of the studies, including a recent meta-analysis [56], found no correlation between having experienced prior mental health problems and the development of symptoms during the pandemic [57], while a few found grounds to support such a connection [9, 36].

Undoubtedly, pregnant women endured several additional stressors and found themselves deprived of the support from their formal and unformal network. In detail, women had only limited or no access to their informal social network, especially during the lockdown periods, reporting a significant decrease in perceived social support [51, 58, 59]. This situation also led to the increase of household and caregiving tasks, self-isolation, and to a higher risk of financial instability [40, 46]. One of the greatest worries reported by pregnant women was actually related to job and financial insecurity [56]. Overall, the COVID-19 outbreak led to an increase in women unemployment rates, thus exposing them to a higher likelihood of becoming poor [60].

Moreover, the lockdowns and restrictions to physical mobility posed several women in greater danger of being exposed to domestic abuse and violence; such restrictions also made it harder for victims to seek help [40].

Lastly, several studies also reported a significant decrease in pregnant women's physical activity, especially during the lockdown periods, which in turn may have had detrimental effects on both their physical and psychological well-being [42, 61].

While the Coronavirus' spread has undoubtedly negatively impacted on pregnant women's lives, there have also been some positive effects: First, several women could count on a greater presence of their partners [46], which sometimes also led to a more equal distribution of family chores [62].

Secondly, the reorganization of obstetric services led many facilities to adopt telehealth solutions [48]. Online interactions with practitioners made healthcare more accessible and promoted self-management among women. The wide spread of mobile phones, even in remote areas of the globe, also made it possible to combine telehealth appointments with app-based self-monitoring, which resulted in women having greater control over their health and being able to interact with care providers at a regular basis [63, 64].

Lastly, while some of the changes that happened in maternal hospital units seem to have led to adverse pregnancy outcomes, others have brought about positive novelties for expectant mothers: For example, several studies reported a decrease in the length of postpartum hospital stay [48, 65] as well as an increase in breastfeeding both during and after hospitalization [66].

To sum up, while it is undoubtedly true that the pandemic introduced an additional stress factor for mothers-to-be, it is also true that both women and care providers have proven capable of adaptation and resilience, and their assets can teach us a lesson on how to structure better facilities and develop policies at the service of those who struggle.

19.3 Guidelines and Implications for Practice

Research on the psychological impact of the pandemic confirmed that expectant mothers may be a vulnerable population, liable to develop symptoms that may affect their well-being and that of their offspring. Our review pinpointed a list of risk and protective factors that can help draw some implications for practice and formulate practical recommendations for policymakers and healthcare workers.

In our opinion, actions to be undertaken should focus on four main areas: *information*, *promotion*, *care*, and *coordination*.

First, it has been demonstrated that women who were more knowledgeable about COVID-19, its risks, and its treatment were less prone to develop anxiety symptoms. Having trust in the authorities and in the medical staff also constituted an important protective factor [36]. In this perspective, it would be extremely important to provide women with consistent, authoritative, and updated information about both the potential impact of COVID-19 on their health and on that of their babies as well as about the medical and obstetric procedures and care provision modalities used in each care facility. Such information should be provided by means of different media (e.g., television, social media, leaflets) so to reach as many women as possible and to reinforce the message. Applications allowing pregnant women to interact with healthcare professionals (medical doctors, midwifes, psychologists, etc.), pose them questions, and share their concerns should be provided in order to foster a sense of trust and promote women's direct involvement with their own care. Information on psychological symptoms and on how to prevent them should also be spread. In this respect, several countries have activated free psychological hotlines to provide consultations to people struggling with pandemic-related stress. It could be useful to activate hotlines exclusively devoted to pregnant and postpartum women involving trained professionals, capable to address the specific questions and concerns of such population. Such hotlines might involve gynecologists, midwives, and doulas along with mental health professionals.

With regard to promotion, telehealth should be promoted and healthcare facilities should provide professionals with the necessary instruments and training to deliver teleconsultations. Promoting telehealth also means for governments to invest on bridging the digital divide that makes telemedicine inaccessible to some. Specifically, broadband connection should be made available to all, especially those living in rural areas or low-income households, and when this is not possible, mobile/landline consultations should substitute online visits. Policymakers should also organize campaigns to improve people's digital literacy and to raise awareness on the importance of monitoring their health and attending to medical appointments. Finally, telehealth instruments should grant accessibility to everyone, while particular care should be placed in designing devices, websites, or applications in order to foster an equitable access to health. Similarly to teleconsultations, applications allowing the monitoring of one's pregnancy and general health have proven to be extremely useful increasing patients' access to care [36, 61]. We believe that such applications should become widespread and their use encouraged by family doctors. Such applications might also include some nutritional and training programs to help expectant mothers maintain a balanced diet and an active lifestyle.

With respect to care, coordination and constant communication between maternal health and mental health professionals should be fostered. Specifically, screening for mental health disorders should be compulsory for each woman both during pregnancy and at postpartum. Medical staff should be informed of the importance of such screenings and trained to recognize signs of depression, trauma, or anxiety in order to provide timely help and referral. Taking care of pregnant women also means guaranteeing their access to their formal and informal support network. Research findings confirmed the crucial role of social support as a protective factor for pregnant women's mental health during the pandemic. Specifically, different sources of support might serve different purposes: While support from one's partner and family has been proven to reduce depression and anxiety and to facilitate labor and delivery [14], support from friends was found to be associated with both symptom reduction and an increase in life satisfaction [51]. In turn, support from the medical staff, also in terms of a good communication and guidance, has been found to be associated with less anxiety symptoms and greater feelings of empowerment and an overall more positive birthing experience [15, 45]. In light of such results and also in compliance with the WHO guidelines [67], every woman, even if positive to COVID-19, should be granted the right to a companion of choice during labor and childbirth. From healthcare providers, to policymakers, from local communities to women's networks, everyone can play a crucial role in advocating for the importance of labor companionship. Furthermore, we can hypothesize that new technologies and social media could help in facilitating pregnant women's relationship with friends and family as well as foster the development of new ties and the birth of informal support networks. Indeed, social media friends are an increasingly important source of support [68]. Finally, research has also shown that the COVID-19 outbreak led to an increase in demands for obstetric and midwifery care [34, 61], especially at home. This is not necessarily a worrying sign, as it means that an increasing number of women are seeking support and guidance and desire a more direct, more intime and one-on-one relationship with the medical staff. Home assistance should be promoted to ensure more regular screenings of the women's condition and to provide them with the practical and emotional support they need. In this perspective, doula and midwifery services should be implemented and their costs—at least partially—covered by health insurance policies.

Finally, coordination is much needed at several levels: Among nations to close the gap of information regarding COVID-19, its implications on maternal health and the methods and strategies to provide expectant women with the best possible care; among researchers, in order to share the most recent and updated findings and to build on previous data to conduct more advanced and complete studies; among care facilities, to develop shared protocols for the care and treatment of expectant women as well as for the training of their staff members.

The effort and commitment of all interested stakeholders is crucial to promote the application of the existing WHO guidance and offer all prospective mothers a "woman-centred, respectful, skilled care" (67, pp. 54).

References

1. Biaggi A, Conroy S, Pawlby S, Pariante CM. Identifying the women at risk of antenatal anxiety and depression: a systematic review. J Affect Disord. 2016;191:62–77. https://doi.org/10.1016/j.jad.2015.11.014.
2. Nasreen HE, Rahman JA, Rus RM, Kartiwi M, Sutan R, Edhborg M. Prevalence and determinants of antepartum depressive and anxiety symptoms in expectant mothers and fathers: results from a perinatal psychiatric morbidity cohort study in the east and west coasts of Malaysia. BMC Psychiatry. 2018;18:195. https://doi.org/10.1186/s12888-018-1781-0.
3. Molgora S, Fenaroli V, Saita E. Psychological distress profiles in expectant mothers: what is the association with obstetric and relational variables? J Affect Disord. 2020;262:83–9. https://doi.org/10.1016/j.jad.2019.10.045.
4. van de Loo KFE, Vlenterie R, Nikkels SJ, Merkus PJFM, Roukema J, Verhaak CM, et al. Depression and anxiety during pregnancy: the influence of maternal characteristics. Birth. 2018;45:478–89. https://doi.org/10.1111/birt.12343.
5. Molgora S, Fenaroli V, Prino LE, Rollé L, Sechi C, Trovato A, et al. Fear of childbirth in primiparous Italian pregnant women: the role of anxiety, depression, and couple adjustment. Women Birth. 2018;31:117–23. https://doi.org/10.1016/j.wombi.2017.06.022.
6. Dennis CL, Falah-Hassani K, Shiri R. Prevalence of antenatal and postnatal anxiety: systematic review and meta-analysis. Br J Psychiatry. 2017;210:315–23. https://doi.org/10.1192/bjp.bp.116.187179.

7. O'Connell MA, Leahy-Warren P, Khashan AS, Kenny LC, O'Neill SM. Worldwide prevalence of tocophobia in pregnant women: systematic review and meta-analysis. Acta Obstet Gynecol Scand. 2017;96:907–20. https://doi.org/10.1111/aogs.13138.
8. Guzzo KB, Hayford SR. Pathways to parenthood in social and family contexts: decade in review, 2020. J Marriage Fam. 2020;82:117–44. https://doi.org/10.1111/jomf.12618.
9. Molgora S, Accordini M. Motherhood in the time of coronavirus: the impact of the pandemic emergency on expectant and postpartum women's psychological well-being. Front Psychol. 2020;11:567155. https://doi.org/10.3389/fpsyg.2020.567155.
10. Molgora S, Fenaroli V, Saita E. The association between childbirth experience and mother's parenting stress: the mediating role of anxiety and depressive symptoms. Women Health. 2020;60:341–51. https://doi.org/10.1080/03630242.2019.1635563.
11. Fenaroli V, Saita E, Molgora S, Accordini M. Italian women's childbirth: a prospective longitudinal study of delivery predictors and subjective experience. J Reprod Infant Psychol. 2016;34:235–46. https://doi.org/10.1080/02646838.2016.1167864.
12. Fekadu DA, Miller ER, Mwanri L. Antenatal depression and its association with adverse birth outcomes in low and middle-income countries: a systematic review and meta-analysis. PLoS One. 2020;15(1):e0227323. https://doi.org/10.1371/journal.pone.0227323.
13. Figueiredo B, Canário C, Tendais I, Pinto TM, Kenny DA, Field T. Couples' relationship affects mothers' and fathers' anxiety and depression trajectories over the transition to parenthood. J Affect Disord. 2018;238:204–12. https://doi.org/10.1016/j.jad.2018.05.064.
14. Racine N, Zumwalt K, McDonald S, Tough S, Madigan S. Perinatal depression: the role of maternal adverse childhood experiences and social support. J Affect Disord. 2020;263:576–81. https://doi.org/10.1016/j.jad.2019.11.030.
15. Friedman LE, Gelaye B, Sanchez SE, Williams MA. Association of social support and antepartum depression among pregnant women. J Affect Disord. 2020;264:201–5. https://doi.org/10.1016/j.jad.2019.12.017.
16. Huschke S, Murphy-Tighe S, Barry M. Perinatal mental health in Ireland: a scoping review. Midwifery. 2020;89:102763. https://doi.org/10.1016/j.midw.2020.102763.
17. Carvalho CE, Cardoso Antunes JCV, Carvalho DJ, Castro PV, Balula Chaves CM, Batista Nelas PA. Benefits for the father from their involvement in the labour and birth sequence. Procedia Soc Behav Sci. 2016;217 435–42. https://doi.org/10.1016/j.sbspro.2016.02.010.
18. Milgrom J, Hirshler Y, Reece J, Holt C, Gemmill AW. Social support-a protective factor for depressed perinatal women? Int J Environ Res Public Health. 2019;16(8):1426. https://doi.org/10.3390/ijerph16081426.
19. Tani F, Castagna V. Maternal social support, quality of birth experience, and post-partum depression in primiparous women. J Matern Fetal Neonatal Med. 2017;30(6):689–92. https://doi.org/10.1080/14767058.2016.1182980.
20. River LM, Narayan AJ, Atzl VM, Rivera LM, Lieberman AF. Romantic partner support during pregnancy: the discrepancy between self-reported and coder-rated support as a risk factor for prenatal psychopathology and stress. J Soc Pers Relat. 2020;37(1):27–45. https://doi.org/10.1177/0265407519850333.
21. Ilska M, Przybyła-Basista H. Partner support as a mediator of the relationship between prenatal concerns and psychological well-being in pregnant women. Health Psychol Rep. 2017;5(4):285–95. https://doi.org/10.5114/hpr.2017.68235.
22. Battulga B, Benjamin MR, Chen H, Bat-Enkh E. The impact of social support and pregnancy on subjective well-being: a systematic review. Front Psychol. 2021;12:710858. https://doi.org/10.3389/fpsyg.2021.710858.
23. Fitzgerald E, Parent C, Kee MZL, Meaney MJ. Maternal distress and offspring neurodevelopment: challenges and opportunities for pre-clinical research models. Front Hum Neurosci. 2021;15:635304. https://doi.org/10.3389/fnhum.2021.635304.
24. Ludwig A, Miani C, Breckenkamp J, Sauzet O, Borde T, Doyle IM, et al. Are social status and migration background associated with utilization of non-medical antenatal care? Analyses from two German studies. Matern Child Health J. 2020;7:943–52. https://doi.org/10.1007/s10995-020-02937-z.

25. Kacperczyk-Bartnik J, Bartnik P, Symonides A, Sroka-Ostrowska N, Dobrowolska-Redo A, Romejko-Wolniewicz E. Association between antenatal classes attendance and perceived fear and pain during labour. Taiwan J Obstet Gynecol. 2019;54(4):492–6. https://doi.org/10.1016/j.tjog.2019.05.011.
26. Barimani M, Forslund Frykedal K, Rosander M, Berlin A. Childbirth and parenting preparation in antenatal classes. Midwifery. 2018;57:1–7. https://doi.org/10.1016/j.midw.2017.10.021.
27. Nolan ML, Mason V, Snow S, Messenger W, Catling J, Upton P. Making friends at antenatal classes: a qualitative exploration of friendship across the transition to motherhood. J Perinat Educ. 2012;21(3):178–85. https://doi.org/10.1891/1058-1243.21.3.178.
28. Ługowska K, Kolanowski W. The nutritional behavior of pregnant women attending antenatal classes and non-attendees. Br Food J. 2020;122(4):1268–88. https://doi.org/10.1108/BFJ-10-2019-0754.
29. Bittner A, Peukert J, Zimmermann C, Junge-Hoffmeister J, Parker LS, Stöbel-Richter Y, et al. Early intervention in pregnant women with elevated anxiety and depressive symptoms. J Perinat Neonatal Nurs. 2014;28(3):185–95. https://doi.org/10.1097/JPN.0000000000000027.
30. Wadephul F, Jones C, Jomeen J. The impact of antenatal psychological group interventions on psychological well-being: a systematic review of the qualitative and quantitative evidence. Healthcare (Basel). 2016;4(2):32. https://doi.org/10.3390/healthcare4020032.
31. Broberg L, De Wolff MG, Anker L, Damm P, Tabor A, Hegaard HK, Midtgaard J. Experiences of participation in supervised group exercise among pregnant women with depression or low psychological well-being: a qualitative descriptive study. Midwifery. 2020;85:102664. https://doi.org/10.1016/j.midw.2020.102664.
32. Favieri F, Forte G, Tambelli R, Casagrande M. The Italians in the time of coronavirus: psychosocial aspects of unexpected COVID-19 pandemic. Front Psych. 2021;12:551924. https://doi.org/10.3389/fpsyt.2021.551924.
33. Rajkumar RP. COVID-19 and mental health: a review of the existing literature. Asian J Psychiatr. 2020;52:102066. https://doi.org/10.1016/j.ajp.2020.102066.
34. Ahmad M, Vismara L. The psychological impact of COVID-19 pandemic on women's mental health during pregnancy: a rapid evidence review. Int J Environ Res Public Health. 2021;18(13):7112. https://doi.org/10.3390/ijerph18137112.
35. Thapa SB, Mainali A, Schwank SE, Acharya G. Maternal mental health in the time of the COVID-19 pandemic. Acta Obstet Gynecol Scand. 2020;99(7):817–8. https://doi.org/10.1111/aogs.13894.
36. Suwalska J, Napierała M, Bogdański P, Łojko D, Wszołek K, Suchowiak S, et al. Perinatal mental health during COVID-19 pandemic: an integrative review and implications for clinical practice. J Clin Med. 2021;10:1–16. https://doi.org/10.3390/jcm10112406.
37. CIGNA. Cigna Covid-19 global impact study. 2020. https://www.cignaglobalhealth.com/static/docs/pdfs/covid-19-global-impact-study-future-uncertainty-hangs-heavy.pdf.
38. APA. Stress and decision-making during the pandemic. 2021. https://www.apa.org/news/press/releases/stress/2021/october-decision-making.
39. Ravaldi C, Wilson A, Ricca V, Homer C, Vannacci A. Pregnant women voice their concerns and birth expectations during the COVID-19 pandemic in Italy. Women Birth. 2021;34(4):335–43. https://doi.org/10.1016/j.wombi.2020.07.002.
40. Shah PS, Diambomba Y, Acharya G, Morris SK, Bitnun A. Classification system and case definition for SARS-CoV-2 infection in pregnant women, fetuses, and neonates. Acta Obstet Gynecol Scand. 2020;99(5):565–8. https://doi.org/10.1111/aogs.13870.
41. Arab W, Atallah D. Cesarean section rates in the COVID-19 era: false alarms and the safety of the mother and child. Eur J Midwifery. 2021;5:1–2. https://doi.org/10.18332/ejm/134998.
42. Zaigham M, Andersson O. Maternal and perinatal outcomes with COVID-19: a systematic review of 108 pregnancies. Acta Obstet Gynecol Scand. 2020;99(7):823–9. https://doi.org/10.1111/aogs.13867.
43. Lobel M, DeLuca RS. Psychosocial sequelae of cesarean delivery: review and analysis of their causes and implications. Soc Sci Med. 2007;64(11):2272–84. https://doi.org/10.1016/j.socscimed.2007.02.028.

44. Davis-Floyd R, Gutschow K, Schwartz DA. Pregnancy, birth and the COVID-19 pandemic in the United States. Med Anthropol Q. 2020;39(5):413–27. https://doi.org/10.1080/01459740.2020.1761804.
45. Coxon K, Turienzo CF, Kweekel L, Goodarzi B, Brigante L, Simon A, Lanau MM. The impact of the coronavirus (COVID-19) pandemic on maternity care in Europe. Midwifery. 2020;88:102779. https://doi.org/10.1016/j.midw.2020.102779.
46. Stampini V, Monzani A, Caristia S, Ferrante G, Gerbino M, De Pedrini A, et al. The perception of Italian pregnant women and new mothers about their psychological wellbeing, lifestyle, delivery, and neonatal management experience during the COVID-19 pandemic lockdown: a web-based survey. BMC Pregnancy Childbirth. 2021;21:473. https://doi.org/10.1186/s12884-021-03904-4.
47. Gregory ECW, Osterman MJK, Valenzuela CP. Changes in home births by race and hispanic origin and state of residence of mother: United States, 2018-2019 and 2019-2020. Natl Vital Stat Rep. 2021;70(15):1–10.
48. Townsend R, Sileo FG, Allotey J, Dodds J, Heazell A, Jorgensen L, et al. Prediction of stillbirth: an umbrella review of evaluation of prognostic variables. BJOG. 2021;128(2):228–50. https://doi.org/10.1111/1471-0528.16525.
49. Hodnett ED, Gates S, Hofmeyr GJ, Sakala C. Continuous support for women during childbirth. Cochrane Database Syst Rev. 2013;7:CD003766. https://doi.org/10.1002/14651858.CD003766.pub5.
50. Hermann A, Fitelson EM, Bergink V. Meeting maternal mental health needs during the COVID-19 pandemic. JAMA Psychiat. 2021;78(2):123–4. https://doi.org/10.1001/jamapsychiatry.2020.1947.
51. Corno G, Villani D, de Montigny F, Pierce T, Bouchard S, Molgora S. The role of perceived social support on the pregnant women's mental health during the Covid19 pandemic. J Reprod Infant Psychol. 2022. https://doi.org/10.1080/02646838.2022.2042799.
52. Cameron EE, Joyce K, Delaquis C, Reynolds K, Protudjer J, Roos LE. Maternal psychological distress & mental health service use during the COVID-19 pandemic. J Affect Disord. 2020;276:765–74. https://doi.org/10.1016/j.jad.2020.07.081.
53. Ceulemans M, Hompes T, Foulon V. Mental health status of pregnant and breastfeeding women during the COVID-19 pandemic: a call for action. Int J Gynecol Obstet. 2020;151:146–7. https://doi.org/10.1002/ijgo.13295.
54. Lebel C, MacKinnon A, Bagshawe M, Tomfohr-Madsen L, Giesbrecht G. Elevated depression and anxiety symptoms among pregnant individual during the COVID-19 pandemic. J Affect Disord. 2020;277:5–13. https://doi.org/10.1016/j.jad.2020.07.126s.
55. Saccone G, Florio A, Aiello F, Venturella R, De Angelis MC, Locci M, et al. Psychological impact of coronavirus disease 2019 in pregnant women. Am J Obstet Gynecol. 2020;223:293–5. https://doi.org/10.1016/j.ajog.2020.05.003.
56. Robinson GE, Benders-Hadi N, Conteh N, Brown KM, Grigoriadis S, Nadelson CC, et al. Psychological impact of COVID-19 on pregnancy. J Nerv Ment Dis. 2021;209(6):396–7. https://doi.org/10.1097/NMD.0000000000001339.
57. Broberg L, Ron AL, de Wolff MG, Høgh S, Nathan NO, Paarlberg LD, et al. Psychological well-being and worries among pregnant women in the first trimester during the early phase of the COVID-19 pandemic in Denmark compared with a historical group: a hospital-based cross-sectional study. Acta Obstet Gynecol Scand. 2022;101(2):232–40. https://doi.org/10.1111/aogs.14303.
58. Matvienko-Sikar K, Pope J, Cremin A, Carr H, Leitao S, Olander EK, et al. Differences in levels of stress, social support, health behaviours, and stress-reduction strategies for women pregnant before and during the COVID-19 pandemic, and based on phases of pandemic restrictions, in Ireland. Women Birth. 2021;34:447. https://doi.org/10.1016/j.wombi.2020.10.010.
59. Pope J, Olander EK, Leitao S, Meaney S, Matvienko-Sikar K. Prenatal stress, health, and health behaviours during the COVID-19 pandemic: an international survey. Women Birth. 2021;35:272. https://doi.org/10.1016/j.wombi.2021.03.007.

60. FEMM Committee. COVID-19 and its economic impact on women and women's poverty. 2021. https://www.europarl.europa.eu/RegData/etudes/STUD/2021/693183/IPOL_STU(2021)693183_EN.pdf.
61. Biviá-Roig G, La Rosa VL, Gómez-Tébar M, Serrano-Raya L, Amer-Cuenca JJ, Caruso S, et al. Analysis of the impact of the confinement resulting from COVID-19 on the lifestyle and psychological wellbeing of Spanish pregnant women: an internet-based cross-sectional survey. Int J Environ Res Public Health. 2020;17(16):5933. https://doi.org/10.3390/ijerph17165933.
62. Biroli P, Bosworth S, Della GM, Di Girolamo A, Jaworska S, Vollen J. Family life in lockdown. Front Psychol. 2021;12:687570. https://doi.org/10.3389/fpsyg.2021.687570.
63. Hill I, Burroughs E. Maternal telehealth has expanded dramatically during the COVID-19 pandemic. Robert Wood Johnson Foundation; 2020.
64. Shu C, Han S, Li L, Xu P, Bai Y. The clinical application and prospect of smart prenatal care and postpartum recovery. J Healthc Eng. 2021;2021:3279714. https://doi.org/10.1155/2021/3279714.
65. Bornstein E, Gulersen M, Husk G, Grunebaum A, Blitz MJ, Rafael TJ, et al. Early postpartum discharge during the COVID-19 pandemic. J Perinat Med. 2020;48(9):1008–12. https://doi.org/10.1515/jpm-2020-0337.
66. Noddin K, Bradley D, Wolfberg A. Delivery outcomes during the COVID-19 pandemic as reported in a pregnancy mobile app: retrospective cohort study. JMIR Pediatr Parent. 2021;4(4):e27769. https://doi.org/10.2196/27769.
67. WHO. 2021. https://apps.who.int/iris/bitstream/handle/10665/338882/WHO-2019-nCoV-clinical-2021.1-eng.pdf.
68. Baker B, Yang I. Social media as social support in pregnancy and the postpartum. Sex Reprod Healthc. 2018;17:31–4. https://doi.org/10.1016/j.srhc.2018.05.003.

Chapter 20
Ethical Issues of COVID-19 During Pregnancy and Childhood

Daniele De Luca, Alexandra Benachi, and Renzo Pegoraro

20.1 Background

The SARS-CoV-2 pandemic is the first of the century and a major public health problem. COVID-19, the disease caused by SARS-CoV-2, preferentially affects adults and has more severe consequences in the elderly, while it does not seem particularly aggressive in young people and children, although severe cases may be seldom possible as well as the development of paediatric inflammatory multiorgan syndrome. Nonetheless, knowledge about this new disease has been increasing, and we now know that young adults, including pregnant women, children and even neonates can develop COVID-19. These patients may not significantly contribute to the public health emergency but may be individually affected by severe COVID-19 and are subjected to particular ethical concerns.

These ethical issues are linked to the clinical features of this patient population, as COVID-19 may be more severe during pregnancy, while pregnant women and children have particular outcomes that are not of concern in the general population (i.e. pregnancy outcome, growth or neurodevelopmental issues), and our knowledge of COVID-19 treatment options for these patients is limited, as trials specifically

D. De Luca (✉)
Neonatology Department, APHP-University of Paris-Saclay, Le Kremlin-Bicêtre, France

A. Benachi
Obstetrics and Gynecology Department, APHP-University of Paris-Saclay,
Le Kremlin-Bicêtre, France
e-mail: alexandra.benachi@aphp.fr

R. Pegoraro
Pontifical Academy for Life, Vatican State, Rome, Italy
e-mail: cancelliere@pav.va

© The Author(s), under exclusive license to Springer Nature
Switzerland AG 2023
D. De Luca, A. Benachi (eds.), *COVID-19 and Perinatology*,
https://doi.org/10.1007/978-3-031-29136-4_20

recruiting them are scarce. Since severe COVID-19 is less common in these patients than in other populations, the different risk dimension also contributes to ethical uncertainty.

While the medical community is fighting the global pandemic, ethical issues should not be forgotten as they are relevant at an individual level, for the clinical care of any patient and particularly of those who are more vulnerable, such as pregnant women and children. We examine these ethical issues, in the clinical context of these patients, based on the most recent literature, and offer thoughts on how to address them and how to guide future clinical research in the field.

20.2 COVID-19 Can Be More Severe in Pregnant Women

20.2.1 *Clinical Context*

It is now known that COVID-19 is more severe in pregnant women infected by SARS-CoV-2 than in age-matched, non-pregnant patients [1, 2]. The maximum reported rates of maternal death and of admission to intensive care are roughly 11% and 28.5%, respectively [3]. This points to the need for particularly strong preventive measures for pregnant women or for those wishing to become pregnant. More severe COVID-19 may endanger the mother's life and have negative effects on the offspring [4]. Several studies have reported that pregnant women affected by COVID-19 have an increased rate of prematurity (which according to available systematic reviews, might reach 61% of pregnancies [3]) compared to noninfected pregnant women, and delivery is often induced in order to improve maternal conditions [5]. Interestingly, similar findings are reported when considering coronavirus infections as a whole [6]. The picture is complicated by results that differ between geographical areas, suggesting that other factors, such as healthcare quality, public health measures and the availability of accurate data may influence the detection of the real impact of COVID-19 on pregnancies [7, 8]. Be that as it may, prematurity is associated with increased admission to neonatal intensive care, several short- and long-term comorbidities and increased burden of care and costs, so the effect of COVID-19 in this setting should not be underestimated. Observational real-world data suggest that vaccination is safe and effective [9], and so it is considered extremely advisable in pregnant women [10, 11]. This is very interesting because the transplacental passage of anti-SARS-CoV-2 antibodies is less effective than that observed for antibodies against other respiratory viruses or bacteria, but this seems to be partially compensated by increased IgG and antibody receptors following SARS-CoV-2 placental infection [12]. Moreover, RNA vaccines induce the production of IgG, IgM and IgA, which are found in significant concentrations in human milk for several weeks [13, 14]. These findings, taken together, highlight the importance of maternal vaccination during pregnancy.

20.2.2 Ethical Issues

There is an urgent need for dedicated studies about the treatment of pregnant women with COVID-19, as this patient population has been much less studied than the general population with COVID-19. A search of the PubMed, clinicaltrial.gov and IRSCTN registries (on May 16, 2021) retrieved only five trials (2 of which were withdrawn) specifically dedicated to pregnant women, compared to several hundred focused on the general population. As the design and conduct of randomized clinical trials in pregnant women, and particularly in the perinatal period, are objectively more difficult that in non-pregnant patients, regulatory authorities worldwide have reaffirmed the importance of well-controlled, high-quality observational studies, as they may add to knowledge and inform clinical policies [15]. Clinical researchers of different disciplines are urged to invest in this direction. However, given the publicized retractions of hospital database studies investigating COVID-19 therapies at the beginning of the pandemic, specifically dedicated methodological guidelines should be issued and followed in order to increase the quality of data and facilitate their interpretation in the pandemic context [16].

There is a need to take difficult clinical decisions while balancing maternal and foetal-neonatal health. A preterm caesarean section may be needed to improve maternal conditions, and its delay may increase the risk of worsening respiratory failure. However, the effects on the neonate should also be considered: gestational age should be factored in, and appropriate measures should be taken to optimize the conditions of preterm delivery, i.e., adequate foetal monitoring and antenatal steroids and magnesium sulphate. This may not be possible in some emergency situations, but a collegial decision, involving obstetricians, adult and neonatal critical care physicians is always advisable (see also chap. 1). Maternal care has evolved along the pandemic course. In early 2020, maternal respiratory distress was considered as an indication for caesarean section in many cases, while today the use of non-invasive ventilation support has allowed to follow the mother through the acute phase of the disease and to avoid premature delivery in at least some cases.

Maternal well-being should also be considered, since preterm delivery, newborn care and COVID-19 itself may negatively impact on the mother's psychological status. Appropriate counselling and support should be provided: this may be long-lasting and require human resources that may be difficult to find, especially when the healthcare system is under pressure during a pandemic. Prenatal counselling should be honest and informative and based on the best knowledge available at that particular moment. It should be clearly explained that the maternal and foetal risks are low (compared to older populations), but not zero, and that anxiety related to these risks should be minimized in order to avoid increasing maternal psychological distress. A recent study has shown that birth during the COVID-19 pandemic but not maternal SARS-CoV-2 infection was associated with difference in neurodevelopment at age 6 months of the offspring [17]. COVID-19-related stress could be considered as a potential underlying mechanism, although other mechanisms may co-exist. Many things are most probably still to be studied and discovered on the side effect of the pandemic on maternal and child sides.

Finally, vaccination in pregnant women also raises important ethical issues. As pregnancy constitutes a period of vulnerability, increased scepticism may be faced when it comes to promoting vaccination. After 1.5 year of experience with worldwide use of mRNA COVID-19 vaccines, the US Centers for Disease Control and Prevention [10], the World Health Organization [18] and many scientific societies worldwide agree that vaccination should be offered to pregnant women with no difference compared to the general population, given the reassuring data coming from preliminary animal studies, reports of vaccinated women [9] and the risk/benefit ratio in favour of vaccination. The latter should be particularly well explained to each woman who should get vaccinated considering her risk of being infected whatever the predominant variant is, the aforementioned consequences for maternal and foetal health and the available reassuring data. The same considerations apply to lactating women. A particular effort should be made to provide suitable counselling and education to avoid any vaccine refusal that is no more ethically acceptable at this point in time.

20.3 SARS-COV-2 Can Be Transmitted from Mother to Foetus/Neonate

20.3.1 Clinical Context

After initial scepticism and several suspected cases reported worldwide, mother-to-child transmission of SARS-CoV-2 was confirmed in July 2020 by Vivanti et al. [19]. As the World Health Organization released the clinical definition of foetal and neonatal SARS-CoV-2 infections [20], this virus has been added to the group of vertically transmitted infectious agents, the most recent of which was Zika virus.

The clinical and biological details of vertical SARS-CoV-2 transmissions are covered in this book in Chapters 6, 7, 8 and 9. Vertical SARS-CoV-2 transmission is a rare event whose mean prevalence is 1–3% [21] (reported range 0%–10% [3]) of women infected during the third trimester. Earlier infections associated with still-birth and foetal demise have also been described, but the data are scanty although rapidly accumulating [22, 23]. SARS-CoV-2 actively infects the placenta and chronic histiocytic intervillositis and necrosis of the syncytiotrophoblast seem to be the typical, albeit non-specific hallmarks [24]. Moreover, placentas from women infected by SARS-CoV-2 during pregnancy show evidence of both maternal and foetal vascular malperfusion [25]. ACE-II proteins (i.e. the main receptors used by the virus to enter cells) are expressed in placental tissue [26]. However, the molecular mechanisms of SARS-CoV-2 passage are complex [27] and described in Chapter 9 details.

No congenital malformations have been attributed to COVID-19, so far, and drugs generally used in COVID-19 patients seem safe for the offspring [28–30]. However, neonates infected by SARS-CoV-2 present the same distribution of clinical manifestations observed in adults: about 50% are totally asymptomatic, while the other half may present mainly with respiratory manifestations but also cardiovascular and neurological signs [31]. As in adults, these clinical features are similar to those of other diseases, the distinction may not be easy, and a high suspicion index is required in order not to miss the diagnosis. Severe cases are rare but possible: In fact, cases of severe neonatal COVID-19 appearing as neonatal ARDS [32], with neurological or hemodynamic compromise, have been described [19, 33, 34]. These clinical manifestations have a pathobiological background in the expression of viral receptors in several tissues and organs already during foetal life [35, 36].

20.3.2 Ethical Issues

There is a need to inform parents about a rare but possible event, that is mother-to-child SARS-CoV-2 transmission, which they should be aware of, but without increasing anxiety or triggering other negative consequences. The balance between the need to inform and the need to avoid excessive anxiety may not be easy to achieve, also because pandemics directly or through the introduction of strict public health measures, reduce psychological well-being in various settings [37–41]. As mental problems vary significantly between countries, depending on their healthcare system and socio-economic status, they may increase disparities between different populations [42].

Dedicated studies about possible foetal and neonatal consequences of COVID-19 are scarce, and these consequences are regrettably still unknown to many, as the scientific community is especially vested in investigating COVID-19 in adult patients. Severe disease during pregnancy and adversely affected offspring are major events that influence the well-being of the whole family, and they should be adequately addressed.

Given the rarity of severe neonatal infections, it is logical to ask if this low prevalence constitutes an ethically sound reason not to protect the baby with preventive measures used for any other person at risk. In other terms, should parents be trained in preventive, although cumbersome, hygiene measures while taking care of the baby? This may imply the need to be helped by other family members or caregivers with important logistic consequences. Inevitably, this question goes along with the issue of mother-neonate separation, which is an extreme preventive measure. There is huge variability between guidelines issued by authorities and scientific societies around the world on this topic [43]. For instance, the majority of western scientific societies reject mother-neonate separation, which has, however, been strictly enforced in China and in some other Asian countries. The US Centers for Disease Control and Prevention advise mothers and healthcare providers to discuss this issue prenatally, considering risks and benefits on a case-by-case basis [43]. Thus, these considerations lead us to the questions: 'what is the best way to protect the neonate and to promote mother-neonate bonding?' and 'is it more important to protect the neonate or to support an optimal mother-neonate relationship?' or 'should we care more about maternal well-being or baby's health?' These questions may not have an easy and single ethically sound answer for each case and may require personalized decision-making on a case-by-case basis. Also, the diffusion of vaccination, fortunately reduced the contingency of this problem. The participation of parents to infants' care should be considered, whenever possible. As our knowledge on COVID-19 increases, guidelines should be updated and consider different ethical scenarios. Parents' opinions and social conditions should always be considered together with clinical data and risk estimation. The counselling provided by a clinical bioethicist or appropriate ethical review boards might be useful for more difficult cases.

20.4 COVID-19 Can Severely Affect Paediatric Patients

20.4.1 Clinical Context

Although they are undoubtedly less common than in the elderly, severe and critical forms of COVID-19 are seen in children as well [44]. The clinical manifestations of SARS-CoV-2 infection in children are similar to those observed in adults and may appear as paediatric ARDS, neurological and cardiovascular manifestations or multi-organ system failure and, as in adults, seem to be dependent on viral load and on the presence of comorbidities [45]. On top of this, children who had been infected by SARS-CoV-2 may develop severe paediatric inflammatory multi-organ syndrome several weeks after the original infection [46]. This condition may appear as macrophage activation, Kawasaki syndrome, myocarditis or a combination of clinical features typical of these disorders [47]. The rarity of severe paediatric COVID-19 and the fact that some of these complications may appear well after the infection, even in originally asymptomatic patients, has delayed full understanding of their pathophysiology. It is not clear which age range is actually more at risk, since infants initially seemed to be more affected by severe COVID-19 forms [48], but then severe cases have been described at any age [46]. Moreover, some children have been anecdotally treated using drugs and techniques adequately investigated only in adult populations, and this obviously raises several medical and ethical questions. Some of these issues may be clarified by appropriate epidemiological studies, and this is why the European Society of Paediatric and Neonatal Intensive Care launched the international paediatric and neonatal COVID-19 registry called EPICENTRE, which is collecting data from more than 100 hospitals around the globe [49].

20.4.2 Ethical Issues

There is a need for dedicated studies to increase understanding of the pathophysiology, clinical picture and epidemiology of COVID-19 in paediatric populations of different ages. These data can be used to inform decisions in terms of public health and particularly regarding the opening of schools and vaccination policies.

Children affected by COVID-19 are usually treated with therapeutics originally designed and tested in adults. This is not a new problem in paediatrics and, particularly, in paediatric critical care, but it becomes even more important during pandemics. In fact, specific paediatric studies and paediatric drug development plans are needed, but this cannot delay the application of promising and reasonable treatments in critically ill children. Compassionate and emergency off-label use of drugs and techniques should be promoted in children as in older patients. This applies to all types of therapeutics, including vaccines, monoclonal antibodies, antiviral and anti-inflammatory agents.

This latter point is also highly relevant to vaccination. While vaccination campaigns are progressing at different rates worldwide, all countries have faced unreasonable scepticism, at least in some contexts. The common belief that COVID-19 is a harmless disease in infancy may reduce even further the parental interest in vaccination of their children. Nonetheless, paediatric vaccination is crucial in reaching sufficient population coverage, and the existence of severe paediatric forms of COVID-19, coupled with the lack of age-specific approved treatments, demonstrates that there is also an urgent clinical interest in protecting children. Paediatric vaccines have been eventually developed taking into account particular characteristics of paediatric population aged more than 5 years [50]. Nonetheless, while paediatric vaccination advances, there is a gradually more evident need to protect also toddlers and infants (i.e. children less than 5 years old). In fact, with the advancement of vaccinations worldwide, children (and particularly the younger ones) have started to represent a significant portion of the susceptible population, given the lack of specific vaccine and immunization program. As a consequence, paediatric cases have increased including those needing critical care. Vaccination has proved efficient in reducing severe COVID-19 cases in children and adolescents as well as late-onset paediatric inflammatory multiorgan syndrome [51]. During the northern hemisphere 2021/2022 winter season, this has represented a real stress test for paediatric and neonatal intensive care units. These wards were sometimes already understaffed and lacking resources before the pandemics and have also contributed to take care of adults COVID-19 patients and their offspring, but their resources have not been increased as the public attention is mostly dedicated to adult critical care. The final strike has been represented by the respiratory syncytial virus (RSV) outbreak that came back in 2021, while it was significantly flattened by 2020 lockdowns: thus, many infants have needed intensive care for RSV bronchiolitis at the same moment of COVID-19 surge, creating huge logistic problems. The consequences of interplay between the seasonal surges of two very contagious respiratory viruses such as SARS-CoV-2 and RSV are still to be fully understood, but it is sure that this creates relevant ethical problems. A higher attention to paediatric and neonatal (critical) care, at least until children of all ages might be vaccinated against SARS-CoV-2 infections, will be needed to protect them from RSV more efficaciously.

20.5 Indirect Ethical Consequences of COVID-19 for Pregnancy and Paediatric Care

All the aforementioned points demonstrate the direct ethical consequences of COVID-19 for pregnancy and childhood care. However, as a pandemic, COVID-19 also seems to have indirect effects on obstetrics, neonatology and, more generally, paediatrics.

As COVID-19 preferentially affects adults and the elderly, many healthcare and research resources are being focused on these demographic categories, and attention to other groups may be reduced. This problem has affected many healthcare fields but is particularly relevant for pregnancy and paediatric care. In fact, some pregnant women have been very sick, and their offspring may need neonatal critical care even during pandemics. It has been quite difficult to explain why perinatal staff members cannot help in other departments because of the risk of jeopardizing the quality of maternal, neonatal and paediatric healthcare, particularly in some regions or settings.

As pregnancy and childhood are crucial moments in life, this shift may have negative long-lasting consequences that should not be forgotten by clinicians, researchers and healthcare policymakers. The complexity of care during pandemics may lead to shortage of human resources and hence difficulties in providing multidisciplinary care, as nurses and physicians of various specialties are redirected to the care of COVID-19 patients. This is potentially important for pregnant women with COVID-19, as clinical decisions may need input from obstetricians, infectious disease specialists, clinical bioethicists and critical care physicians who manage adults and neonates. The importance of a multidisciplinary approach appears important in order to identify the various ethical issues and be able to develop responses to them.

On another plan, COVID-19 also had relevant ethical consequences in terms of communication. Classical and new media were not ready to provide a correct and rightful information. Pandemics occurred in an era of redundant and extremely diffused information tools. This has allowed the diffusion of misleading or wrongful information creating potentially severe damages to the management of this worldwide emergency. Healthcare authorities had to create systems and action to identify and fight the diffusion of fake news and the consequences of what has been called "infodemics" [52]. Nonetheless, this has not been well prepared in advance and demonstrate as adequate resources should be dedicated to this issue. The acknowledgement of specialist competency and of its ethical value must be recognised and adequately promoted. This would require a worldwide effort and is of utmost importance for the management of the next pandemics.

Conflict of Interest Authors have no conflict of interest to declare.

References

1. Allotey J, Stallings E, Bonet M, et al. Clinical manifestations, risk factors, and maternal and perinatal outcomes of coronavirus disease 2019 in pregnancy: living systematic review and meta-analysis. BMJ. 2020;370:m3320.
2. Badr DA, Mattern J, Carlin A, et al. Are clinical outcomes worse for pregnant women at ≥20 weeks' gestation infected with coronavirus disease 2019? A multicenter case-control study with propensity score matching. Am J Obstet Gynecol. 2020;223:754–8.
3. Vergara-Merino L, Meza N, Couve-Pérez C, et al. Maternal and perinatal outcomes related to COVID-19 and pregnancy: an overview of systematic reviews. Acta Obstet Gynecol Scand. 2021;2021:14118.
4. Metz TD, Clifton RG, Hughes BL, et al. Disease severity and perinatal outcomes of pregnant patients with coronavirus disease 2019 (COVID-19). Obstet Gynecol. 2021. https://doi.org/10.1097/AOG.0000000000004539.
5. Di Toro F, Gjoka M, Di Lorenzo G, et al. Impact of COVID-19 on maternal and neonatal outcomes: a systematic review and meta-analysis. Clin Microbiol Infect. 2021;27:35–46.
6. Di Mascio D, Khalil A, Saccone G, et al. Outcome of Coronavirus spectrum infections (SARS, MERS, COVID-19) during pregnancy: a systematic review and meta-analysis. Am J Obstet Gynecol. 2020;2020:100107.
7. Magee LA, von Dadelszen P, Khalil A. COVID-19 and preterm birth. Lancet Glob Health. 2021;9:e117.
8. Kc A, Gurung R, Kinney MV, et al. Effect of the COVID-19 pandemic response on intrapartum care, stillbirth, and neonatal mortality outcomes in Nepal: a prospective observational study. Lancet Glob Health. 2020;8:e1273–81.
9. Shimabukuro TT, Kim SY, Myers TR, et al. Preliminary findings of mRNA Covid-19 vaccine safety in pregnant persons. N Engl J Med. 2021;2021:2104983.
10. https://www.cdc.gov/coronavirus/2019-ncov/vaccines/recommendations/pregnancy.html.
11. Stock SJ, Carruthers J, Calvert C, et al. SARS-CoV-2 infection and COVID-19 vaccination rates in pregnant women in Scotland. Nat Med. 2022. https://doi.org/10.1038/s41591-021-01666-2.
12. Atyeo C, Pullen KM, Bordt EA, et al. Compromised SARS-CoV-2-specific placental antibody transfer. Cell. 2021;184:628–42.
13. Gray KJ, Bordt EA, Atyeo C, et al. COVID-19 vaccine response in pregnant and lactating women: a cohort study. Am J Obstet Gynecol. 2021;2021:S0002937821001873.
14. Golan Y, Prahl M, Cassidy A, et al. Immune response during lactation after anti-SARS-CoV2 mRNA vaccine. Pediatrics. 2021. https://doi.org/10.1101/2021.03.09.21253241.
15. https://www.ema.europa.eu/en/news/global-regulators-commit-cooperate-observational-research-context-covid-19.
16. Fell DB, Dimitris MC, Hutcheon JA, et al. Guidance for design and analysis of observational studies of fetal and newborn outcomes following COVID-19 vaccination during pregnancy. Vaccine. 2021;39:1882–6.
17. Shuffrey LC, Firestein MR, Kyle MH, et al. Association of birth during the COVID-19 pandemic with neurodevelopmental status at 6 months in infants with and without in utero exposure to maternal SARS-CoV-2 infection. JAMA Pediatr. 2022;2022 e215563.
18. https://www.youtube.com/watch?v=19J9Hbpt114.
19. Vivanti A, Vauloup-Fellous C, Prevot S, et al. Transplacental transmission of SARS-CoV-2 infection. In Review. 2020. https://doi.org/10.21203/rs.3.rs-28884/v1.
20. https://www.who.int/publications/i/item/WHO-2019-nCoV-mother-to-child-transmission-2021.1.
21. Kotlyar AM, Grechukhina O, Chen A, et al. Vertical transmission of coronavirus disease 2019: a systematic review and meta-analysis. Am J Obstet Gynecol. 2020 https://doi.org/10.1016/j.ajog.2020.07.049.

22. Shende P, Gaikwad P, Gandhewar M, et al. Persistence of SARS-CoV-2 in the first trimester placenta leading to transplacental transmission and fetal demise from an asymptomatic mother. Hum Reprod. 2020;2020:367.
23. Baud D, Greub G, Favre G, et al. Second-trimester miscarriage in a pregnant woman with SARS-CoV-2 infection. JAMA. 2020;323:2198.
24. Schwartz DA, Baldewijns M, Benachi A, et al. Chronic histiocytic intervillositis with trophoblast necrosis are risk factors associated with placental infection from coronavirus disease 2019 (COVID-19) and intrauterine maternal-fetal severe acute respiratory syndrome coronavirus 2 (SARS-CoV-2) transmission in liveborn and stillborn infants. Arch Pathol Lab Med. 2020. https://doi.org/10.5858/arpa.2020-0771-SA.
25. Sharps MC, Hayes DJL, Lee S, et al. A structured review of placental morphology and histopathological lesions associated with SARS-CoV-2 infection. Placenta. 2020;101:13–29.
26. Gengler C, Dubruc E, Favre G, Greub G, de Leval L, Baud D. SARS-CoV-2 ACE-receptor detection in the placenta throughout pregnancy. Clin Microbiol Infect. 2020. https://doi.org/10.1016/j.cmi.2020.09.049.
27. Facchetti F, Bugatti M, Drera E, et al. SARS-CoV2 vertical transmission with adverse effects on the newborn revealed through integrated immunohistochemical, electron microscopy and molecular analyses of Placenta. EBioMedicine. 2020;59:102951.
28. Rizzi S, Wensink MJ, Lindahl-Jacobsen R, Tian L, Lu Y, Eisenberg ML. Risk of pre-term births and major birth defects resulting from paternal intake of COVID-19 medications prior to conception. BMC Res Notes. 2020;13:509.
29. Giampreti A, Eleftheriou G, Gallo M, et al. Medications prescriptions in COVID-19 pregnant and lactating women: the Bergamo Teratology Information Service experience during COVID-19 outbreak in Italy. J Perinat Med. 2020;48:1001–7.
30. Louchet M, Sibiude J, Peytavin G, Picone O, Tréluyer J-M, Mandelbrot L. Placental transfer and safety in pregnancy of medications under investigation to treat coronavirus disease 2019. Am J Obstet Gynecol. 2020;2:100159.
31. Raschetti R, Vivanti AJ, Vauloup-Fellous C, Loi B, Benachi A, De Luca D. Synthesis and systematic review of reported neonatal SARS-CoV-2 infections. Nat Commun. 2020;11:5164. https://doi.org/10.1038/s41467-020-18982-9.
32. De Luca D, van Kaam AH, Tingay DG, et al. The Montreux definition of neonatal ARDS: biological and clinical background behind the description of a new entity. Lancet Respir Med. 2017;5:657–66.
33. Frauenfelder C, Brierley J, Whittaker E, Perucca G, Bamford A. Infant With SARS-CoV-2 infection causing severe lung disease treated with remdesivir. Pediatrics. 2020;146:e20201701. https://doi.org/10.1542/peds.2020-1701.
34. Hosier H, Farhadian SF, Morotti RA, et al. SARS-CoV-2 infection of the placenta. J Clin Invest. 2020;130:4947–53.
35. Varma P, Lybrand ZR, Antopia MC, Hsieh J. Novel targets of SARS-CoV-2 spike protein in human fetal brain development suggest early pregnancy vulnerability. Front Neurosci. 2021;14:614680.
36. Li M, Chen L, Zhang J, Xiong C, Li X. The SARS-CoV-2 receptor ACE2 expression of maternal-fetal interface and fetal organs by single-cell transcriptome study. PLoS ONE. 2020;15:e0230295.
37. Kola L, Kohrt BA, Hanlon C, et al. COVID-19 mental health impact and responses in low-income and middle-income countries: reimagining global mental health. Lancet Psychiatry. 2021;2021:S2215036621000250.
38. Rogers JP, Chesney E, Oliver D, et al. Psychiatric and neuropsychiatric presentations associated with severe coronavirus infections: a systematic review and meta-analysis with comparison to the COVID-19 pandemic. Lancet Psychiatry. 2020;7:611–27.
39. Mansfield KE, Mathur R, Tazare J, et al. Indirect acute effects of the COVID-19 pandemic on physical and mental health in the UK: a population-based study. Lancet Digit Health. 2021;3:e217–30.

40. Varga TV, Bu F, Dissing AS, et al. Loneliness, worries, anxiety, and precautionary behaviours in response to the COVID-19 pandemic: a longitudinal analysis of 200,000 Western and Northern Europeans. Lancet Reg Health Eur. 2021;2:100020.
41. Pierce M, McManus S, Hope H, et al. Mental health responses to the COVID-19 pandemic: a latent class trajectory analysis using longitudinal UK data. Lancet Psychiatry. 2021;2021:S2215036621001516.
42. Nochaiwong S, Ruengorn C, Thavorn K, et al. Global prevalence of mental health issues among the general population during the coronavirus disease-2019 pandemic: a systematic review and meta-analysis. Sci Rep. 2021;11:10173.
43. Yeo KT, Oei JL, De Luca D, et al. Review of guidelines and recommendations from 17 countries highlights the challenges that clinicians face caring for neonates born to mothers with COVID-19. Acta Paediatr. 2020. https://doi.org/10.1111/apa.15495.
44. Castagnoli R, Votto M, Licari A, et al. Severe acute respiratory syndrome coronavirus 2 (SARS-CoV-2) infection in children and adolescents: a systematic review. JAMA Pediatr. 2020. https://doi.org/10.1001/jamapediatrics.2020.1467.
45. Pinninti SG, Pati S, Poole C, et al. Virological characteristics of hospitalized children with SARS-CoV-2 infection. Pediatrics. 2021;2021:e2020037812.
46. Belot A, Antona D, Renolleau S, et al. SARS-CoV-2-related paediatric inflammatory multisystem syndrome, an epidemiological study, France, 1 March to 17 May 2020. Eur Secur. 2020;25:2001010. https://doi.org/10.2807/1560-7917.ES.2020.25.22.2001010.
47. Toraih EA, Hussein MH, Elshazli RM, et al. Multisystem inflammatory syndrome in pediatric COVID-19 patients: a meta-analysis. World J Pediatr. 2021. https://doi.org/10.1007/s12519-021-00419-y.
48. Dong Y, Mo X, Hu Y, et al. Epidemiological characteristics of 2143 pediatric patients with 2019 coronavirus disease in China. Pediatrics. 2020;2020:e20200702.
49. De Luca D, Rava L, Nadel S, et al. The EPICENTRE (ESPNIC Covid pEdiatric Neonatal Registry) initiative: background and protocol for the international SARS-CoV-2 infections registry. Eur J Pediatr. 2020. https://doi.org/10.1007/s00431-020-03690-9.
50. Callaway E. COVID vaccines and kids: five questions as trials begin. Nature. 2021;592:670–1.
51. Levy M, Recher M, Hubert H, et al. Multisystem inflammatory syndrome in children by COVID-19 vaccination status of adolescents in France. JAMA. 2022;327:281.
52. https://www.who.int/health-topics/infodemic#tab=tab_1.

Printed by Printforce, United Kingdom